Techniques of measurement in medicine: 6
Series Editor: Professor B. Watson
Department of Medical Electronics
St Bartholomew's Hospital, London
Consultant Editor: Professor J. Rotblat

£17-50

A manual of electroencephalographic technology

D1825007

Clwyd North Health District – Libraries	
Hospital NWH	Class WL 150
Dept. E.E.G.	Acc. No. 09329

Dr C. D. Binnie and Thea Gutter are at the Instituut voor Epilepsiebestrijding, Heemstede, The Netherlands. Dr Binnie is Head of Clinical Neurophysiology Service and Thea Gutter is Chief EEG Technician.

Dr A. J. Rowan is Professor of Neurology at The Mount Sinai School of Medicine, New York City, and Chief of the Neurology Service at the Bronx Veterans Administration Medical Center.

A manual of electroencephalographic technology

C. D. BINNIE, A. J. ROWAN AND TH. GUTTER

Medical Library
N. WALES HOSPITAL
DENBIGH

Cambridge University Press

CAMBRIDGE
LONDON   NEW YORK   NEW ROCHELLE
MELBOURNE   SYDNEY

Published by the Press Syndicate of the University of Cambridge
The Pitt Building, Trumpington Street, Cambridge CB2 1RP
32 East 57th Street, New York, NY 10022, USA
296 Beaconsfield Parade, Middle Park, Melbourne 3206, Australia

©Cambridge University Press 1982

First published 1982

Printed in Great Britain at the University Press, Cambridge

British Library Cataloguing in Publication Data
Binnie, C. D.
A manual of electroencephalographic technology –
(Techniques of measurement in medicine; 6)

1. Electroencephalography
I. Title II. Rowan, A. J. III. Gutter, Th.
IV. Series
616.8'047547   RC386.6.E43   80-42003
ISBN 0 521 23847 1 hard covers
ISBN 0 521 28257 8 paperback

Contents

Medical Library
N. WALES HOSPITAL
DENBIGH

Preface

The investigation of the human brain, by whatever method, is generally found to be both exhilarating and frustratingly difficult. The discovery that it was possible to record the electrical activity of brain cells (the electroencephalogram or EEG) through the intact scalp of a conscious human being appeared to offer fascinating possibilities for understanding how the brain works in health and in disease. The reality has proved more mundane. The EEG is so complex that, depending upon one's point of view, it may be seen either as a code which cannot be cracked or conversely as random noise containing little or no information. Moreover, while it is technically quite easy to record the EEG badly, it is extremely difficult to record it in a precise and carefully controlled manner which may make detailed analysis worthwhile. There are therefore basically two schools of thought about EEG recording. The one holds that, as the EEG provides little useful information anyway, it is not worthwhile devoting much effort to recording it carefully. Adherents of this school do indeed find that their records are of little value, which in their eyes justifies their views. A radically different approach is to endeavour to achieve the highest possible standard of recording and interpreting the EEG at the limits currently imposed by 'the state of the art'. Provided the investigation is directed to the solution of worthwhile clinical or scientific problems and is not for instance used as a substitute for careful neurological examination and history taking, those who adopt this approach find their endeavours to be worthwhile and their work professionally rewarding. It should be obvious from the above and will become clear in the chapters that follow where the sympathies of the present authors lie.

In trying to write a book about how to record EEGs we had several different groups of readers in mind and in trying to meet all their needs we have included material which for one or other group may be superfluous. Firstly, we have tried to provide a text for EEG technologists, upon whose skills the quality of EEG practice ultimately depends. For them we have also included an introductory chapter on the basic anatomy and physiology of the brain and some information concerning abnormal EEGs and the diseases which the EEG is most often used to investigate. Many neuro-biologists (psychologists, pharmacologists and the like) use the EEG for research purposes. Often they do so in an academic environment remote from any clinical EEG service and without ready access to trained EEG technologists or electroencephalographers. These readers may require a practical guide to EEG recording and may also have some use for a brief account of abnormal EEG phenomena if only because these will from time to time be found in their supposedly healthy experimental subjects. The increasing use of technology in medicine has lead to the creation and rapid growth of departments of medical electronics and of bio-medical data processing, which clinicians expect to provide expert and detailed advice on instrumentation and analysis of biological signals. We have tried to cater for their needs with a fairly detailed account of specifications, calibration and use of the EEG equipment, a summary of the current status of EEG data processing, and again some background information to set the biological and clinical context of electroencephalography. Finally, since a knowledge of technology is an essential qualification for the head (usually medically qualified) of any EEG department, we have included some material (on EEG reports and setting up a department) which may be of particular use to trainee electroencephalographers.

We are indebted to many present and past colleagues who have read various parts of the text; they cannot be blamed for its deficiencies but have at least helped to eliminate many errors. Most of the illustrations were prepared by H. Musscher at the Instituut voor Epilepsiebestrijding. Rosemary Slater of St Bartholomew's Hospital drew the figures of electrodes and D.S.L. Lloyd provided many of the computer graphics. We are also grateful: for textual criticism, to Colleen Darby, Marion Smith, D.S.L. Lloyd, Dr P.F. Prior, R. Billings, F. Stubbe and T. Wisman; for bibliographic assistance, to Joyce Apeldoorn-Bastiaenen and Helma Bennett-Kip; for accurately typing multiple drafts of a technical manuscript in a language not their own, Minke van Taarling-Wassenaar and Marian Vink; for detailed advice on the technical sections, T. Wisman and on data-processing, D.S.L. Lloyd. Finally we are grateful to our teachers, particularly the late Dr J.H. Margerison, Drs D.F. Scott, E. Goldensohn and G. Pampiglione, for their insistence that a high standard of technological practice is prerequisite to useful clinical or research work in electroencephalography.

1. The basis of the electroencephalogram

The electroencephalogram (EEG) is a recording of the electrical activity of the brain. Bioelectrical signals can be registered from many organs, for electrical activity is generated by the cell membranes of every living tissue. The electrocardiogram or ECG, arising from the heart, is commonplace and easily obtained. However, the EEG is considerably more difficult either to record or to interpret than the ECG. The electrical potentials from the brain are very much smaller than those from the heart – a hundred times smaller in fact. Furthermore, the potentials generated by the brain are very much more complex than those generated by other organ systems. These factors create enormous technical problems. It is the solution of these problems and the resultant contributions that EEG can make to our understanding of the function and disease processes of the brain that form the basis for this book. The EEG technologist plays an important and often undervalued role in electroencephalography and in diagnosis of neurological disease. This book is therefore dedicated to the recognition of this importance and the development of expertise in a complicated but rewarding technical field.

1.1. History
In the early years of this century Dr Hans Berger, a psychiatrist working in Germany, became fascinated with the function of the brain. In particular, he was determined to find some physiological basis for psychiatric illness. The work of earlier physiologists on the electrical activity of the brains of animals was well known to him, particularly that of Caton who in 1875 first recorded electrical activity from the exposed brains of rabbits. The technical difficulties were overwhelming, and indeed today it is hard to imagine how Berger managed to record anything at all from the scalp of a human being, considering the equipment available to him. Since there were no powerful amplifiers at that time he had to record the minute brain potentials with a string galvanometer connected to two scalp electrodes. He pursued his experiments with remarkable tenacity over nearly three decades until in 1929 he published his first paper on the human EEG ('Uber das Elektroenkephalogramm des Menschen'). Berger was able to demonstrate a low-amplitude rhythmic waveform with a frequency of about 10 cycles per second (hertz or Hz) which was present in the occipital areas when the subject (actually his son) was resting with his eyes closed. Later Berger named this activity the alpha rhythm to distinguish it from other, faster (beta) activity. Even today, the

alpha rhythm is considered the single most important characteristic of the EEG, and in spite of technical advances in the recording of brain potentials, modern descriptions of the alpha
rhythm are little different from that of Berger. Hans Berger
published many papers between 1929 and 1938, describing for
the first time such important phenomena as the abnormal paroxysmal brain activity seen during epileptic seizures. His careful and
painstaking work stands as an admirable model of the clinical
exploitation of new technology.

It is ironic that Berger's discovery was generally dismissed. It
was felt that the waves he described were not truly cerebral in
origin and were probably produced by vibrations due to passing
trams. Indeed, there were many possibilities for artefact production considering the primitive nature of the recording equipment, and in any case no one had ever seen such a rhythmic
waveform produced by other living tissues such as muscle or
peripheral nerve. Nonetheless workers in other countries attempted
to reproduce Berger's findings. In 1934 Adrian and Matthews
confirmed the presence of the electroencephalogram using a
much more sophisticated amplification system based on the
vacuum tube or valve. In America, Davis and Gibbs quickly
followed suit. This period marked the true beginning of the
recognition and use of electroencephalography from which has
grown an enormously productive scientific and clinical field.

1.2. Basic anatomy

A solid background of anatomy and physiology is essential for an
understanding of the origin of the brain's electrical potentials and
the proper application of EEG studies to the solution of clinical
problems. This knowledge is needed if the technologist is to take
his or her proper place as a member of the diagnostic team rather
than functioning as an unthinking 'knob turner', a situation that
unfortunately obtains in many EEG laboratories today. Regardless
of how competent the electroencephalographer may be, he is
dependent on the technologist's expertise in order to exercise his
own skills.

1.2.1. The skull

Fortunately the brain is enclosed in a hard, bony box, providing
excellent protection for its substance which has the consistency
of a soft pudding. The skull is actually constructed of several
individual bones which, in the years after birth, gradually unite

at irregular lines of demarcation known as sutures. Fig. 1.1 demonstrates the various bones of the skull. Although it is thick and strong there are vulnerable areas that assume importance in head injuries. An example is the temporal bone, parts of which are extremely thin. The overlying temporal muscle provides protection, but a fracture here may readily occur with severe damage to underlying brain tissue.

The bottom or base of the skull is a complicated structure which cradles the brain as a glove the hand (Fig. 1.2). It is thick and irregular and contains many holes or foramina which provide pathways for nerves and blood vessels. Like Gaul, it is conveniently divided into three parts called the anterior, middle and posterior fossae. The frontal lobes of the brain fit nicely into the anterior fossa, the temporal lobes into the middle, and the cerebellum and brain stem into the posterior fossa. The large foramen, the foramen magnum, accommodates the lower brain stem which at that point changes character and becomes the spinal cord. Through the brain stem run nerve pathways serving many neurological functions both sensory and motor, and even more importantly this region contains structures controlling consciousness. These aspects will be further examined in Section 1.3.5.

Fig.1.1. Lateral view of the skull.

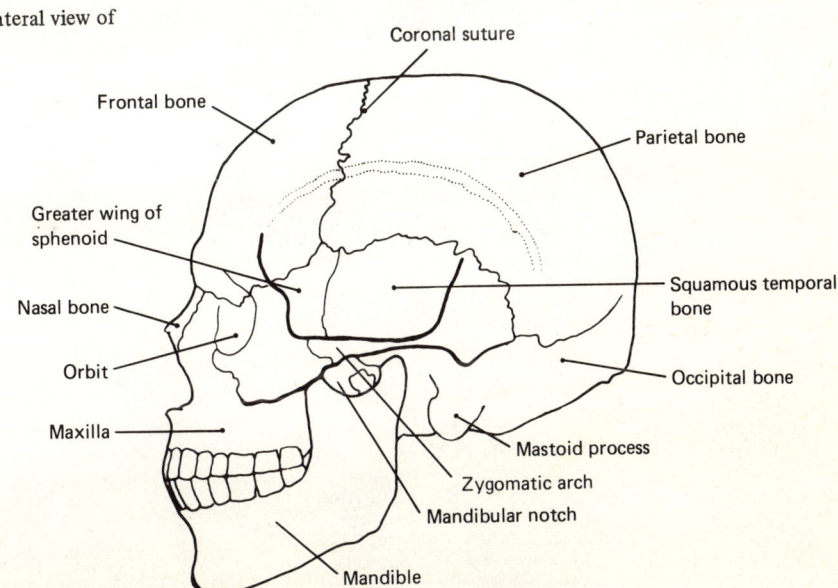

1.2.2. The meninges

The brain itself is clothed in three layers of tissue, each of which is anatomically and functionally distinct. These are known collectively as the *meninges*, and individually as the *dura, arachnoid* and *pia* (Fig. 1.3). The dura is the tough fibrous outer layer, whereas the arachnoid (from Latin for spidery) is thin and filmy. The innermost layer, pia, closely conforms to the surface of the brain and is clinically the least important. The dura and arachnoid, on the other hand, are often of great clinical significance. For example, a blow to the head may result in bleeding from torn veins so that blood collects between the dura and the brain (subdural haematoma – see Section 2.3.2). Another type of bleeding results from the rupture of the arteries outside the brain and is

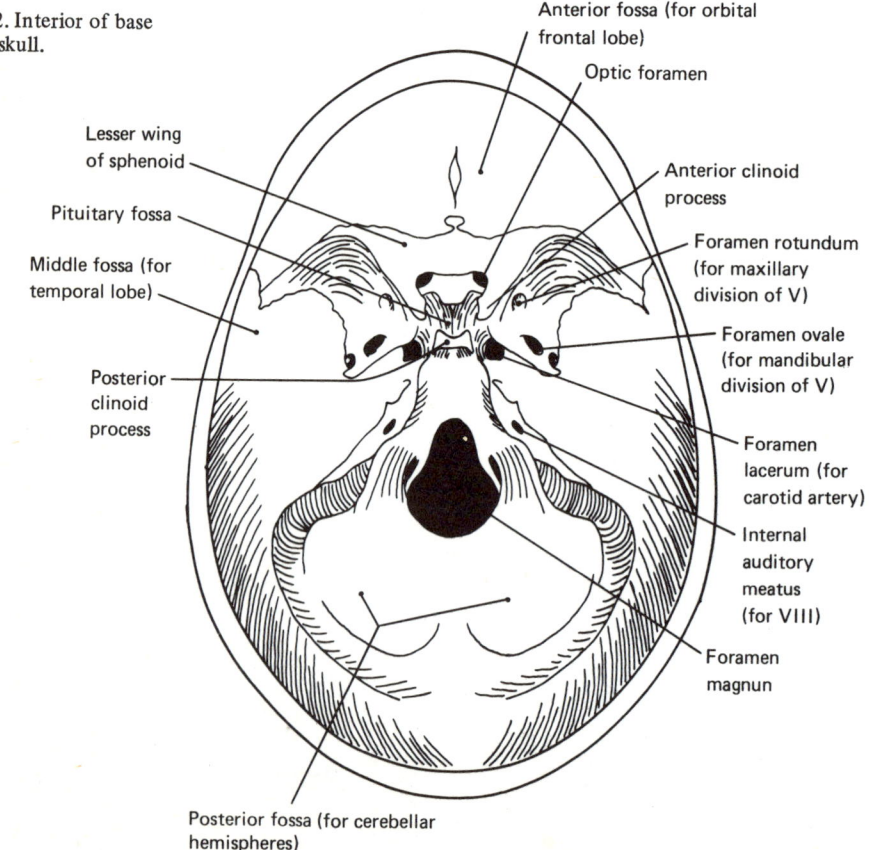

Fig. 1.2. Interior of base of the skull.

Anterior fossa (for orbital frontal lobe)

Optic foramen

Lesser wing of sphenoid

Anterior clinoid process

Pituitary fossa

Foramen rotundum (for maxillary division of V)

Middle fossa (for temporal lobe)

Foramen ovale (for mandibular division of V)

Posterior clinoid process

Foramen lacerum (for carotid artery)

Internal auditory meatus (for VIII)

Foramen magnun

Posterior fossa (for cerebellar hemispheres)

vigorous and rapid. The blood collects beneath the arachnoid as a subarachnoid haemorrhage (Section 2.3.2). In both these conditions the EEG may provide important and sometimes life-saving diagnostic information.

1.2.3. The cerebrum

The three main divisions of the brain are the cerebrum, the cerebellum and the brain stem. The most remarkable of these structures is the cerebrum, the source of the electroencephalogram and the structure that most clearly differentiates man from lower animals. Its surface is convoluted and largely folded inwards in grooves, or sulci. The outer layer of the cerebrum, the cerebral cortex, is composed of grey matter, which is rich in nerve cells; the deep part, or white matter, is mostly made up of nerve fibres. The cerebrum is divided into two similar halves, the cerebral hemispheres, and these in turn are divided by deep fissures into four or more less distinct parts known as lobes (Fig. 1.4). The technologist will have occasion to refer to these subdivisions daily, and their anatomy and major functions must be known.

Fig. 1.3. The meninges: cross-section through the region of the saggital sinus at the vertex.

   The *frontal* lobe is the largest of the four and comprises about half of the entire hemisphere. It is the most forward or anterior portion and extends backwards or posteriorly to the central

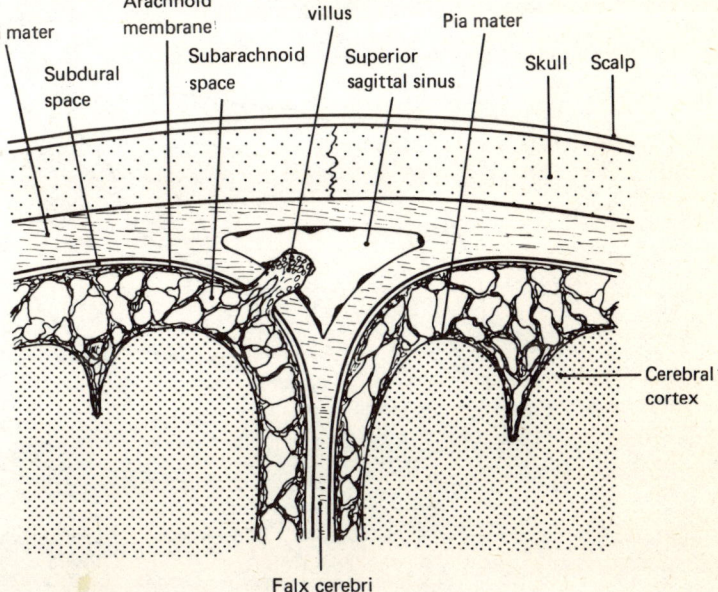

sulcus (fissure of Rolando). One of the most important features of the frontal lobe is that it contains the primary motor area which is the major cerebral centre for voluntary movement. Cerebral centres for eye movement and the function of elaborating the human personality are also contained in this lobe.

Directly behind the central sulcus and extending to the more posterior portion of the cerebrum is the *parietal* lobe. Here are contained the primary cerebral centres for sensation and for perception and spatial orientation.

The *temporal* lobe is a prominent feature of the inferolateral aspect of the cerebrum and lies beneath the frontal and parietal lobes. Memory depends in part on normal temporal lobe functioning. It is also, as we shall see later, a common location for epileptic activity, producing seizures of a distinct type (the complex partial or psychomotor seizure).

The *occipital* lobe occupies the most posterior region of the cerebrum and is the primary visual centre.

Fig. 1.5 demonstrates the medial view of a cerebral hemisphere. In their uppermost aspect, the two hemispheres are separated from each other by a fold of the dura known as the falx. Another prominent feature of the medial aspect is the corpus callosum, a large structure composed of nerve fibres which connects the two hemispheres both anatomically and functionally.

Fig.1.4. The left cerebral hemisphere, lateral aspect.

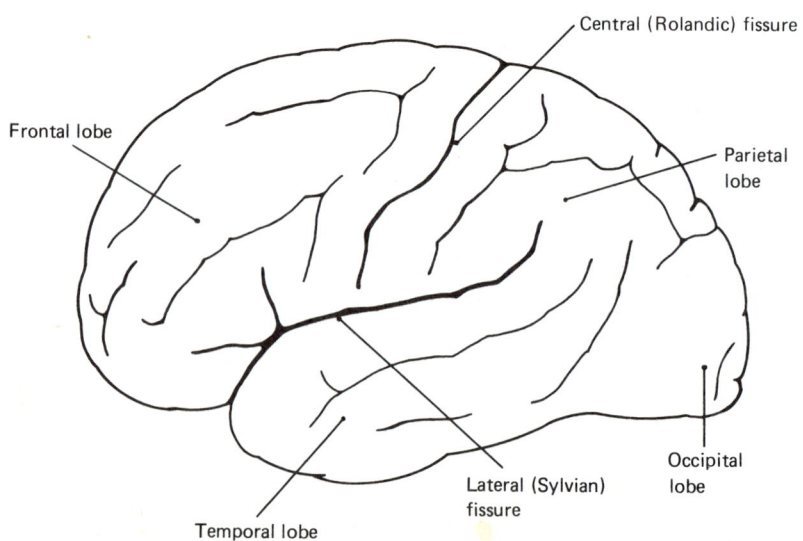

Central (Rolandic) fissure

Frontal lobe

Parietal lobe

Occipital lobe

Lateral (Sylvian) fissure

Temporal lobe

Deep in the cerebrum are a number of important structures with diverse functions. These are composed mainly of grey matter and include the *basal ganglia*, groups of nerve cells which have complex motor control functions, the *hypothalamus* which regulates the production of hormones via its influence on the pituitary gland, and the *thalamus* (Fig. 1.6). The thalamus is the major relay station for many impulses travelling between the spinal cord and the cerebral cortex. For example, nerve fibres serving primary sensory function have a relay station (synapse) in a particular collection of thalamic nerve cells called the ventral posterior lateral (VPL) nucleus. Other nuclei serve auditory or visual functions. There are also thalamic nuclei which project fibres diffusely to the cerebral cortex and serve the maintenance of consciousness (nonspecific thalamic projection system (Section 1.3.5)).

1.2.4. The brain stem

The brain stem contains the cranial nerve nuclei and numerous fibre tracts running between the cerebrum and spinal cord. The brain stem lies in the posterior fossa just under the cerebellum, and both the brain stem and cerebellum are separated from the cerebral hemispheres by a thick extension of the dura known as the tentorium. A large hole in the centre of the tentorium, the tentorial notch, surrounds the junction of the brain stem with the diencephalon. As Fig. 1.6 demonstrates, there are three distinct component parts to the brain stem, the midbrain or mesen-

Fig.1.5. The medial aspect of the left cerebral hemisphere and midline section through the corpus callosum, brain stem and cerebellum.

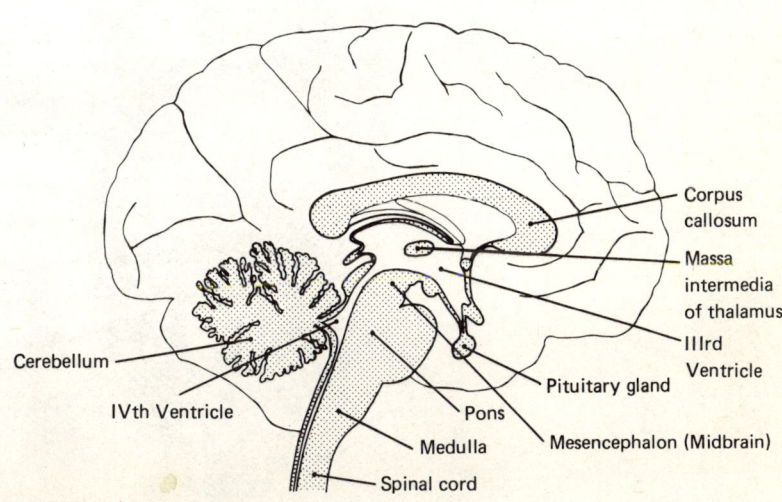

Corpus callosum

Massa intermedia of thalamus

IIIrd Ventricle

Pituitary gland

Mesencephalon (Midbrain)

Pons

Medulla

Spinal cord

IVth Ventricle

Cerebellum

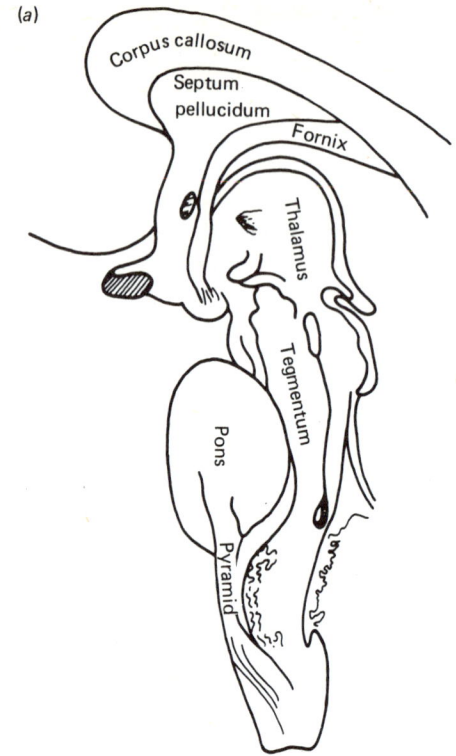

(a)

Corpus callosum

Septum pellucidum

Fornix

Thalamus

Tegmentum

Pons

Pyramid

Fig. 1.6. The brain stem and diencephalon. (a) Longitudinal section. (b) Ventral view.

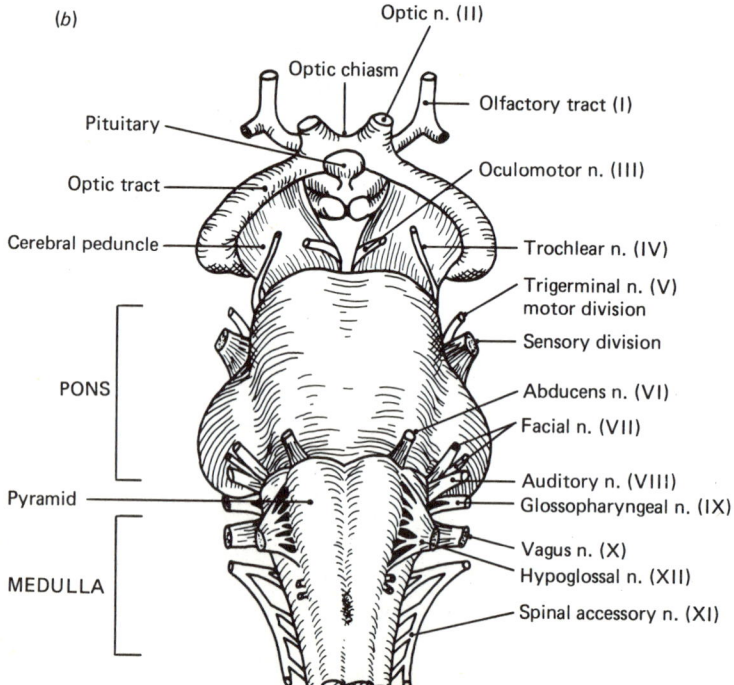

(b)

Optic n. (II)

Optic chiasm

Pituitary

Optic tract

Cerebral peduncle

Olfactory tract (I)

Oculomotor n. (III)

Trochlear n. (IV)

Trigerminal n. (V) motor division

Sensory division

Abducens n. (VI)

Facial n. (VII)

Auditory n. (VIII)

Glossopharyngeal n. (IX)

Vagus n. (X)

Hypoglossal n. (XII)

Spinal accessory n. (XI)

PONS

Pyramid

MEDULLA

cephalon, the pons and the medulla. Each contains the origins of several cranial nerves. These nerves serve motor and sensory functions of the structures of the head and neck such as eye movements, pupillary reflexes, chewing, facial and tongue movements, and sensation from the face and pharynx. The cranial nerves exit the skull through the various foramina at its base as noted in Fig. 1.2. Among other structures of great importance in the brain stem are the reticular formation, a core of nerve cells with multiple interconnections which runs throughout its length, and respiratory and cardiac control centres which are contained in the medulla.

1.2.5. The ventricular system

Within the brain there are inter-communicating cavities or ventricles, which together make up the ventricular system. A fluid fills the ventricles and also bathes the surface of the brain and spinal cord. This *cerebrospinal fluid* (CSF) is actually an ultrafiltrate of the blood serum and contains various electrolytes such as sodium and potassium, and protein and sugar. The CSF is constantly secreted by structures within the ventricular system known as the *choroid plexus* and is reabsorbed into the venous system at the surface of the dura through the bodies known as arachnoid villi or Pacchionian bodies. The ventricles are four in number: two large ventricles within the cerebral hemispheres, the IIIrd ventricle which is surrounded by the diencephalon and the IVth ventricle which travels through the medulla (Fig. 1.7). The lateral ventricles are connected with the IIIrd ventricle via the foramen of Monro while the IIIrd and IVth ventricle are united by the acqueduct of Sylvius. From the IVth ventricle, the CSF reaches the surface of the spinal cord via several small foramina.

1.2.6. Cerebrospinal fluid

The CSF contributes important information in the diagnosis of various neurological conditions. Certain diseases cause changes in the constituents of the fluid, for example, the sugar content is decreased if the patient suffers from bacterial meningitis (inflammation of the meninges). Another characteristic finding is an increase in the protein content which occurs frequently in patients with cerebral tumours.

The CSF is very easily obtained for diagnostic purposes by a needle that is introduced into the spinal subarachnoid space (lumbar puncture or LP) between the lumbar vertebrae, usually

the 3rd and 4th. The procedure is quick and generally painless.
The flow of CSF is a dynamic process and is associated with a
fluid pressure which can be measured via the LP needle with a
simple manometer. If a pathological process interrupts the flow
of CSF, whether due to blockage at the base of the brain or at
the site of reabsorption, the pressure will be elevated. Elevation
of CSF pressure is an ominous sign, and the patient requires
urgent treatment of the underlying condition (Section 2.3.2).

1.2.7. Vascular supply
The brain is one of the most metabolically active organs in the
human body. It must have a vigorous and constant blood supply
in order to provide the requisite nutrients, mainly sugar and

Fig.1.7. The circulation
of the CSF (for the
purposes of this diagram
the brain stem is shown
disproportionately
large and the spinal
cord foreshortened).

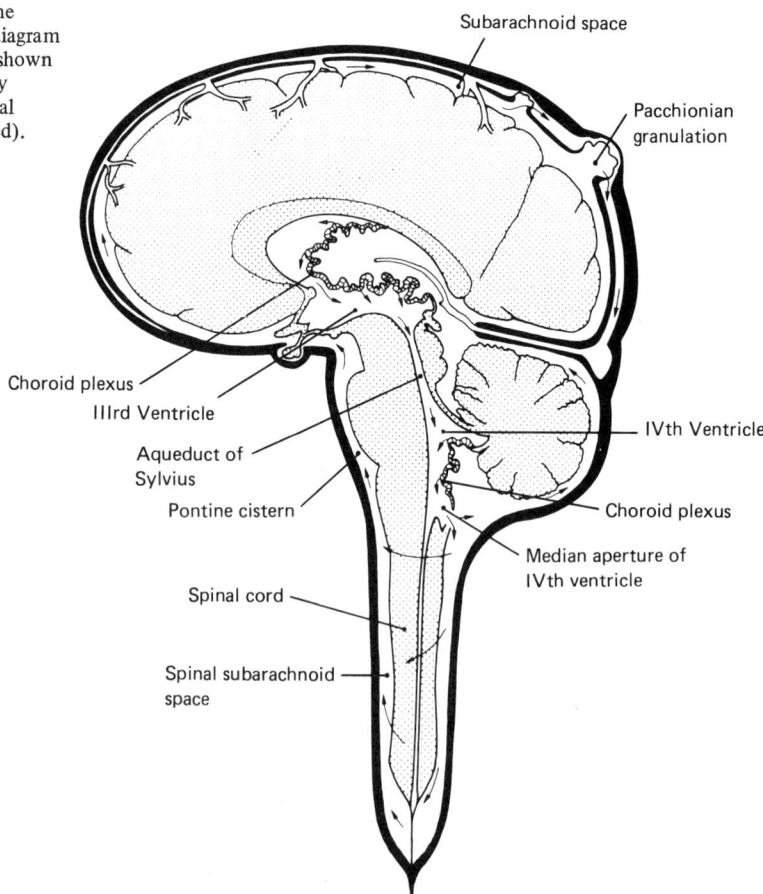

oxygen, which serve its metabolic processes. The brain in fact receives approximately 25% of the entire output of the heart. The blood is supplied by the four great vessels which originate at the aortic arch: the right and left carotid arteries and the right and left vertebral arteries. The carotid arteries run in the anterior portion of the neck while the vertebral arteries pass through foramina in the cervical vertebral bodies. After the four arteries enter the skull they converge on a structure at the base of the brain known as the *Circle of Willis* (Fig. 1.8). As can be seen, the major cerebral arteries originate at the circle and travel to various portions of the brain.

The *anterior* and *middle cerebral* arteries together with the *carotid* arteries constitute the anterior circulation (Fig. 1.9). The anterior cerebral artery runs over the frontal lobe and supplies the most anterior and superior portions of this structure. The middle cerebral artery is actually an extension of the carotid and supplies a large portion of the frontal, parietal and temporal lobes.

Fig. 1.8. Basal view of the brain with the Circle of Willis.

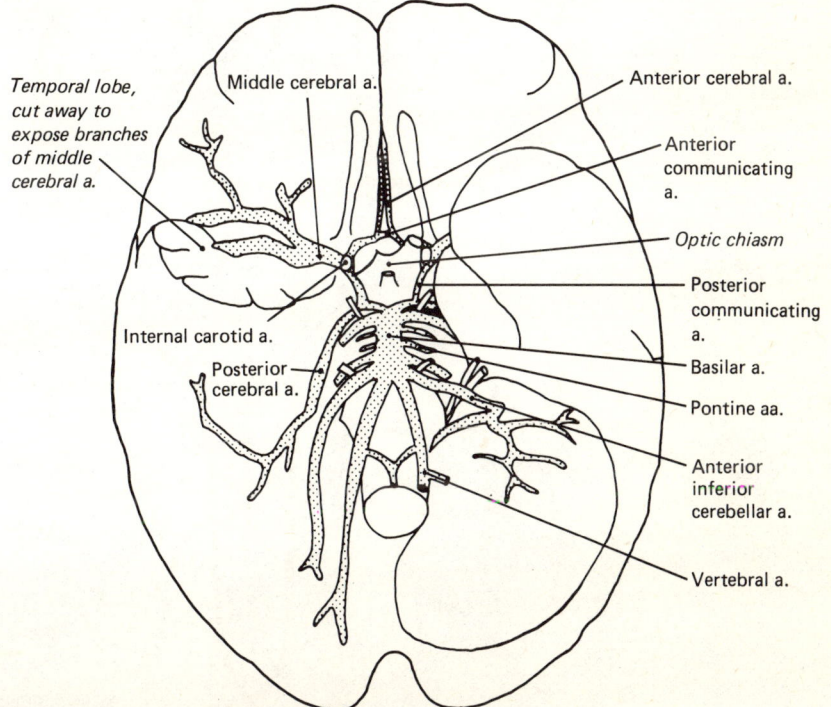

Temporal lobe, cut away to expose branches of middle cerebral a.

Middle cerebral a.

Anterior cerebral a.

Anterior communicating a.

Optic chiasm

Posterior communicating a.

Internal carotid a.

Posterior cerebral a.

Basilar a.

Pontine aa.

Anterior inferior cerebellar a.

Vertebral a.

The posterior circulation derives from the *vertebral* arteries which unite to form the *basilar* artery. Branches of the basilar and the vertebral arteries provide most of the blood supply for the cerebellum and brain stem. The basilar artery divides to form the posterior cerebral arteries which supply the occipital lobes, the posterior portions of the temporal lobes and some of the deep

Fig. 1.9. The blood supply of the (*a*) lateral and (*b*) medial aspects of the left cerebral hemisphere.

(*a*)

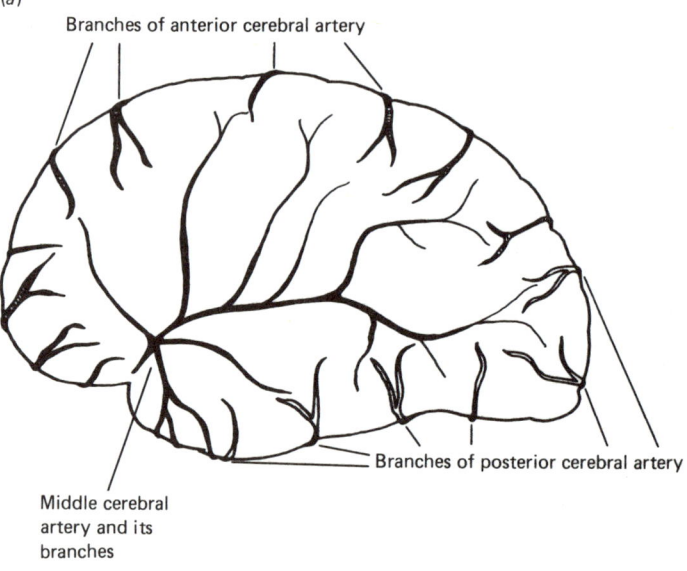

Branches of anterior cerebral artery

Branches of posterior cerebral artery

Middle cerebral artery and its branches

(*b*)

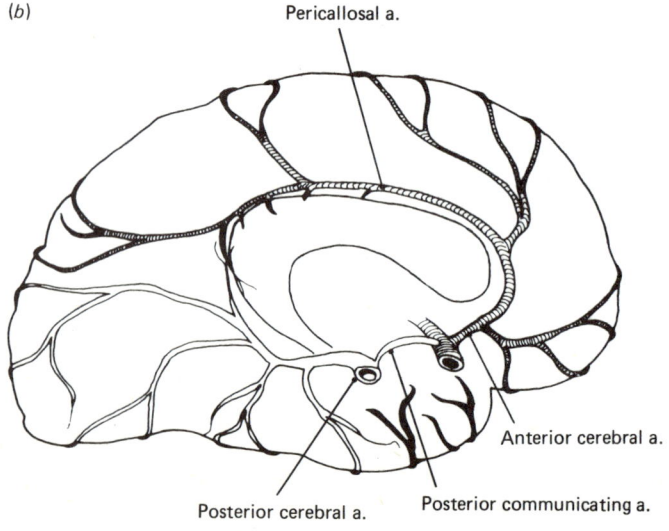

Pericallosal a.

Anterior cerebral a.

Posterior cerebral a.

Posterior communicating a.

nuclear structures. It can be seen that occlusion of one of the major cerebral arteries above the Circle of Willis will result in death of cerebral tissue in the area it serves (Section 2.3.3).

1.3. Basic physiology

1.3.1. The neurone

Nerve cells, or *neurones*, vary greatly in detailed structure but typically comprise a cell-body, containing a nucleus, a long nerve fibre or *axon* which carries nerve-impulses away from the cell-body, and many short branching processes, *dendrites*, which carry impulses towards the cell-body (Fig. 1.10). There are a number of varieties of neurones each having a configuration appropriate to its function (Fig. 1.10*b*).

Fig.1.10. (*a*) A neurone (after Schmidt, 1978). (*b*) Various types of neurones. (After Ramon y Cajal.)

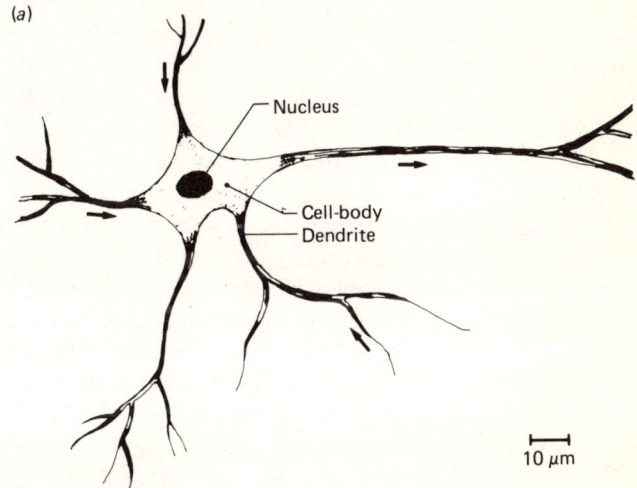

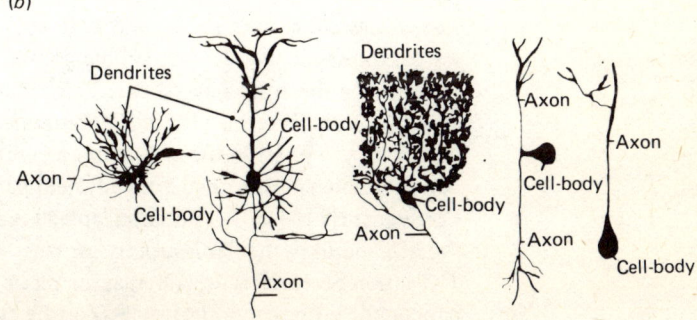

Inside the neurone there is a high concentration of potassium ions (K^+), whilst outside the potassium concentration is low. The reverse is true of sodium (Na^+) which has a much lower concentration within the nerve cell than in extracellular fluid. These ions have a natural tendency to diffuse down their concentration gradients, that is for potassium to leak out of the cell and sodium inwards. However, the cell membrane has the property of being selectively much more permeable to potassium ions than to sodium. Consequently potassium diffuses out of the cell but sodium cannot so readily diffuse inwards. This imbalance of ionic movements causes a net loss of positive charge from the cell, setting up a difference of electrical potential across the cell membrane. An equilibrium is established when the negative potential inside the membrane with respect to the outside becomes large enough to prevent the continued escape of K^+ ions. This occurs at about -70 mV (the *resting potential*) and the membrane is said to be 'polarized'.

1.3.2. The action potential

Under certain circumstances the membrane potential may locally be reduced ('depolarized'); how this happens physiologically is considered in the next section but it can be studied in the laboratory by passing a current through the membrane of an isolated nerve cell. When the membrane potential is reduced (becoming less negative) beyond a certain threshold the selective ionic permeabilities change: suddenly, the membrane becomes impermeable to potassium but sodium can move freely inwards down its concentration gradient. The local flow of positively charged sodium ions into the cell reverses the membrane potential at this point (Fig. 1.11). When the inside of the membrane has become some 30 mV positive with respect to the outside, the selective permeabilities abruptly revert to their previous states. The inflow of sodium ceases and potassium again diffuses outwards, thus restoring the original membrane potential, and indeed producing a short-lived overshoot. This sequence of events lasts about 1 ms and is termed the *action potential*. An action potential occurring at a point in the cell membrane sets up local electric currents which in turn depolarize adjacent parts of the membrane. Consequently the action potential spreads across the surface of the cell and in particular is rapidly propagated down the axon. The action potential is described as an 'all or none' event: it either happens or it does not. The process may be likened to the burning of a fuse, but with the difference that a fuse cannot regenerate itself, whereas the nerve cell membrane is again ready to discharge within a few milliseconds of the passage of an action potential. The repeated occurrence of action potentials would tend to cause a gradual accumulation of sodium and loss of potassium within the cell. This is corrected by active transport of these ions across the cell membrane by a mechanism termed the *sodium–potassium pump*. This process consumes a large amount of energy which demands a high level of metabolic activity, and the cell consequently requires an abundant supply of oxygen and glucose for its survival.

1.3.3. The synapse

Though the action potential transmits signals along nerve fibres, communication between nerve cells occurs by a different mechanism. The axon of a neurone typically divides into several terminal branches which make contact with the dendrites and cell-bodies of other neurones. These points of close contact are called 'synapses' (Fig. 1.12). When an action potential passing down the axon reaches the synapse, a chemical substance called a 'neurotransmitter' is released, which diffuses across the very small distance to the membrane of the adjacent 'post-synaptic' neurone and produces changes in the physical properties of its membrane. There are a number of known or suspected neuro-transmitters including such compounds as nor-adrenaline and acetylcholine.

Fig.1.11. The action potential (after Schmidt, 1978).

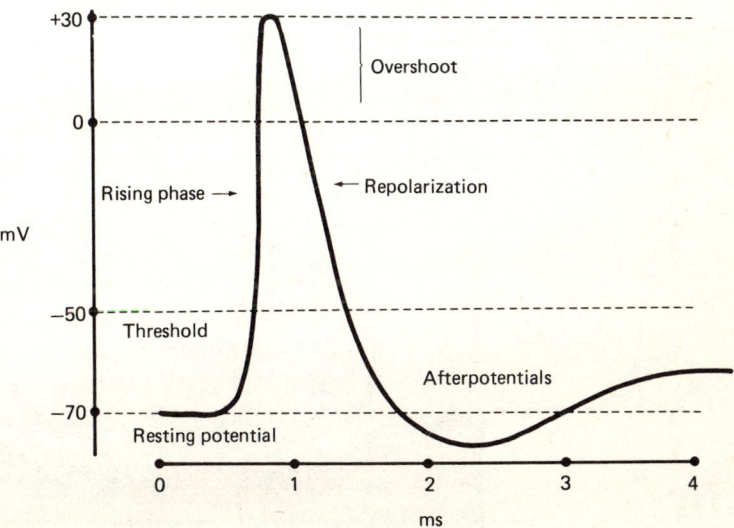

The electrical changes in the post-synaptic membrane are termed *post-synaptic potentials*. They are of lower amplitude than the action potential (some 5–10 mV) but last longer, up to 10 ms. The post-synaptic potentials from several synapses spread over the surface of the cell-body and are averaged out. If the net effect is a depolarization exceeding the necessary threshold, an action potential is set up which is then transmitted down the axon. Some

Fig. 1.12. Synapses. (*a*) A network of inter-connecting neurones. (*b*) The structure of a synapse. (After Schmidt, 1978.)

(*a*)

(*b*)

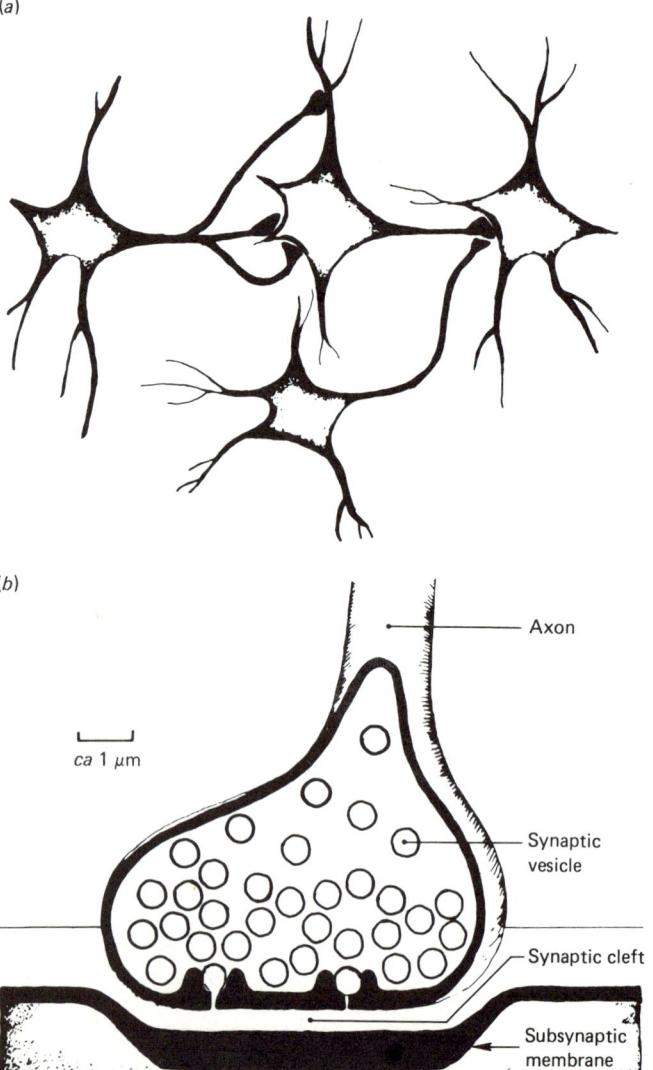

ca 1 μm

Axon

Synaptic vesicle

Synaptic cleft

Subsynaptic membrane

synapses produce depolarizing, or *excitatory post-synaptic potentials* (EPSPs), and these in turn tend to trigger off action potentials (Fig. 1.13). Other synapses produce *inhibitory post-synaptic potentials* (IPSPs) which increase membrane polarization and oppose the effects of the EPSPs. On average there are about 1000 synapses on the dendrites and body of each neurone in the central nervous system; some of these are inhibitory and some excitatory. The balance between EPSPs and IPSPs determines the rate of firing of action potentials by each neurone.

1.3.4. The origin of the EEG

An EEG electrode, about 100 mm^2 in area and recording through the thickness of skull and meninges, picks up the averaged electrical activity from a substantial volume of underlying cortex. It was originally thought that EEG waves might be made up of summated action potentials, but these are too sharply localized to be registered by distant electrodes. It is now known from simultaneous recordings of the activity of individual neurones and of the overlying EEG, that the latter is composed of averaged PSPs (Fig. 1.14). For potentials to appear in the EEG there must be some degree of synchronization of events in different neurones: if the PSPs in all the cells occurred quite independently, the averaged activity recorded as the EEG would not consist of

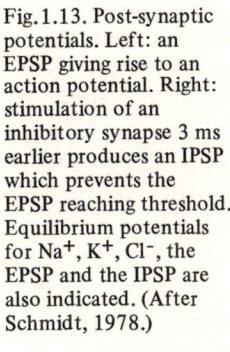

Fig. 1.13. Post-synaptic potentials. Left: an EPSP giving rise to an action potential. Right: stimulation of an inhibitory synapse 3 ms earlier produces an IPSP which prevents the EPSP reaching threshold. Equilibrium potentials for Na$^+$, K$^+$, Cl$^-$, the EPSP and the IPSP are also indicated. (After Schmidt, 1978.)

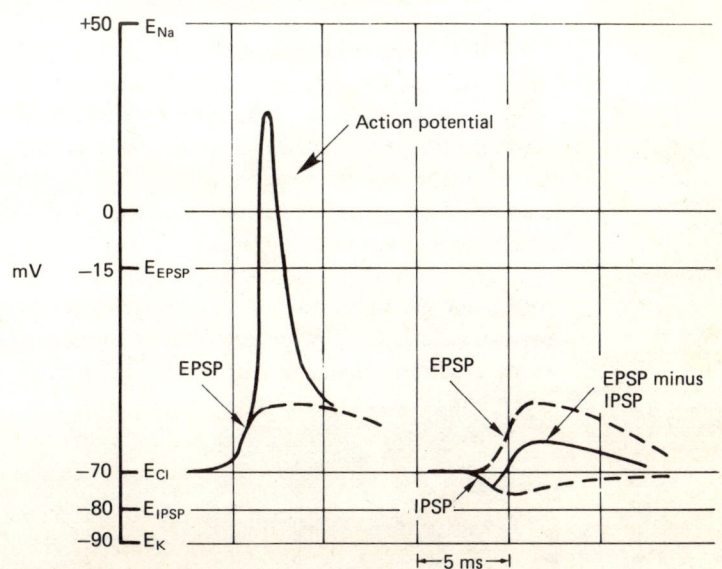

rhythmic, comparatively slow waves, but of low-amplitude random noise. It has however been estimated that synchronous PSPs in only 1% of cortical neurones would be sufficient to account for the signals normally seen in the EEG.

The cause of the rhythmicity of the EEG remains unclear. Isolated groups of interconnected neurones (Fig. 1.12a) certainly have the property of setting up rhythmic patterns of discharge. However there is also good evidence of a pacemaker within the deep midline structures of the brain which can produce rhythmic activity in the cortex. Dempsey and Morison (1942) stimulated certain so-called nonspecific thalamic nuclei in the cat and were able to record cortical slow waves. With repeated stimulation there was a progressive increase in the amplitude of these waves, the *recruiting response*, which then declined in amplitude as the stimulation continued. This activity was similar to spontaneous brain rhythms known as spindles, induced by administering barbiturates. The waves themselves have been shown to correspond to sequential EPSPs and IPSPs. Thus, a thalamic potential which produces a cortical EPSP will itself stimulate adjacent neurones which produce a subsequent IPSP. This sequence will be followed by the next thalamic EPSP, thus setting up a rhythmic process. It should be noted that the various nuclear groups in the thalamus have an intrinsic rhythmicity and do not require 'feedback' from the cortex in order to continue their discharges.

1.3.5. Reticular activating system

The densely packed neurones with numerous interconnections which comprise the core of the brain stem (the *reticular formation*) exert an all-important influence on the cerebral cortex, and it is the reticular formation together with its cortical projections that is known as the reticular activating system (RAS). Bremer in 1935 described the effects of making a cut between the thalamus and midbrain in the cat. This isolated the cerebrum from the brain stem and from most of its sensory input (producing a 'cerveau isolé'). The EEG revealed continuous high-voltage slow waves, a pattern similar to that of natural sleep. Although the

Fig. 1.14. Simultaneous recording from (below) activity of individual neurone and (above) electrocorticogram (the EEG registered directly from the surface of the brain) (reproduced with permission from Creutzfeld, Watanabe and Lux, 1966).

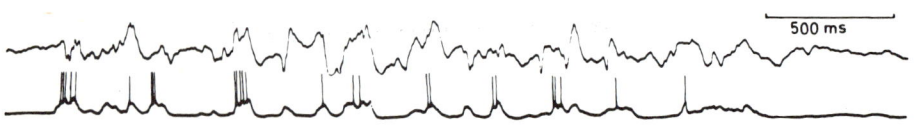

500 ms

animal appeared to be asleep it could not be aroused as the influence of the reticular formation on the cerebral cortex has been
totally interrupted. The mechanism was explained by the classical
studies of Moruzzi and Magoun in 1949. Lesions in the reticular
formation caused drowsiness with the appearance of rhythmic
slow waves in the cortex. Other studies demonstrated that stimulation of the reticular formation in the midbrain of an animal
caused arousal. In fact, any type of sensory input into the reticular
formation, for example auditory or visual, causes activation or
'desynchronization' of cortical activity. The resultant concept
was that proper functioning of the reticular activating system was
necessary in order to maintain consciousness. This is of crucial
clinical importance for many neurological conditions which affect
the brain stem and its reticular formation consequently depressing
consciousness.

Fig. 1.15. The reticular
activating system of
the Macacque monkey.

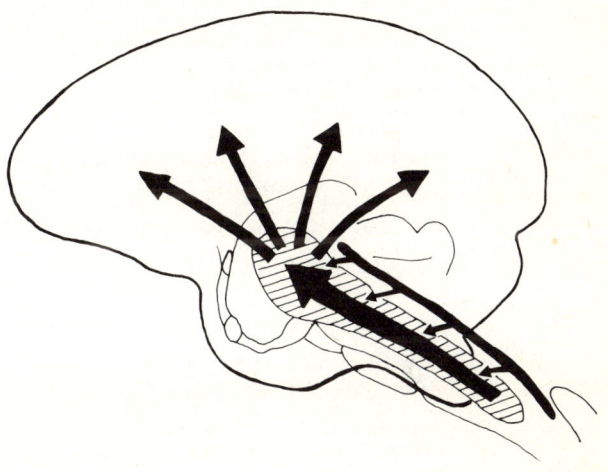

Medical Library
N. WALES HOSPITAL
DENBIGH

2. The EEG and its clinical use

2.1. The normal EEG

The electroencephalogram consists of changing potential differences between one region and another of the scalp; these are generally of low amplitude, not exceeding $150~\mu V$ in a normal waking subject. The signals studied for most clinical and research purposes occupy a frequency range of 0.5–60 Hz, but this may reflect the limitations of the recording systems rather than the actual range of activity present. There is for instance evidence that the EEG contains information at over 200 Hz.

Despite various draft proposals (the most recent by Chatrian *et al.*, 1974) there is not yet an internationally agreed terminology for EEG phenomena. For descriptive purposes, the EEG may be divided into on-going 'background activity' and episodic events or transients which appear suddenly and are of relatively short duration. Most activity in the normal EEG is more or less rhythmic and can therefore be described in terms of frequency and amplitude. By convention, and partly for historical reasons, the signals are classified into four frequency bands:

Delta (δ) – below 4 Hz
Theta (θ) – not less than 4 but less than 8 Hz
Alpha (α) – 8 to 13 Hz inclusive
Beta (β) – more than 13 Hz.

There is some disagreement as to whether the appropriate unit of frequency for EEG activity is cycles/s or Hz, but the latter is currently favoured. The activity recorded differs from one region of the scalp to another and it is therefore generally necessary to record simultaneously from 20 or more electrodes distributed widely over the head. The description of an EEG phenomenon will usually include an account of its topography.

To understand and recognize the pathological features one must first get to know the normal patterns and their variability. The EEG changes continually, both in a random manner, in association with changes in mental activity or emotional state, and with drowsiness or sleep. It also changes gradually over the lifetime of the individual and shows marked differences between one person and another. Only recently has it become possible, with the help of computers, to give detailed objective descriptions of the normal EEG, and the clinical electroencephalographer must still base his criteria of normality on his own experience of looking at EEGs of healthy people. In adults, the limits of normal variation may be learned with no great difficulty but in children the patterns are more varied, for the EEG changes associated with growth and development are as dramatic as those in motor or language skills.

2.1.1. The normal waking adult EEG

A typical sample of the EEG of a normal waking adult is shown in Fig. 2.1. In this example eight recording channels have been used, each displaying the potential difference between a pair of electrodes located as shown on the small head outline to the left of the figure. The most conspicuous activity is at 10 to 11 Hz, i.e. within the alpha range, and is seen mainly on those channels recording from the back of the head (3, 4, 7 and 8). At the point indicated on the tracing, the subject opens her eyes and the alpha activity virtually ceases. Activity of alpha frequency located at the back of the head and responsive to visual attention is designated the *alpha rhythm*.

Though by definition the alpha band is 8–13 Hz, the adult alpha rhythm is commonly between 9 and 11 Hz. A higher alpha frequency is of no significance but an alpha rhythm at only 8 Hz, though not necessarily abnormal, may raise a suspicion of a diffuse disturbance of brain function, especially if a higher frequency has previously been found in the same subject. Certain drugs and metabolic disturbances may lower the alpha frequency before producing any clear abnormality, as can early cerebral degenerations. Alpha slowing may also occur in drowsiness, and the technologist must carefully note the behavioural state of the subject whenever a slow alpha rhythm is seen.

The amplitude of alpha activity varies, typically from 40 to 100 μV, and its amount and persistence are very variable indeed. Fig. 2.2*a* and *b* are also from young normal adults and give some impression of the range of normal variation. In Fig. 2.2*a* there is abundant alpha activity only slightly diminished by eye opening, whereas in Fig. 2.2*b* there is minimal alpha activity even when the eyes are closed.

If the amount of alpha activity is of little clinical significance, symmetry is much more important. A 50% difference in amplitude between the two sides of the head is seen in not more than 5% of healthy subjects. In right-handed people the alpha amplitude is often slightly larger on the right than the left. Either a left-sided predominance of alpha activity in a right-handed person or an asymmetry of more than 50% must therefore be regarded as a

Fig.2.1. EEG of
normal waking subject
aged 24, for description
see text. HF and TC
relate to filter settings
(see Chapter 5). The
uppermost trace is a
time marker.

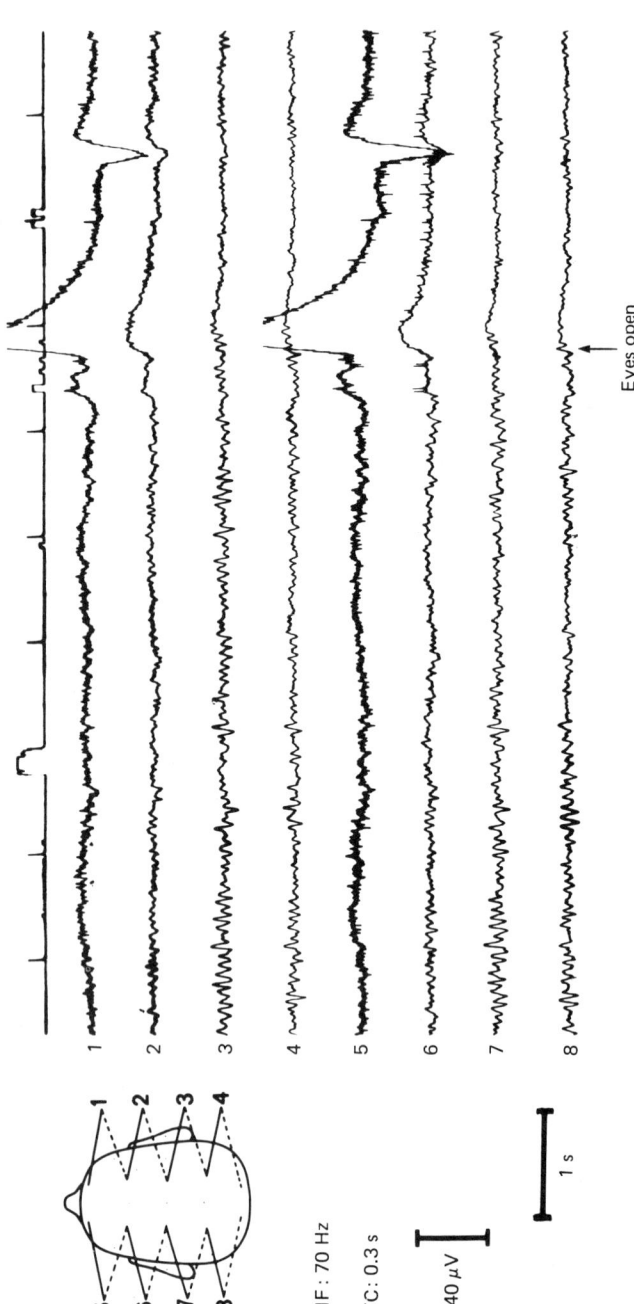

sign of possible disease of that side of the brain on which the alpha rhythm is less well represented.

As seen above, the alpha rhythm may be entirely suppressed ('blocked') or at least attenuated when the subject opens his eyes. *Alpha blocking* is also produced by mental arithmetic and other tasks, and by sudden unexpected stimuli producing arousal or attracting attention. Blocking of the alpha rhythm and its return on eye closure should be prompt and symmetrical. The alpha

Fig. 2.2. Normal variants. (*a*) 'Alpha plus', subject age 22. (*b*) 'Alpha minus', subject aged 23.

(*a*)

(*b*)

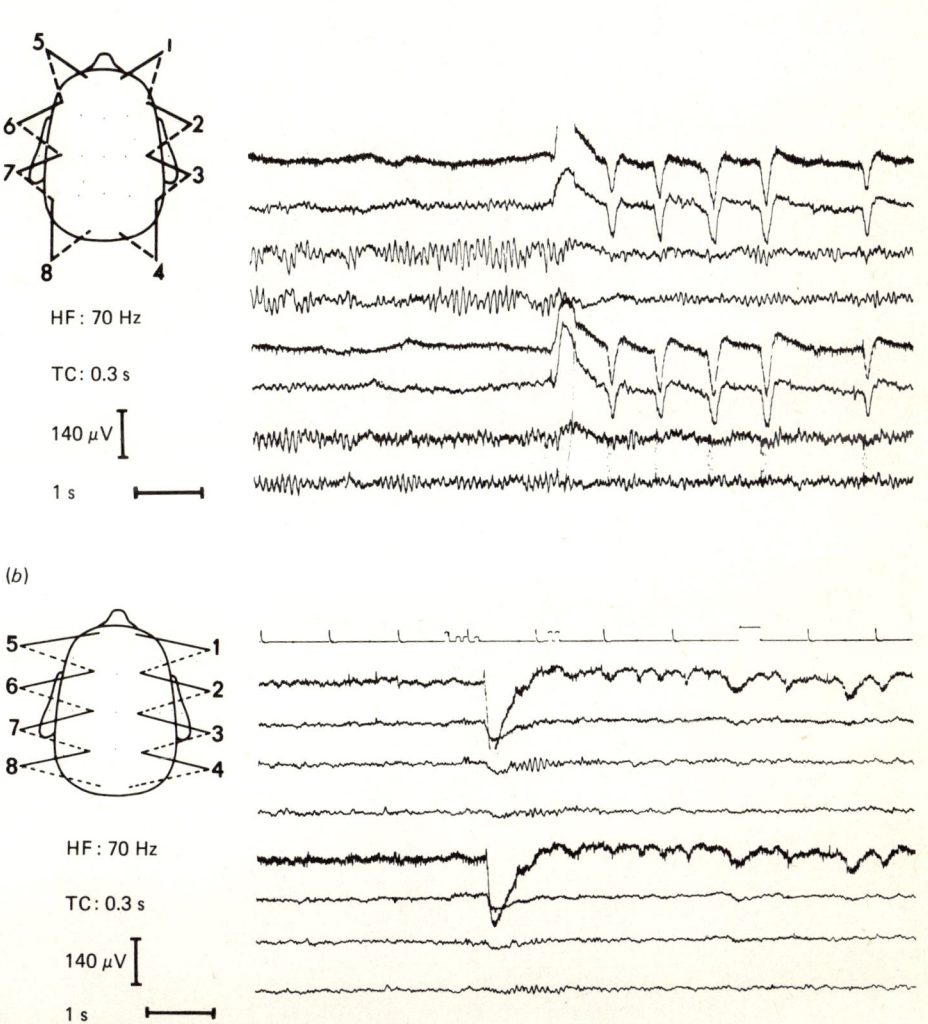

HF: 70 Hz

TC: 0.3 s

140 μV

1 s

Fig. 2.3. Fast alpha variant in normal subject not taking medication.

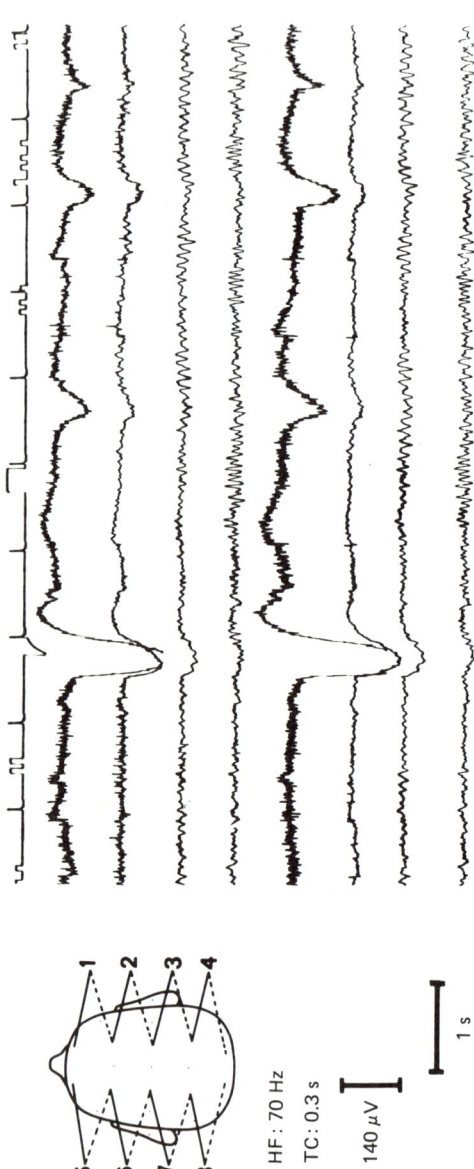

HF: 70 Hz

TC: 0.3 s

140 μV

1 s

rhythm is very sensitive to changes in state of awareness, being attenuated both by arousal and anxiety on the one hand, and by drowsiness on the other. In a drowsy patient showing little alpha activity, opening the eyes may be accompanied by arousal and, instead of blocking, there is a 'paradoxical' return of the alpha rhythm. An unusual normal variation is called 'alpha-squeak', the appearance of alpha activity immediately after eye-closure with a higher frequency than that generally seen. This effect rarely lasts more than one or two seconds and should be symmetrical.

Often the alpha rhythm is intermingled with activity having the same distribution and responsiveness but at a sub-harmonic, for instance half the alpha frequency. Such a *slow alpha variant* is normal in the young but is not conspicuous in adults. Less commonly the alpha rhythm is replaced by activity within the beta frequency band. This *fast alpha variant* may also be a normal finding and occurs particularly in patients taking certain tranquillizers (Fig. 2.3).

In the illustrations above, a number of signals are present which are not of cerebral origin and which for the purposes of electroencephalography may be regarded as noise or artefacts. For instance, because there is a potential difference of some 70 mV between the front and back of the eye, movement, blinking, opening and closure of the eyes produce a changing electrical field which is picked up by the EEG electrodes (see the large excursions on the channels recording from the front of the head in Figs. 2.1 and 2.2). The small short-duration spikes appearing continually on channel 5 and intermittently on channel 6 of Fig. 2.3 are also of non-cerebral origin, arising from the electrical activity of scalp muscles. These and other artefacts can usually be recognized on account of characteristic wave form and distribution. At the least they provide some information about the state and behaviour of the subject which may assist the interpretation of the EEG (see also Section 2.1.3).

Beta activity is rhythmic with a frequency above 13 Hz and typically of greatest amplitude over the anterior regions. It is present in nearly all normal subjects both in wakefulness and sleep with an average amplitude of some 10 to 50 μV. On occasions, the amplitude may be much higher (60 μV or more) either as a normal variant or due to taking certain medications (Fig. 2.4).

Theta activity has by definition a frequency not less than 4 but below 8 Hz. Apart from possible slow alpha variants, theta

Fig. 2.4. Profuse beta
activity induced by
quinalbarbitone. Note
antero-posterior
gradient: this activity
is most prominent in
the frontal channels
(1 to 4) and less in
amount posteriorly
(channels 7 and 8).

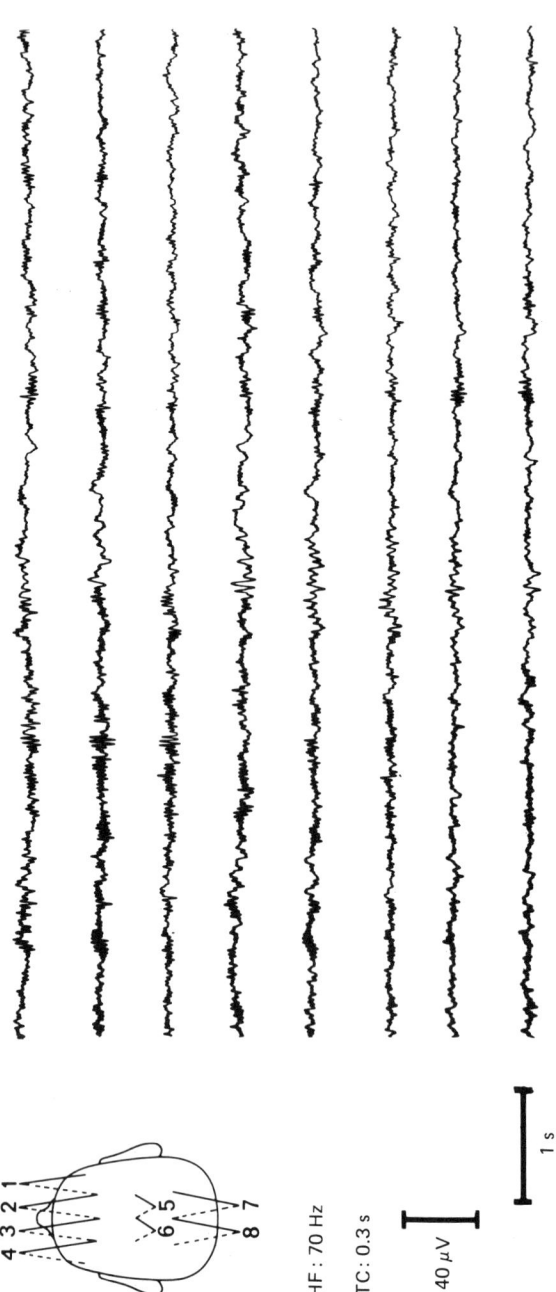

HF : 70 Hz

TC : 0.3 s

140 μV

1 s

activity is not a prominent feature of the waking adult EEG but is generally present in small amounts over the temporal regions.

Delta activity, consisting of rhythmic components below 4 Hz or isolated waves of more than 250 ms duration, is not a usual feature of the waking adult EEG. Small amounts of delta activity may, however, be seen over the posterior temporal regions in young adults and represent the persistence of a component which is conspicuous in childhood.

In association with voluntary changes of visual fixation (saccadic eye movements), small positive or biphasic waves appear over the occipital regions. These *lambda* waves (Fig. 2.5) are most prominent when the subject scans an interesting pattern.

Alpha frequency activity may occur over the central regions with a characteristic outline of alternating sharp and rounded waves (Fig. 2.6). This *mu rhythm* (also called a comb or wicket rhythm or rhythm en arceau) is present with the eyes open but is suppressed by voluntary movement or sensory stimulation of the opposite arm or leg. A mu rhythm may occur in normal subjects and is symmetrical in some instances and unilateral in others. It has no clinical significance.

2.1.2. Effects of age

During childhood and adolescence the EEG changes progressively and also shows marked variability, as cerebral maturation proceeds faster in some children than in others. For a more complete account of what is almost a sub-speciality of EEG, see Gibbs and Gibbs (1950) or Dumermuth (1976).

Fig. 2.5. Lambda waves: note that these appear only when the eyes are open and are closely associated with rapid eye movements in an alert subject.

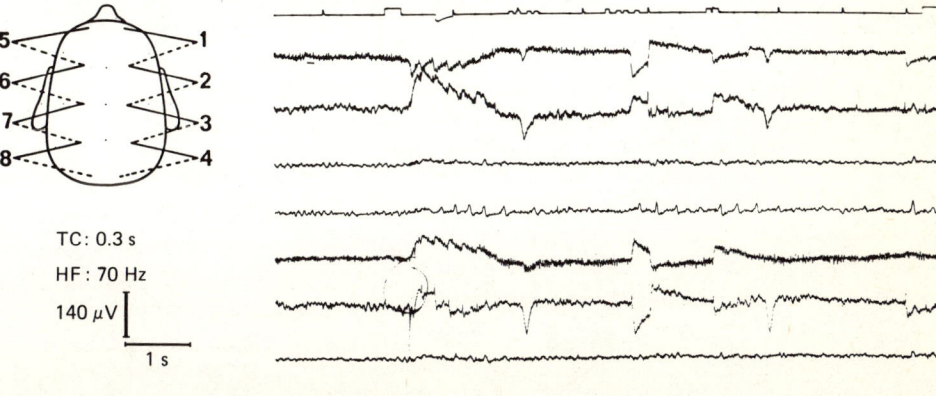

TC: 0.3 s

HF: 70 Hz

140 μV

1 s

Fig. 2.6. Mu rhythm maximal over the central regions. Movement of the right-hand (arrow) blocked the activity.

The record of the newborn is largely made up of irregular theta and delta components and is conspicuously lacking in rhythmic activity (Fig. 2.7a). Indeed rhythmicity may be a sign

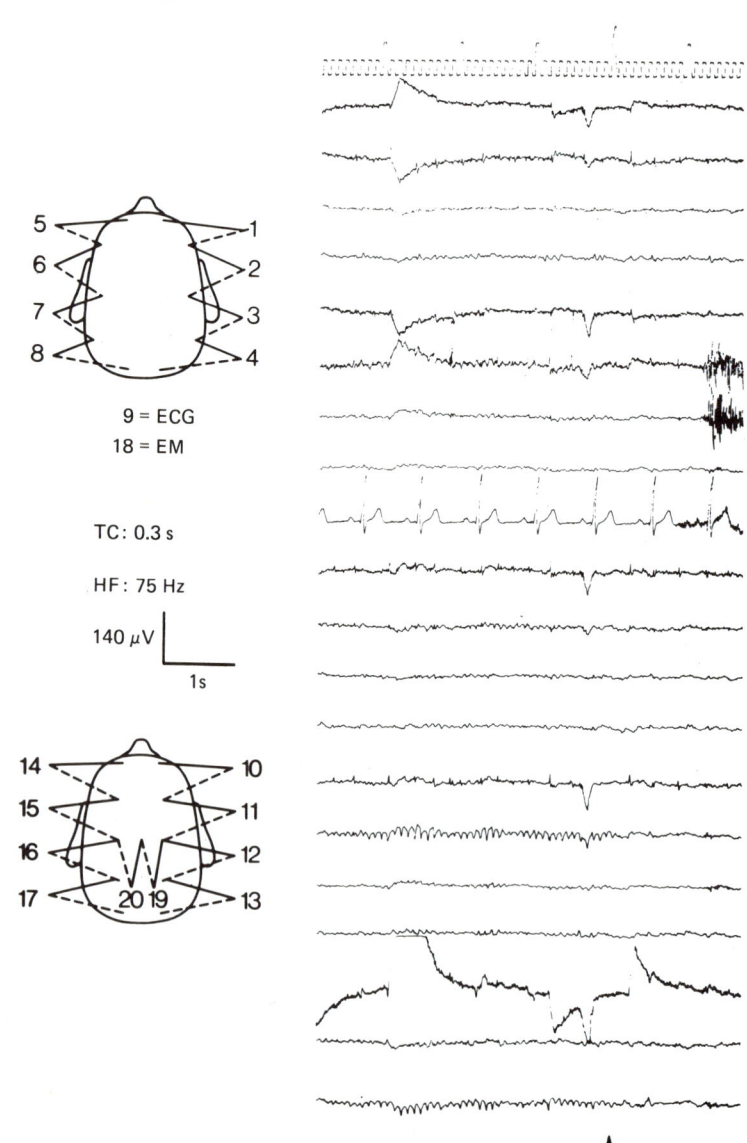

9 = ECG
18 = EM

TC: 0.3 s

HF: 75 Hz

140 μV

1 s

of abnormality in this age group. At 2 to 3 months rhythmic waves appear, first in the delta range, but by 6 months short bursts of rhythmic theta activity are present over the central regions. These become faster and migrate posteriorly so that, by 2 years, an alpha rhythm is beginning to appear at the back of the head. At this age a great deal of irregular theta and delta activity is also present, the latter being maximal over the parieto-temporal regions. During the period of childhood the delta activity becomes increasingly restricted to the posterior temporal regions; the alpha rhythm becomes more regular, faster and greater in amplitude but is still intermixed with large amounts of slow alpha variant. Other theta activities remain prominent over the temporal regions (Fig. 2.7b). These changes continue throughout adolescence, the posterior temporal slow waves and slow alpha variants disappearing and the temporal theta activity being much reduced by the time the adult pattern is established at 18 to 20 years of age. The rate of EEG maturation, like that of social behaviour, is very variable; some 14-year olds already have an EEG like that of an adult, whereas in other individuals posterior slow activity may persist well into the third decade.

The EEG pattern remains essentially unchanged throughout adult life, unless a disease process intervenes. However, in the elderly, gradual brain atrophy and sclerosis of cerebral blood vessels are commonplace, and involvement of the brain in such processes is certainly usual, if not 'normal'. The EEG reflects these pathological changes in several ways. Above the age of 50 two patterns may emerge: often there is a polyrhythmic picture with slowed alpha and increased theta and temporal delta components and occasional sharp waves over the temporal regions; sometimes one sees instead a loss of alpha activity, leaving a low-amplitude record largely composed of beta and theta rhythms (Fig. 2.7c).

2.1.3. Effect of arousal and sleep

The EEG is very sensitive to alterations in state of consciousness. Not only are there gross differences between the waking record and that of light or deep sleep but there are also fluctuations with minimal alterations in attention and alertness. During sleep the EEG follows a very constant pattern and the depth of sleep is classified on the basis of the EEG and other findings. The system most widely used is that of Dement and Kleitman (1957); workers wishing to stage sleep records accurately and consistently often use a manual by Rechtschaffen and Kales (1968).

Fig.2.7. The normal EEG at different ages. (a) 7-day-old baby. (b) 7-year-old child.

The pattern of *wakefulness* was described above. Alpha activity is the most important feature though this may be suppressed by attention and anxiety.

(a)

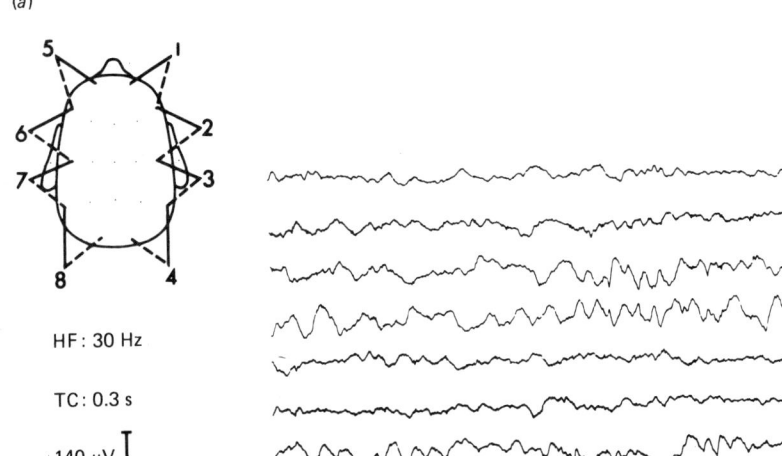

HF: 30 Hz

TC: 0.3 s

140 μV

1 s

(b)

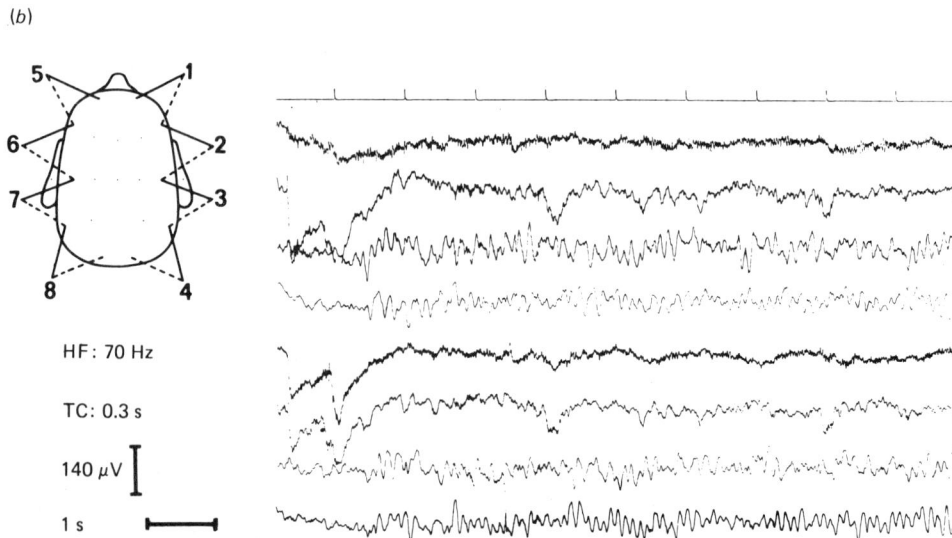

HF: 70 Hz

TC: 0.3 s

140 μV

1 s

The first evidence of *drowsiness* may be an increase of amplitude, slight slowing of the alpha rhythm, reduced blocking and possibly paradoxical increase of alpha activity on eye opening, and often some slowing of heart rate and reduction in muscle artefact.

Sleep *stage I* is characterized by suppression of alpha activity, some increase in beta components and possibly also of rhythmic theta and the appearance of artefacts due to slow lateral eye movements (Fig. 2.8*b*). On slight arousal sharp waves of up to 300 μV appear over the vertex; they are symmetrical and may extend to the frontal and parietal regions.

In *stage II* the background is made up largely of beta and theta activity with some low-amplitude delta components comprising less than 20% of the record. Spindle-shaped bursts of *sigma activity* ('sleep spindles') appear, typically of 12–14 Hz and maximal over the fronto-central regions, but sometimes slower and more widespread (Fig. 2.8*c*). Individual spindles are often asymmetrical but overall there should be no consistent difference in amount between the two hemispheres. Vertex sharp waves continue to occur on arousal and also spontaneously. A new type of arousal response now appears, the *K-complex*. This consists of a sharp wave, followed by a delta component and a sigma burst and is of maximal amplitude at the vertex or midfrontal area. Often positive triangular shaped *lambdoid waves* appear in the occipital regions. These are bilaterally synchronous and usually sym-

Fig.2.7 (cont.)
(*c*) Elderly person aged 95. For description see text.

(*c*)

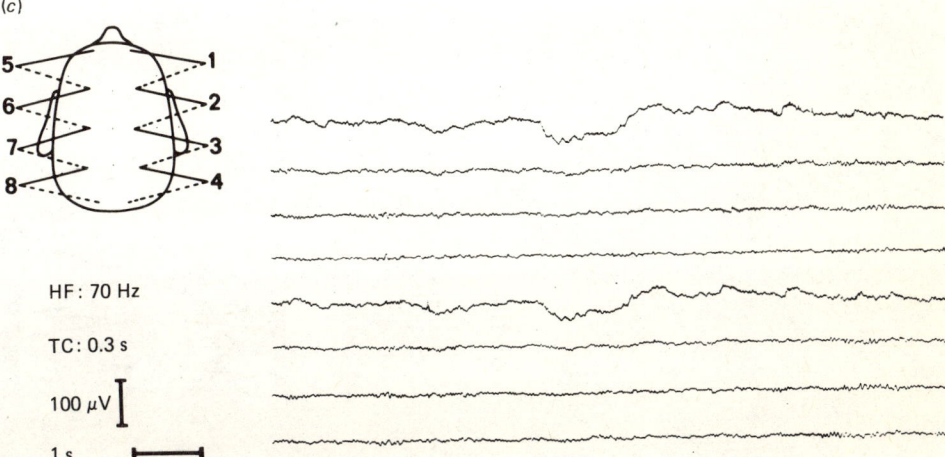

HF: 70 Hz

TC: 0.3 s

100 μV

1 s

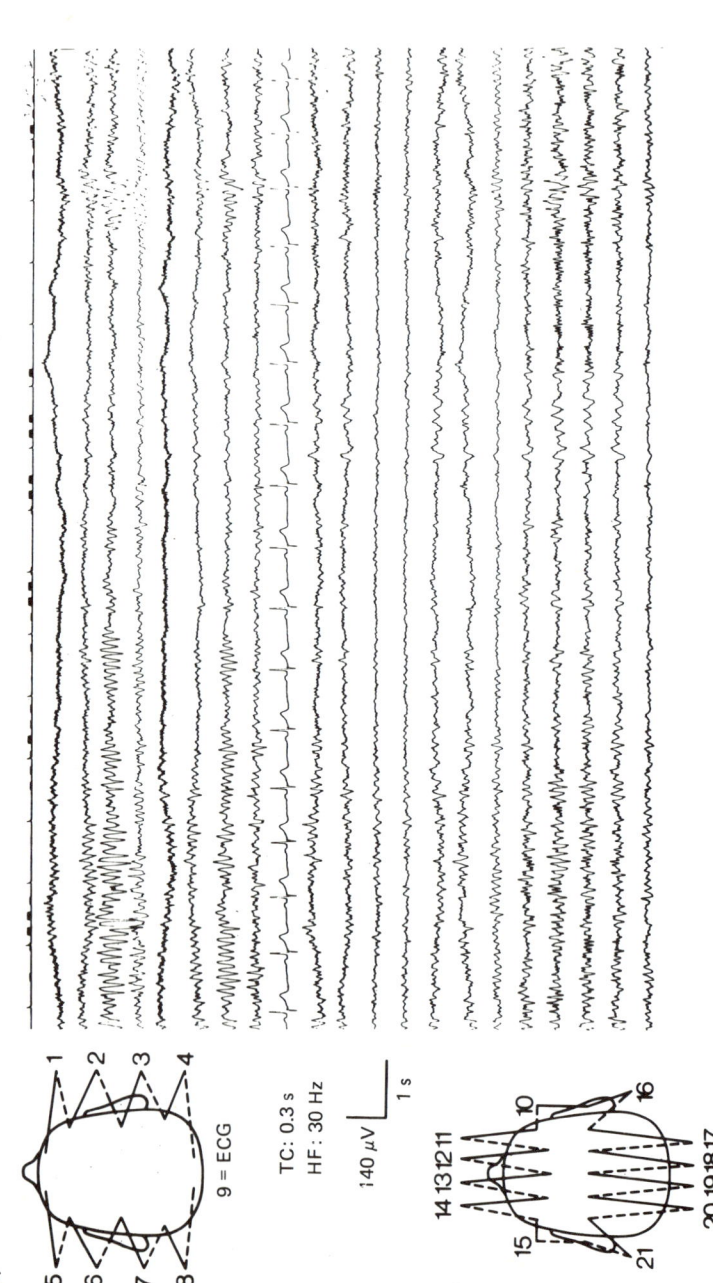

Fig.2.8. Effects of sleep and drowsiness. (a) Early drowsiness note waxing and waning of alpha rhythm.

(b) Sleep stage 1.

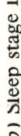

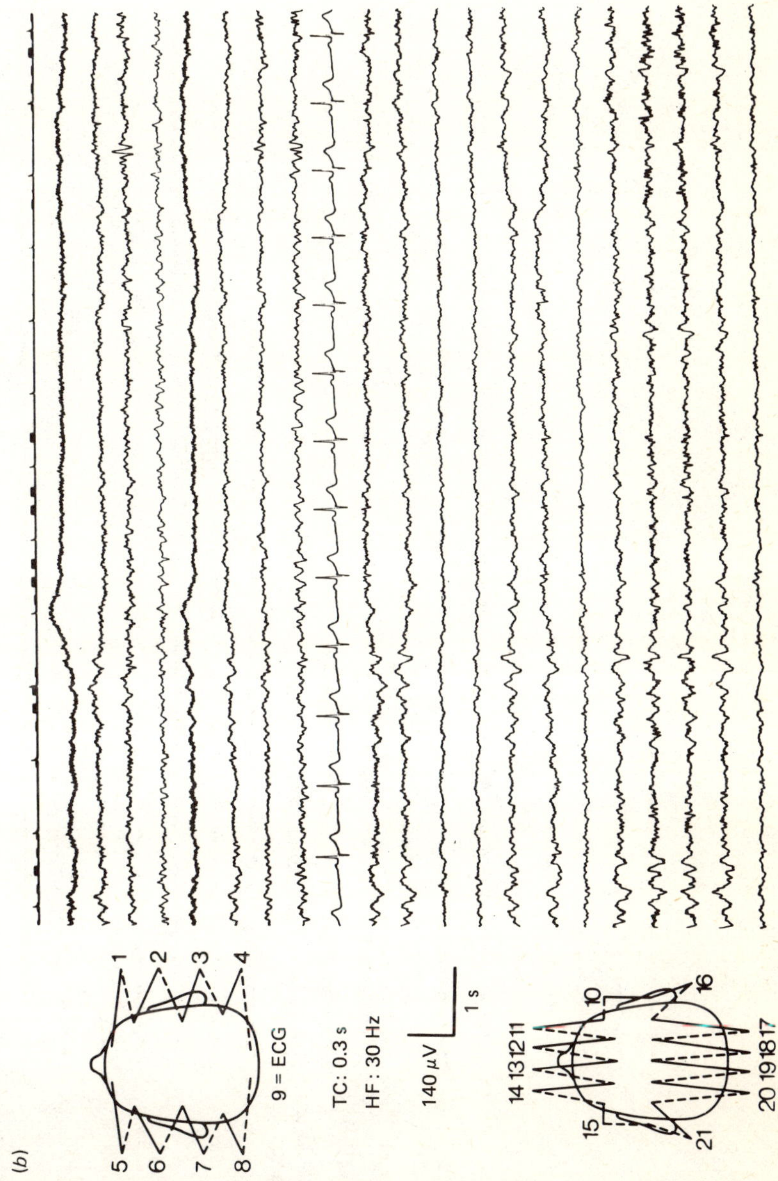

(b)

1
2
3
4

5
6
7
8

9 = ECG

TC: 0.3 s
HF: 30 Hz

140 μV

1 s

10
11
12
13
14

15

16
17
18
19
20

21

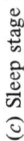

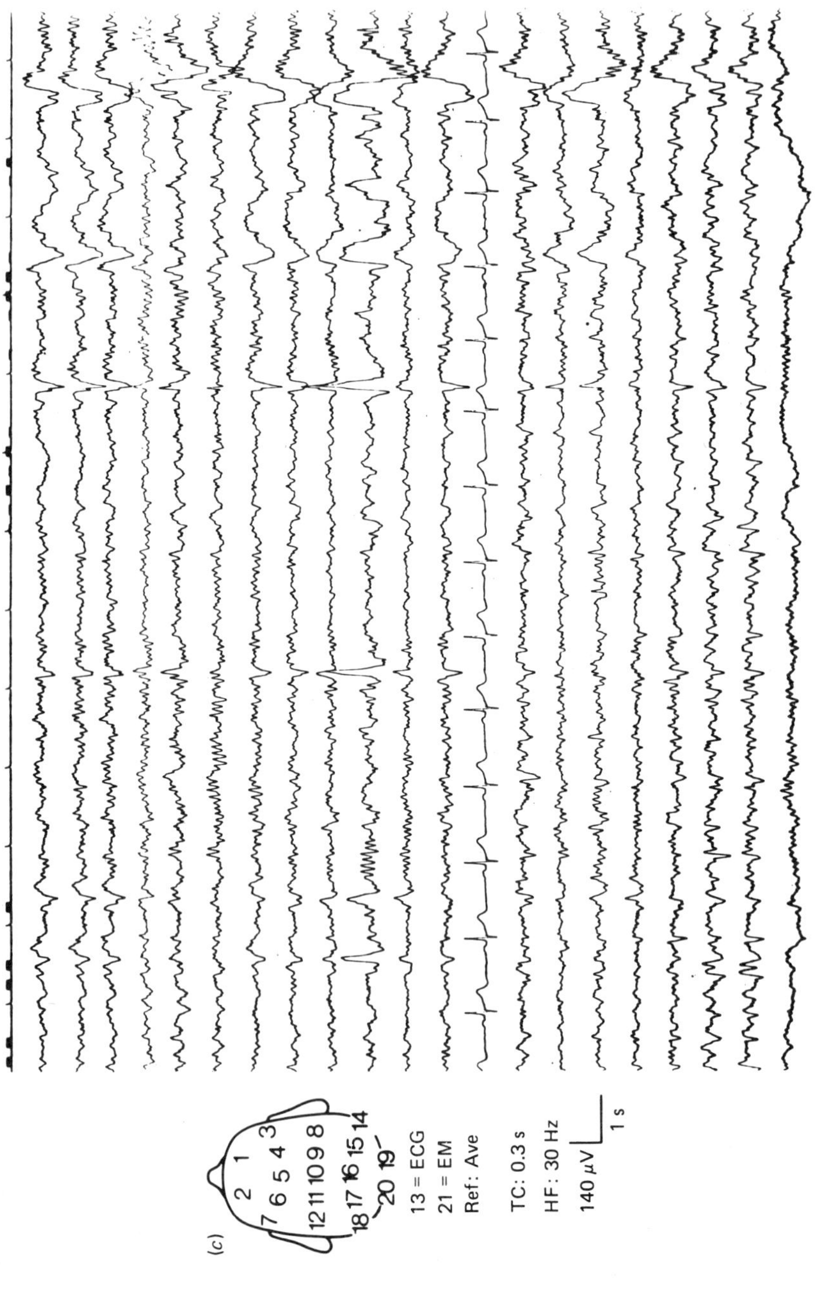

(c) Sleep stage II.

(c)

13 = ECG
21 = EM
Ref: Ave

TC: 0.3 s
HF: 30 Hz

140 µV

1 s

(d) Sleep stage III.

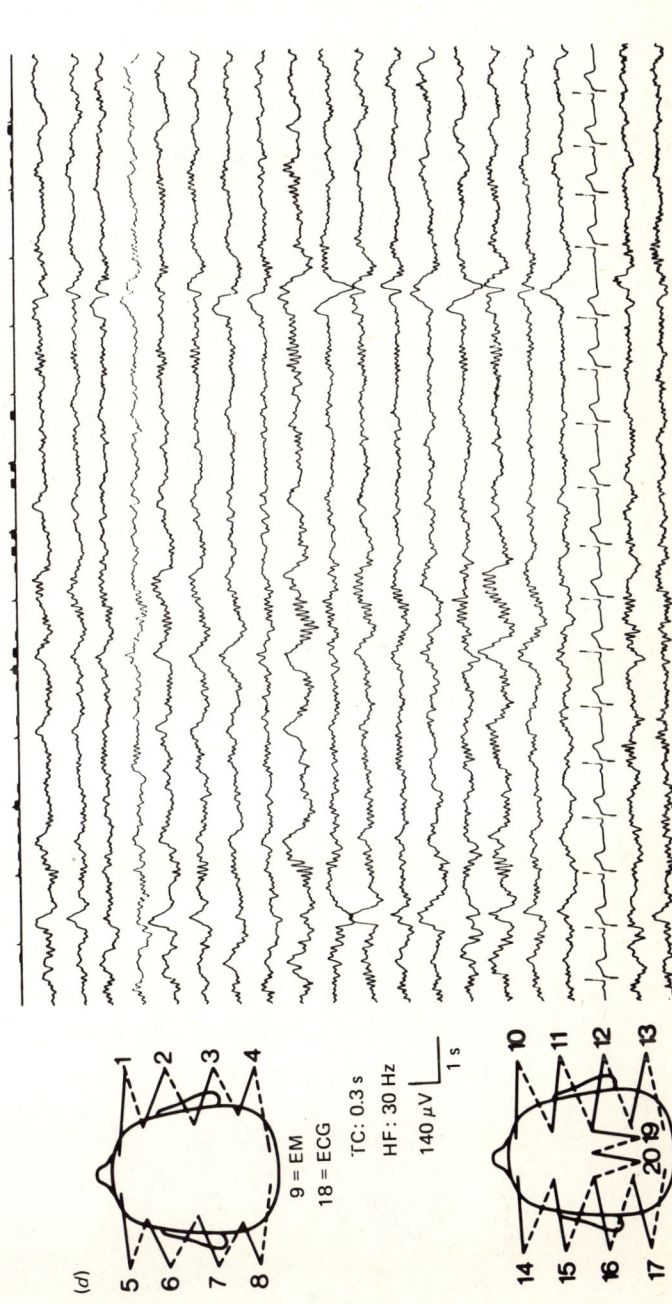

9 = EM
18 = ECG

TC: 0.3 s
HF: 30 Hz

140 μV
1 s

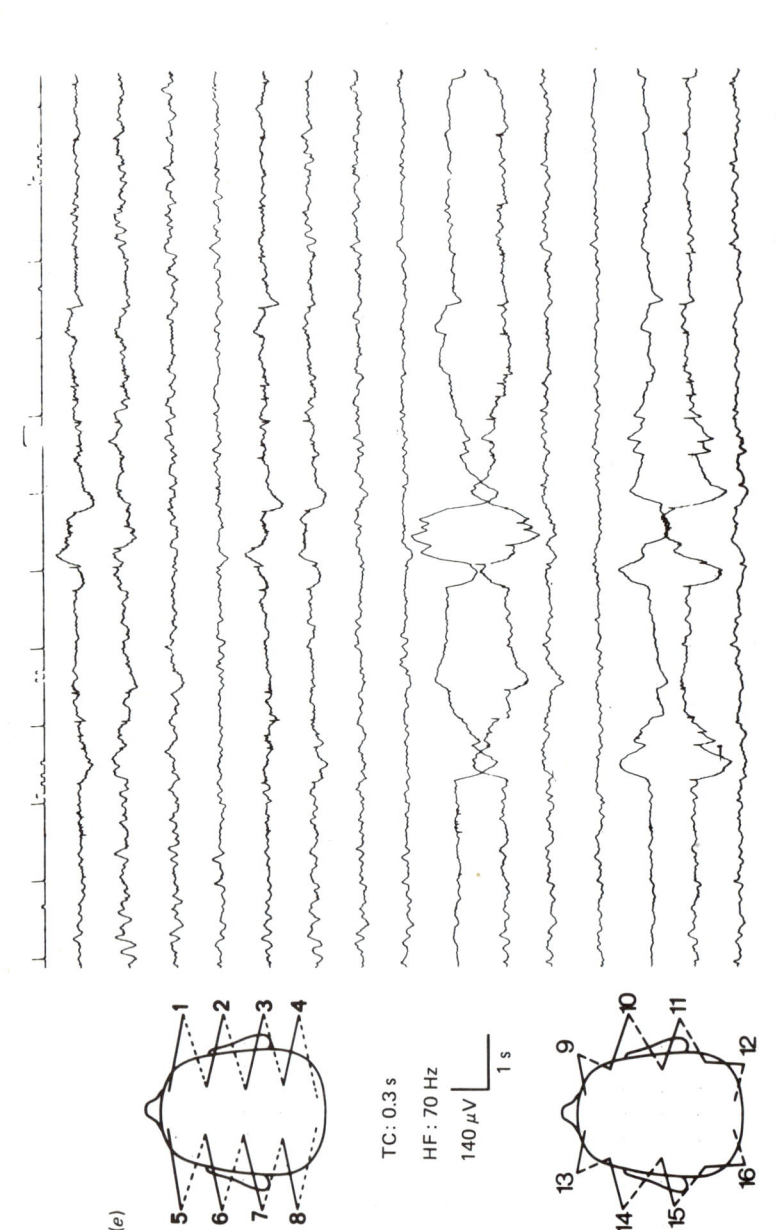

(e) REM sleep, for description see text.

metrical, or may parallel any asymmetry of the alpha rhythm. The slow lateral eye movements of stage I are not seen in stage II sleep.

In *stage III* 20–50% of the recording time is occupied by delta activity below 1 Hz and greater in amplitude than 100 μV. Vertex sharp waves and lambdoid waves decrease and eventually disappear but sleep spindles and K-complexes remain.

Stage IV is characterized by more than 50% slow high-voltage delta activity, occasional K-complexes but no isolated sigma spindles.

Some 1½ hours after the onset of sleep a new pattern emerges, characterized by rapid eye movements and associated with dreaming ('REM'). The background activity has a variable appearance but typically is made up of theta and alpha components of low amplitude, sometimes with central theta bursts (Fig. 2.8*e*). Muscle tone, which can be conveniently monitored by recording the electrical activity of the submental muscles (below the chin), is markedly reduced but spontaneous movements and even grinding of the teeth appear. The ECG may become somewhat irregular. *REM sleep* does not readily occur during routine daytime EEGs and is most conveniently registered at night. It can however be obtained in records of at least 1½ hours duration in the early morning after a night without sleep. It can also be induced with non-barbiturate drugs (for instance flurazepam).

2.1.4. Activation procedures

The EEG changes of sleep often unmask abnormalities of diagnostic significance. Other activation procedures used in routine clinical electroencephalography include asking the subject to breathe extra deeply for a few minutes (hyperventilation) and exposing him to flashing lights (intermittent photic stimulation). These techniques form the subject of Chapter 7 but are mentioned in passing here as they are relevant to the clinical section which follows.

2.2. EEG abnormalities

It is not the purpose of this manual to provide a general account of clinical electroencephalography. However, it is necessary to outline the common EEG abnormalities and the clinical context in which they occur, as the recording of these phenomena is a chief concern of the succeeding chapters. The reader requiring a textbook of electroencephalography is referred to: Kiloh,

McComas and Osselton (1972), Kooi, Tucker and Marstall (1978), Klass and Daly (1979) or (in German) Christian (1975).

As indicated in the previous section, the normal EEG changes with age and with state of awareness and in any case the limits of variation are broad. Abnormalities may appear as changes in the composition of background activity or as transient phenomena and may be generalized, unilateral or focal over a small region of the scalp.

2.2.1. Abnormalities of background activity

As the amplitude of the normal EEG is variable, a *diffuse reduction in amplitude* of background activity may be difficult to recognize unless it is very gross indeed, as in the terminal stages of some cerebral degenerative processes. In the most extreme case, the EEG becomes unrecordable or *isoelectric* (Fig. 2.9). Temporary abolition of EEG activity may occur during intoxication with cerebral depressant drugs or if the body temperature is reduced below 32 °C, a standard procedure during some heart and neurosurgical operations. An isoelectric record is also obtained when the supply of oxygen to the brain is interrupted for more than 15 s. If the anoxia is relieved within a few minutes the patient may recover, but an isoelectric EEG persisting more than 6 hours after an anoxic episode (in the absence of intoxication and with a normal body temperature) indicates that the patient has suffered severe brain damage and is most unlikely to regain consciousness.

As the normal EEG is fairly symmetrical, unilateral or more *localized depression* or flattening of normal activities is easily

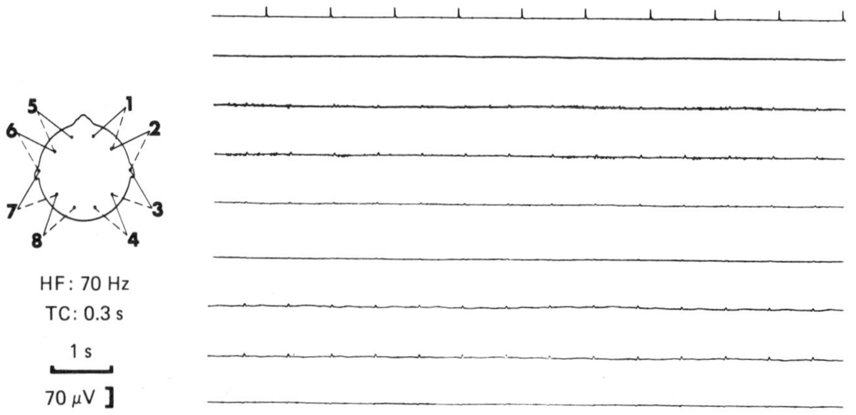

Fig.2.9. Isoelectric EEG (for establishing electro-cerebral silence it would be necessary to record at a higher sensitivity than that shown here).

HF: 70 Hz
TC: 0.3 s

1 s

70 μV]

recognized and is one of the most reliable EEG signs of disease. It may occur because the underlying cerebral cortex has been destroyed or has ceased functioning, as for instance after occlusion of a major cerebral artery. Alternatively, there may be a pathological process intervening between the surface of the brain and the electrodes, for instance a collection of blood in the meninges. From the EEG appearances alone the two mechanisms cannot usually be distinguished. Fig. 2.10 shows an EEG with marked unilateral flattening of normal activities due to blocking of the right middle cerebral artery. This record is virtually diagnostic of right-sided disease but is quite non-specific so far as the nature of the pathology is concerned. Loss of nerve cells due to a severe head injury in the past, or a chronic subdural haematoma (a collection of blood in the space between the dura and the brain) could produce the same picture.

The other common disturbance of background activity is *slowing*. Sometimes normal rhythms are slowed or replaced by activity of lower frequency; this change may be diffuse or localized. Alternatively, distinct theta or delta components, rhythmic or irregular, appear superimposed upon normal activities which may be relatively unaffected or more usually reduced. This type of change is often localized. Metabolic disorders provide an example of *diffuse slowing*. For instance, in early liver failure the alpha rhythm is replaced by rhythmic sinusoidal activity in the upper theta range (Fig. 2.11).

A rapid increase of pressure inside the skull also produces diffuse slowing of the EEG. This can be caused by an expanding

Fig. 2.10. Asymmetrical EEG following occlusion of right middle cerebral artery one month previously.

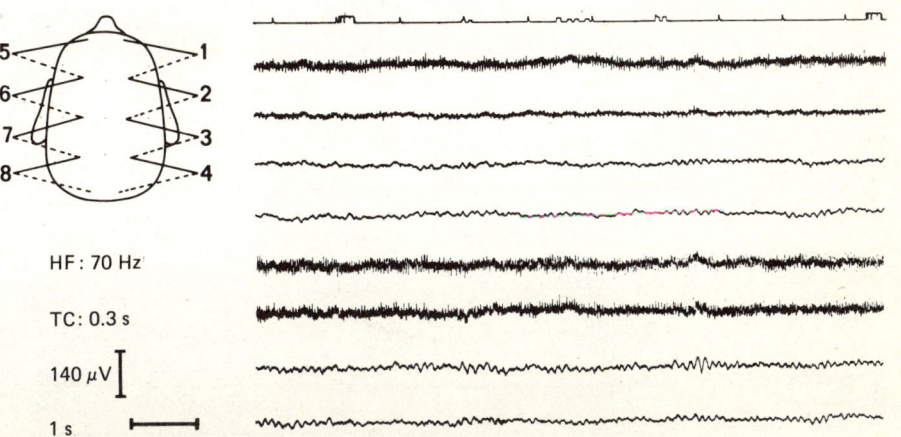

HF: 70 Hz

TC: 0.3 s

140 μV

1 s

mass (a cerebral tumour or a haematoma for instance), by obstruction of the CSF pathway, or by swelling of the brain itself due to infection or reduction of its blood supply. A gradual rise of intracranial pressure causes much less slowing; this may enable one to distinguish slow-growing from more rapidly expanding tumours, and to identify patients with 'benign intracranial hypertension', a condition in which there is a marked but slow rise in CSF pressure producing vomiting and headache but little EEG change.

The combination of generalized slowing and asymmetry of background activity can be difficult to interpret. For instance, a record with a diffuse excess of theta activity higher in amplitude on the right than on the left allows two interpretations: either that there is a generalized disturbance more severe on the right, or that there is a combination of diffuse slowing and left-sided flattening, as could occur in a patient with a left subdural haematoma causing a rise in intracranial pressure. This second possibility may be identified by a reduction in amplitude of normal faster activities on the side where the theta components are also less prominent.

As the frequency composition of the normal EEG is dependent on both age and state of awareness, these two factors must always be taken into account in assessing possible background abnormalities. A useful training exercise for both doctors and technologists is to attempt to determine the age and state of awareness of a subject from a page of EEG presented without further clinical information and to decide whether or not it is abnormal. There are few symmetrical disturbances of background activity which

Fig.2.11. Early hepatic encephalopathy: note slowed dominant rhythm and also rolling lateral eye movements which betray drowsiness. The next day the patient was in coma.

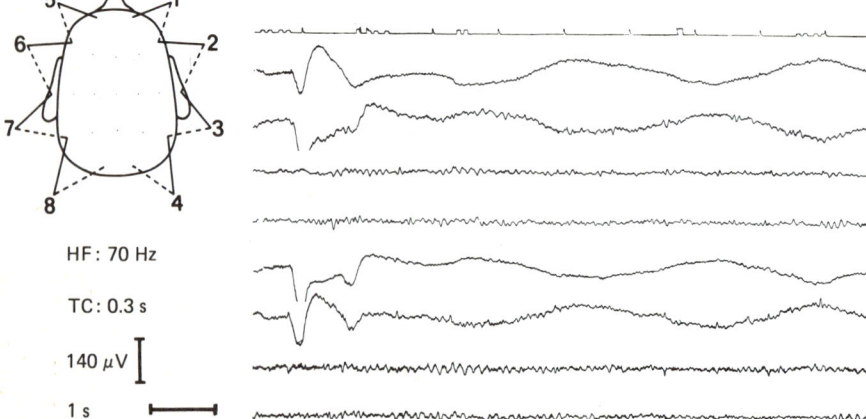

HF: 70 Hz

TC: 0.3 s

140 μV

1 s

produce a picture which could not with a particular combination of age and state of awareness occur in a normal subject.

Localized slow activity in the theta or delta range generally indicates disease of the underlying cortex (but is occasionally 'projected' from deeper structures – see Section 2.2.2). Where brain cells are dead or have been replaced by a mass of some other material (haematoma or tumour for instance) no cerebral electrical activity is generated and one sees flattening. Focal slowing of the EEG arises in surviving cells which are still capable of activity but are malfunctioning. The functional disturbance may arise from the lesion itself, for instance a cerebral contusion (bruise), laceration, or a region of *ischaemia* (impaired blood supply). Alternatively, the malfunctioning cells may be adjacent to the lesion, for instance in the compressed and swollen tissue around a tumour or haemorrhage. The different effects of dysfunction and death of cells are reflected in the evolution of some acute disorders. Fig. 2.12 shows an EEG recorded on the day after a massive right cerebral *infarct* (destruction of tissue due to blockage of an artery). There is a large amount of delta activity over the affected hemisphere, reflecting malfunction of the remaining cells due to brain swelling and impaired blood supply. The patient survived and a year later the EEG showed only a right-sided depression of background activity (as in Fig. 2.10): so far as possible, normal brain function had returned and the residual EEG flattening was due to cell loss. With a tumour the picture is similar to that immediately after a cerebro-vascular accident but slowing (both local, and diffuse due to pressure) is often more marked than the local depression of normal activities.

Fig. 2.12. EEG one day after a massive right cerebral infarct: note gross asymmetry of alpha rhythm, delta activity and sharp waves. There are also slow lateral eye movements due to drowsiness and the patient was in fact stuporous.

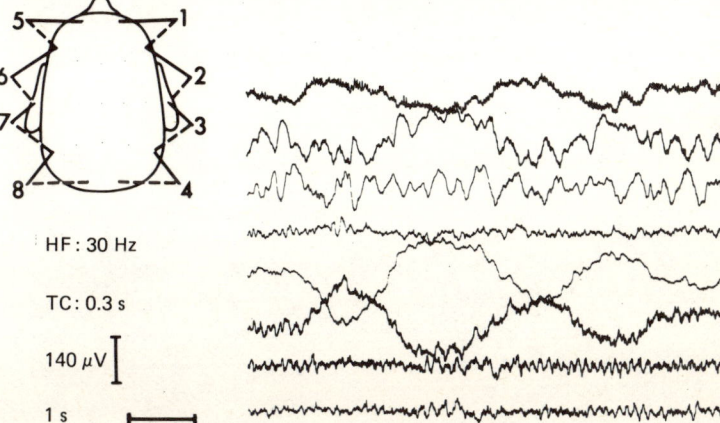

HF : 30 Hz

TC : 0.3 s

140 μV

1 s

Fig. 2.13. Stages in the evolution of a brain abscess. (a) Septic encephalitis preceding the development of a left-sided abscess. Note generalized slowing more prominent on the left. (b) An established left frontal abscess. Note diffuse slowing, left-sided depression of alpha activity and left-frontal triangular delta waves.

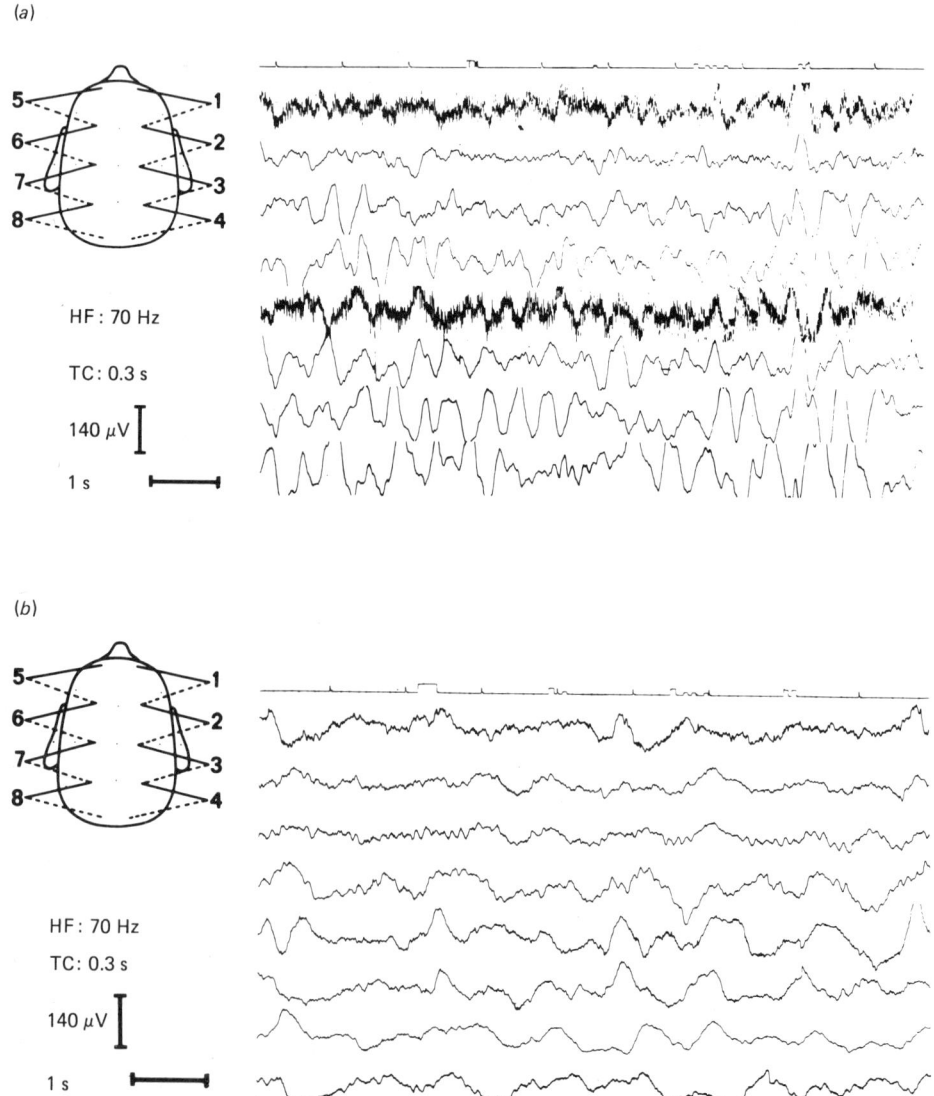

Moreover the changes seen in serial EEGs are quite different, with a tumour the abnormalities steadily increase but after a stroke there is a gradual improvement in the EEG which parallels clinical recovery.

A combination of generalized and local slowing is seen with brain abscess. In the early stages there is diffuse inflammation of the brain and a generalized EEG disturbance (Fig. 2.13a). As the infection progresses there is a reaction of the surrounding tissues producing a localized collection of pus, walled off from the rest of the brain. At this stage, the general EEG disturbance becomes less and there appears a striking focus of very slow triangular delta waves (Fig. 2.13b). After surgical drainage of the abscess the delta focus gradually disappears over six months to a year, but an increase of delta activity usually indicates a recurrence.

Focal theta activity usually implies a less extensive or rapidly progressive process than does delta. On this account it may be more important, as focal theta waves may be the only EEG sign of an early and readily treatable lesion, for instance a meningioma (a tumour of the meninges arising outside the brain itself).

2.2.2. 'Rhythms at a distance'

As indicated in the previous chapter, although the EEG signals themselves arise in cortical neurones, the rhythms are generated

Fig. 2.14. Frontal intermittent rhythmic delta activity (FIRDA) in a patient with anterior thalamic damage due to a ruptured aneurysm of the anterior communicating artery.

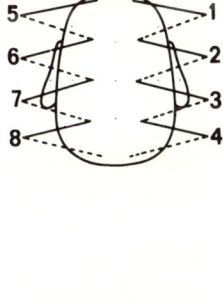

HF: 70 Hz

TC: 0.3 s

140 μV

1 s

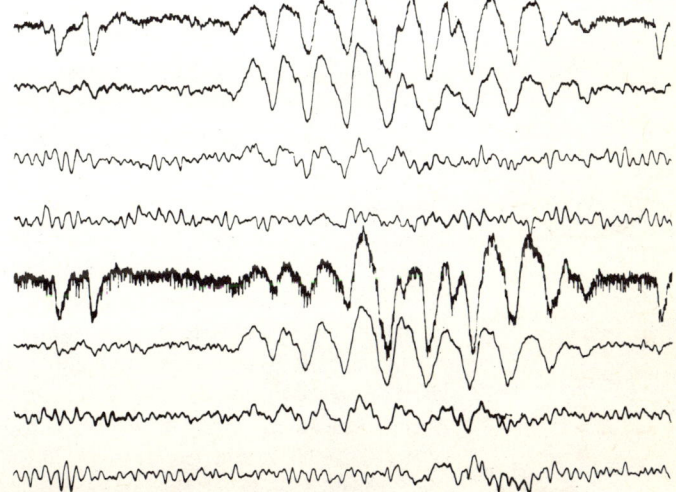

by the interaction of mechanisms located both in the cortex and in deep, particularly diencephalic, structures. EEG abnormalities in general may be produced by malfunction either of the cortex or of deeper parts of the brain and in many instances the under-lying physiological abnormality is imperfectly understood. There is nevertheless a group of disturbances of background activity which is fairly specific to disorders of the brain stem or dien-cephalon.

Frontal intermittent rhythmic delta activity (FIRDA) (Fig. 2.14) is rhythmic bilaterally synchronous delta activity at 1.5–2.5 Hz, generally seen in patients with anterior diencephalic damage and an intact frontal cortex and fronto-thalamic con-nections. Less commonly, FIRDA occurs in metabolic disorders. It is also seen acutely when the fronto-thalamic pathways are disrupted during the neuro-surgical operation of pre-frontal leucotomy. If the frontal lobes are intact this activity is usually symmetrical but in the presence of a deep frontal lesion it may be better developed on the unaffected side. FIRDA at 2–2.5 Hz is generally maximal in amplitude over the frontal poles and extends to the central regions; when the frequency is lower the distribution is more often fronto-temporal. Patients exhibiting this phenomenon usually show some impairment of awareness and FIRDA generally appears in drowsiness. To demonstrate this activity one may therefore need to arouse the patient if he is in stupor or allow him to relax if he has become too alert. FIRDA is blocked by auditory stimuli or eye opening.

Under circumstances similar to those in which FIRDA is seen, bi-temporal theta activity at about 6 Hz may also occur, but this is often difficult to distinguish from normal theta activity of drowsiness. A phenomenon similar to FIRDA, but less common and seldom described, is *'paradoxical arousal'*: this is the oc-currence of bi-frontal delta activity in an alert state, seen in patients with diencephalic or more usually upper brain stem lesions, particularly after head injury. The activity lacks the rhythmicity and the stereotyped waveform and frequency of FIRDA but the most important distinguishing feature is that it occurs, not in drowsiness, but on maximal arousal. The brain stem damage is usually minor and this phenomenon generally carries a good prognosis.

Diencephalic involvement may also influence the waveform of local slow activity. Whereas a tumour in the cerebral cortex pro-duces irregular 'polymorphic' delta activity, often continuous and of variable shape, the waves may become rhythmic and intermittent when deep structures are affected. The combination of both types of slow activity implies that the lesion, or its effects such as swelling and pressure, are extensive, involving both superficial and deep parts of the brain.

Posterior temporal slow activity is normal in the young. It may, however, be exaggerated in a child, or return in adult life, either as a nonspecific abnormality after a variety of cerebral insults, for instance trauma, or more specifically in the presence of brain stem lesions. It is generally bilateral, often of greater amplitude on the right than on the left in right-handed subjects, and of little lateralizing significance. It is generally reduced or blocked by eye opening and greatly increased by hyperventilation.

Another phenomenon associated with brain stem disorders which should probably be included among the 'rhythms at a distance' is *generalized alpha frequency activity in coma* (Fig. 2.15). This differs from the alpha rhythm, in that it often shows no occipital preponderance, is completely unresponsive to eye opening or even painful stimuli, and often has a frequency in the upper alpha range, but most importantly because it is associated with unconsciousness. It is seen in two circumstances, with destructive lesions of the upper brain stem, generally due to vascular disease or trauma, or after severe cerebral anoxia. Patients exhibiting this picture usually die but a few survivals have been reported.

Fig. 2.15. 'Alpha coma', diffuse and unresponsive alpha activity in a 22-year-old youth who was deeply unconscious following an anaesthetic accident. The outcome was fatal.

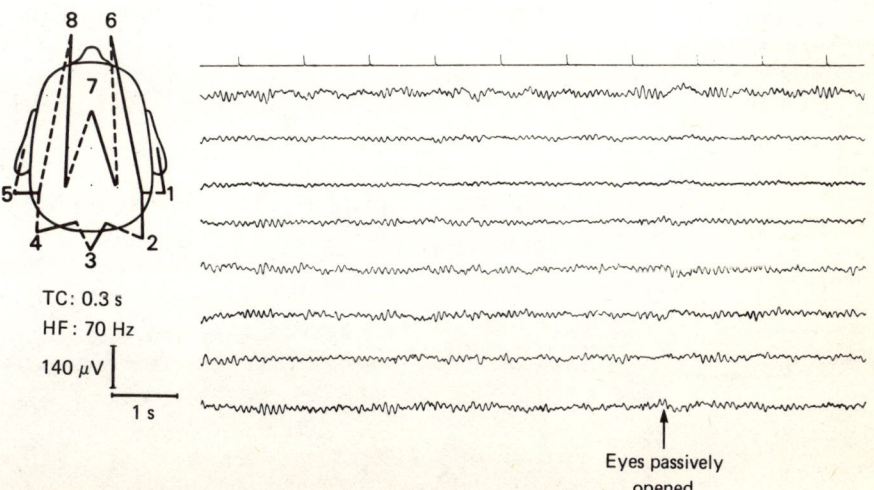

TC: 0.3 s
HF: 70 Hz
140 μV
1 s

Eyes passively
opened

2.2.3. Paroxysmal or epileptiform discharges

During an epileptic seizure various spiky waveforms character-istically appear in the EEG and these are often recorded in smaller amounts in inter-ictal records, i.e. between attacks. Similar activities may also occur in the EEGs of people who do not apparently have seizures. Conversely, a seizure may occasionally be accompanied by an EEG change which is clearly related to the fit but does not have the characteristic waveform. This strong but not entirely consistent association of spiky activity with epilepsy has led to confusion in terminology. Some authors name this activity 'epileptic', stressing its common clinical correlate. Others avoid a term which implies an unwarranted diagnostic conclusion and resort to such names as 'irritative' (which at best is vague and at worst implies speculation about the pathophysi-ology) or 'paroxysmal' (a name which describes any episodic occurrence and could equally be applied to K-complexes or lambda waves). The difficulty lies not in finding a name but in defining the concept. In the present text we use the term 'epilep-tiform' to emphasize the fact that we are referring to the form of the activity rather than its clinical significance. For a more detailed discussion see Zivin and Ajmone Marsan (1968).

The spike is the most typical example of epileptiform activity and is a very sharp transient with a duration less than 80 ms which arises suddenly out of the ongoing background activity. There is a certain flexibility in this definition because the observer's criteria for recognizing spikes will depend upon the amplitude of back-ground beta activity which has of course a similar frequency.

Fig. 2.16. Various epileptiform phenom-ena. In the absence of clear criteria recog-nition of these is highly subjective. Most electro-encephalographers would agree about the sharp waves and spike-wave complex shown in the upper line; there might be some room for doubt as to whether the spikes in the second line are sufficiently con-vincing to allow this activity to be described as a spike-wave dis-charge (compare Fig. 2.17). In the third line there is a short duration spike and wave complex which, though easily recognizable, is a phenomenon unlikely to be related to epilepsy. To the right of the third line is a tiny spike discernible only because the background activity is of very low amplitude. The bottom example illustrates the difficulty of determining criteria of epileptiform activity when the background itself is dominated by diffuse spiky beta components.

HF High   70 μV

TC 0.3 s   1 s

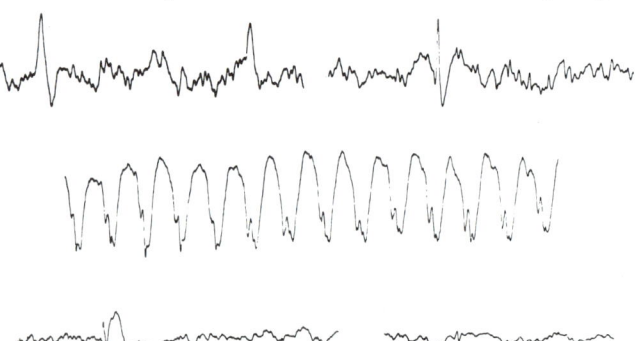

Localized spikes are predominantly surface-negative but may be bounded by positive-going components; the spike is generally followed by a slow wave which may be of very low amplitude and last longer than a second (Fig. 2.16). Spikes may be isolated or occur in runs, which may be irregular or rhythmic. They can be generalized and bilaterally synchronous or be restricted to a small area of brain, often the site of localized cerebral pathology. Spikes may sometimes be confused with muscle action potentials, but these are generally of shorter duration (< 30 ms) and consequently sharper. A number of technical artefacts may superficially resemble spikes (see Chapter 8).

The *sharp wave* resembles the spike but is by definition of longer duration, 80–200 ms, and consequently is less pointed and steep. Focal sharp waves are of somewhat less localizing value than spikes and probably represent a discharge of more extensive origin or arising more deeply located in the network of neurones. However, many patients with focal epileptiform discharges demonstrate both spikes and sharp waves over the same area.

The *spike-wave complex*. Spikes are often accompanied by slow waves but when the slow component is a conspicuous feature, the discharge is called a spike-wave complex. Such complexes may be isolated, in which case the slow wave generally lasts over a half second, or may form continuous rhythmic discharges. This pattern is seen most typically in the generalized regular 3/s spike-wave discharge (Fig. 2.17) which occurs typically during 'absence attacks' (see below).

Fig. 2.17. Generalized spike-wave activity at approximately 3/s during an absence seizure.

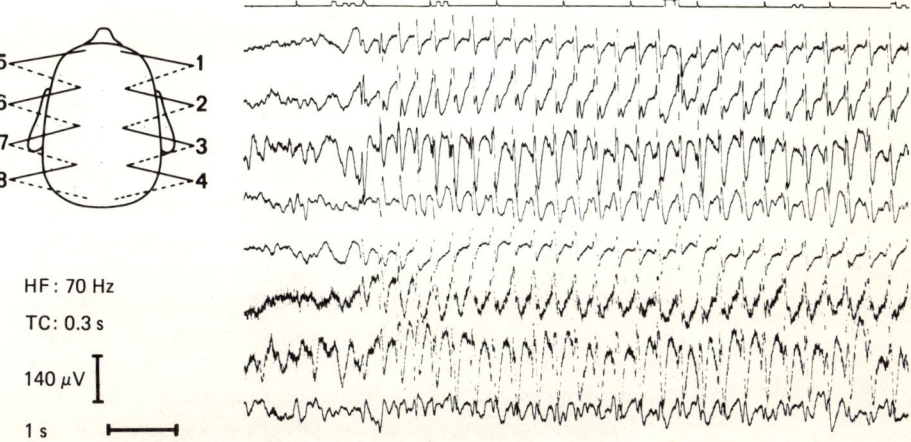

HF : 70 Hz

TC: 0.3 s

140 μV

1 s

The discharge may continue for many seconds with a regular repetition rate, possibly gradually slowing. Generalized spike-wave discharges occur at other frequencies with a different diagnostic significance. Slower generalized spike-wave activity at 1-2/s usually reflects diffuse brain damage and occurs mainly in children. Higher frequency spike-wave discharges at 4-5/s appear chiefly in patients who suffer not only absences but also major convulsive seizures. Spike-wave foci are common and their significance is similar to that of focal spikes or sharp waves.

Epileptiform EEG phenomena are fundamental to concepts of the nature of epilepsy and to classifications of its various forms. Epilepsy is characterized by sudden, usually unpredictable, sustained discharge of nerve cells, producing intermittent clinical symptoms dependent on the part of the brain involved. Such episodes are seizures or fits and there are many variations. Some (such as the 'grand mal' convulsion), are familiar, mainly because of their often dramatic character. Others are less easily recognized and the clinical manifestations may be subtle. The epilepsies are categorized following an international classification which in turn is paralleled by the EEG phenomenology:

Classification of the epilepsies (Merlis, 1970)

I. The generalized epilepsies – epilepsies which involve the brain diffusely
    (a) primary generalized epilepsies (includes petit mal and grand mal)
    (b) secondary generalized epilepsies (includes generalized seizures secondary to diffuse brain disease).
II. Partial (focal, local) epilepsies (includes Jacksonian, temporal lobe and psychomotor seizures).

The *primary generalized epilepsies* have a strong hereditary factor in their origin and are not due to demonstrable structural disease of the brain. They are characterized by two principal types of seizures, the *tonic-clonic convulsion* and the *absence*. The convulsive attack begins with sudden loss of consciousness often accompanied by a cry and a fall to the ground. At the same time there is maximal contraction of all the muscles of the body (tonus) and the patient may become cyanotic due to cessation of respiration. After about half a minute the clonic phase begins characterized by vigorous rhythmic contractions of all the muscles of the body. During the attack the patient often bites his tongue or lips and incontinence of urine and sometimes of faeces occurs. The frequently observed foam around the mouth is actually saliva which has been frothed by forced respirations during the clonic phase. After the convulsion has subsided the patient becomes limp and remains unresponsive for several minutes during which there are deep laboured respirations. He gradually regains consciousness but is confused and disoriented with no recollection of what has happened. He may complain of headache and muscular pain but, except for a painful tongue, he is usually unharmed. The EEG during the convulsion shows generalized epileptiform activity which is of sudden onset and symmetrical (Fig. 2.18). During the tonic phase there is a rapid build-up of generalized rhythmic spike discharges which give way to high-voltage generalized spike-wave complexes at about 3 per second during the clonic phase. In most cases the spike-wave paroxysms are difficult to recognize because of widespread muscle artefact. After clinical seizure activity has subsided the record is dominated by irregular delta activity which, as the patient recovers, is replaced by increasingly faster frequencies.

The absence seizure is common in children with primary generalized epilepsy. As in the tonic-clonic convulsion the initial event is loss of consciousness, but posture is usually retained and the child stares, flutters the eyelids and may make small repetitive movements of the lips or upper extremities. Slight alterations in postural tone are not uncommon. The attack is brief in duration (usually less than 10 s) and has a highly variable frequency of occurrence. Patients having up to a 100 attacks or more a day are not uncommon. At the conclusion of an attack there is no post-ictal confusional state and the patient himself may not recognize that he has been 'absent'. During the seizure the EEG shows the sudden appearance of generalized 3/s spike-wave complexes (Fig. 2.17) which terminate abruptly when the attack is over. There is no post-ictal slowing and background rhythms are immediately reestablished.

The simultaneous appearance of epileptiform activity over all regions of the scalp suggested a trigger in the centre of the brain, and the term 'centrencephalic epilepsy' was coined. Recent research has led many workers to reject this concept (see Gloor 1972 for a review). In an alternative model, an over-excitable state of the cerebral cortex is viewed as the primary abnormality with epileptiform activity being a cortical response to various inputs, themselves not necessarily abnormal, originating from the

Fig. 2.18. Series of EEG
excerpts during a tonic-
clonic seizure. (a) Onset
of the seizure with
abrupt appearance of
generalized spikes; note
also EMG artefact on
ECG channel.

(a)

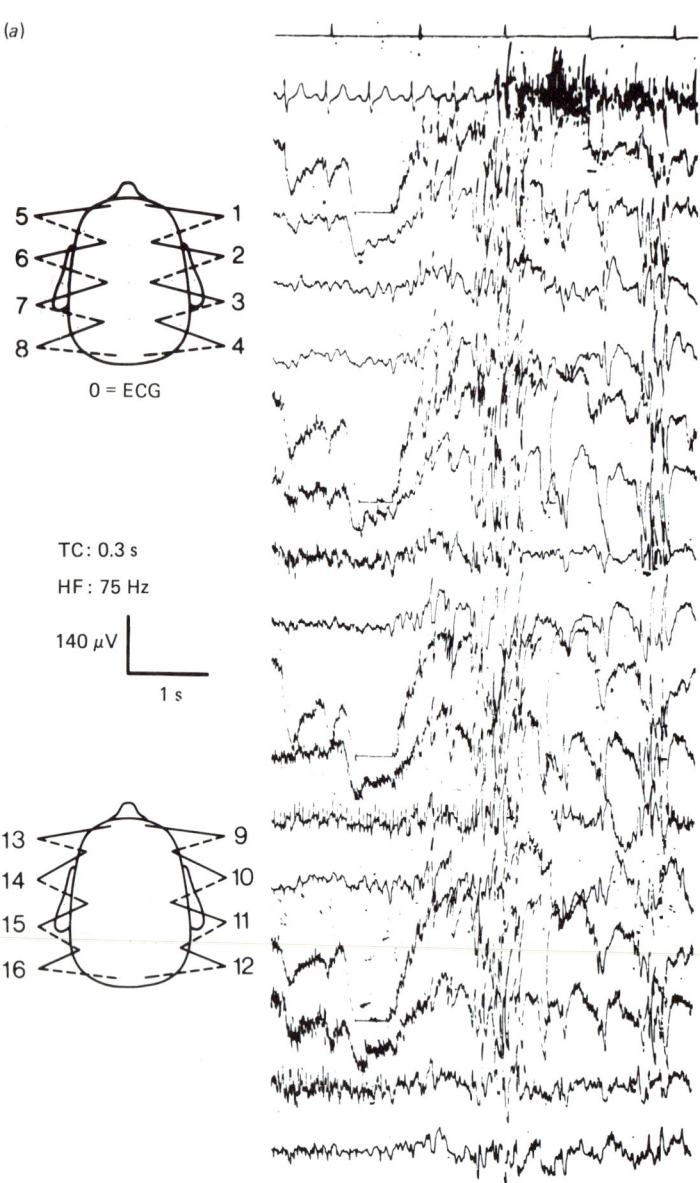

0 = ECG

TC: 0.3 s

HF: 75 Hz

140 μV

1 s

Fig. 2.18. (cont.)
(b) 10 s later: record
composed mostly of
EMG artefact.

(b)

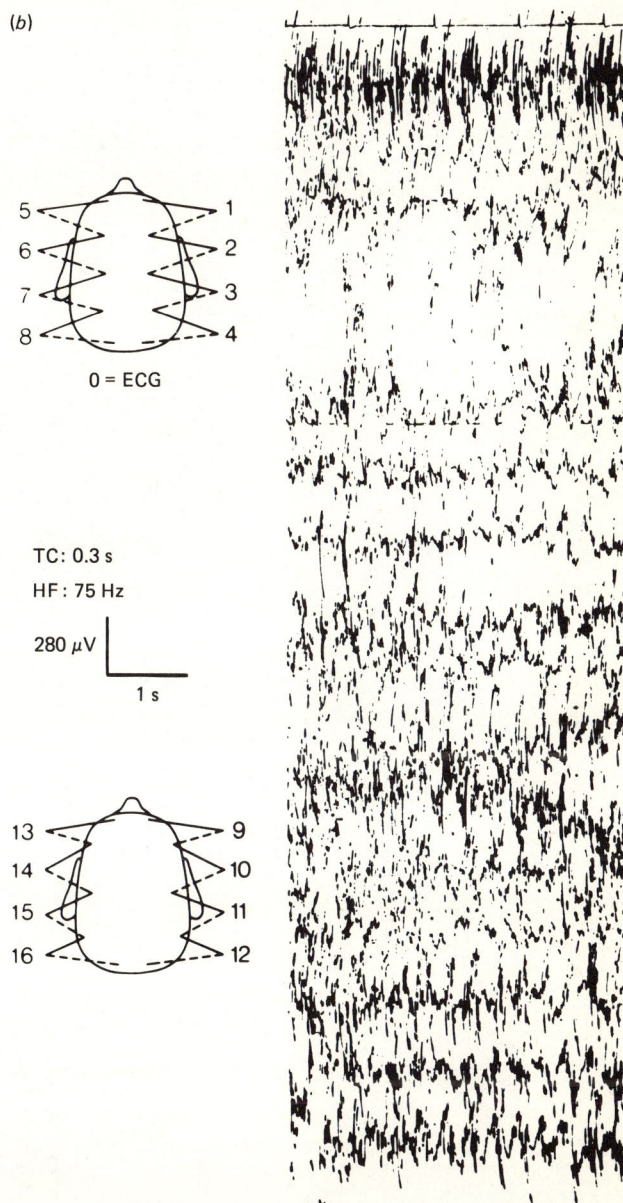

0 = ECG

TC: 0.3 s

HF: 75 Hz

280 μV

1 s

Fig. 2.18. (cont.) (c)
(c) 30 s from start of
seizure: generalized
multiple spike and wave
activity.

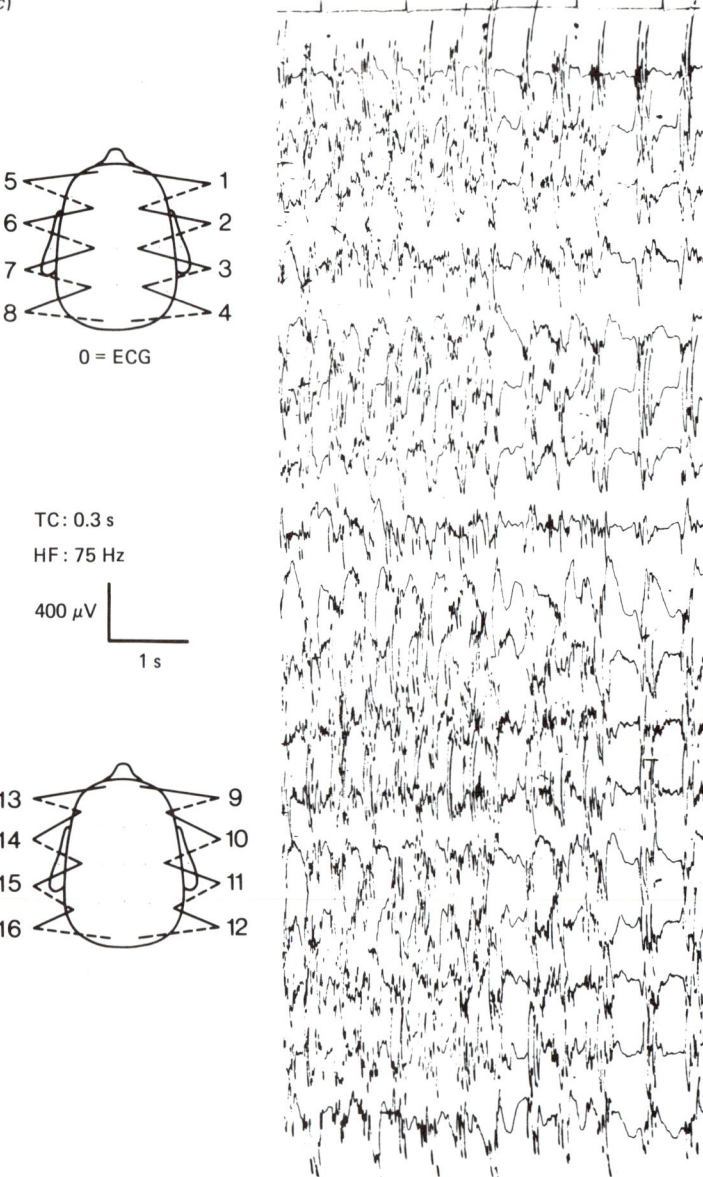

5 ← 1
6 ← 2
7 ← 3
8 ← 4

0 = ECG

TC: 0.3 s

HF: 75 Hz

400 μV

1 s

13 ← 9
14 ← 10
15 ← 11
16 ← 12

thalamus. The reticular activating system influences the level of cortical excitability and this is reflected in the often marked effects of sleep, waking and attention on seizure liability and EEG epileptiform activity.

Partial epilepsies, by contrast, arise from a localized structural cerebral abnormality, for example brain damage during a difficult birth or later in life, a tumour, or a localized infection. The initial symptoms of the seizure reflect the functions of the part of the brain affected. If this is the motor cortex, localized jerking will commence on the opposite side of the body, commonly in the hand or face. The discharge may spread to involve cortical areas serving other muscle groups in a sequence determined by the body's anatomical representation in the motor cortex (Fig. 2.19).

Fig. 2.18. (cont.)
(d) After 60 s: spike-wave activity becoming irregular and disappearing.

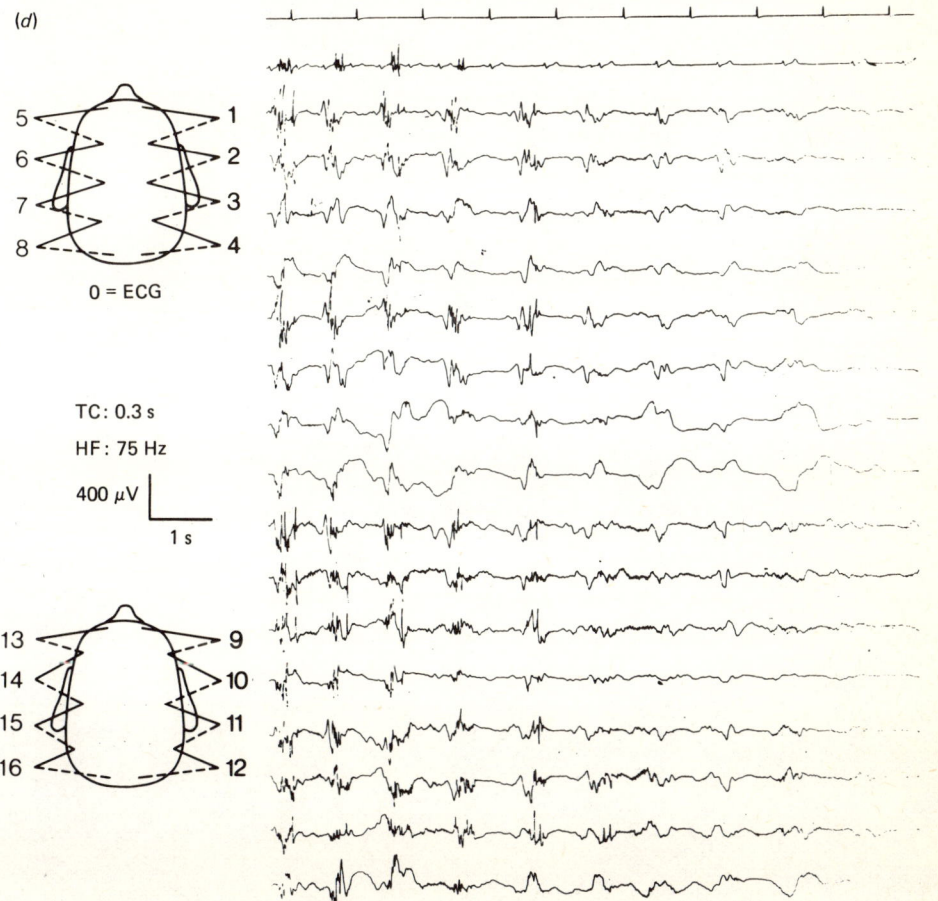

(d)

0 = ECG

TC: 0.3 s

HF: 75 Hz

400 μV

1 s

Fig. 2.18. (cont.)
(e) 5 s later: tracing of
very low amplitude.

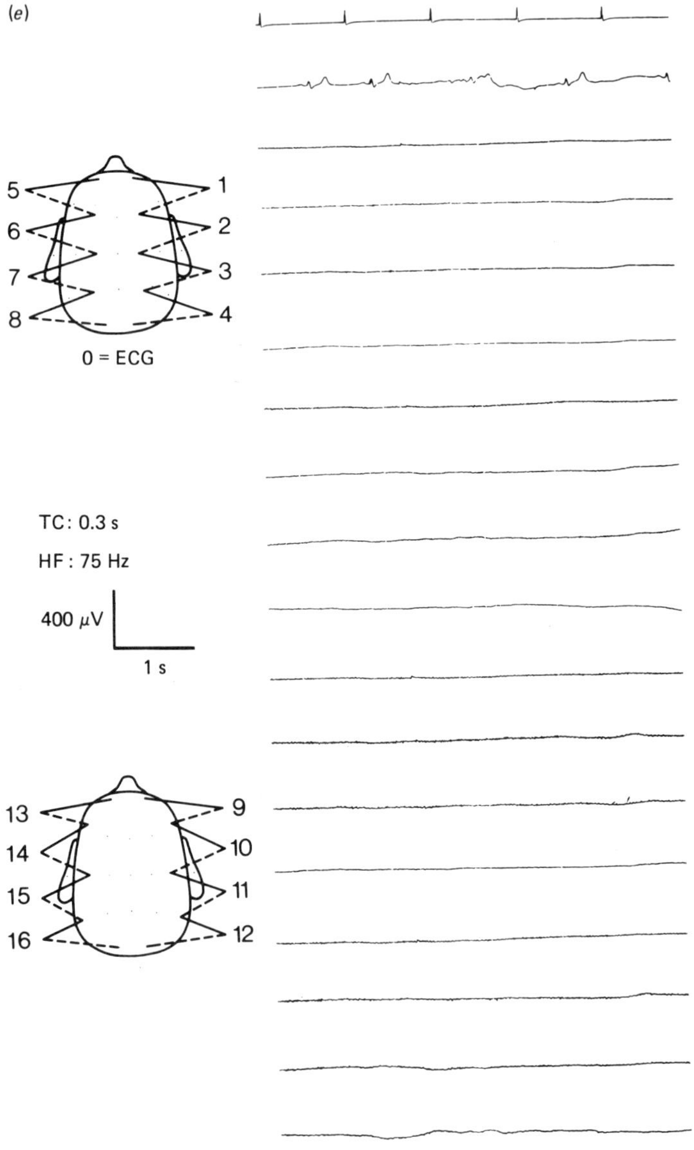

(e)

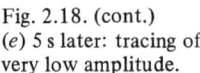

5 ⟵ ⟶ 1
6 ⟵ ⟶ 2
7 ⟵ ⟶ 3
8 ⟵ ⟶ 4

0 = ECG

TC: 0.3 s

HF : 75 Hz

400 μV

1 s

13 ⟵ ⟶ 9
14 ⟵ ⟶ 10
15 ⟵ ⟶ 11
16 ⟵ ⟶ 12

After an initial orderly spread of the discharge the entire brain may eventually become involved resulting in a generalized convulsion. If the site of the initial seizure discharge is the primary sensory area the patient may complain of strange sensations such as tingling in a specific part of his body. Such a discharge may spread in a fashion similar to that of the motor seizure. Attacks characterized principally by motor or sensory symptoms, whether or not there is spread involving successive parts of the body (so-called Jacksonian seizures, named after a nineteenth-century English neurologist who studied them) are known as *partial seizures with elementary symptomatology*. If the epileptogenic focus lies in the region of the brain concerned with psychological functions, for example the temporal lobe, these will be disturbed during the attack and the symptoms could be mistaken for

Fig. 2.18. (cont.) (*f*) 5 minutes from start of seizure: generalized post-ictal disturbance: patient still confused and restless, hence movement artefacts.

(*f*)

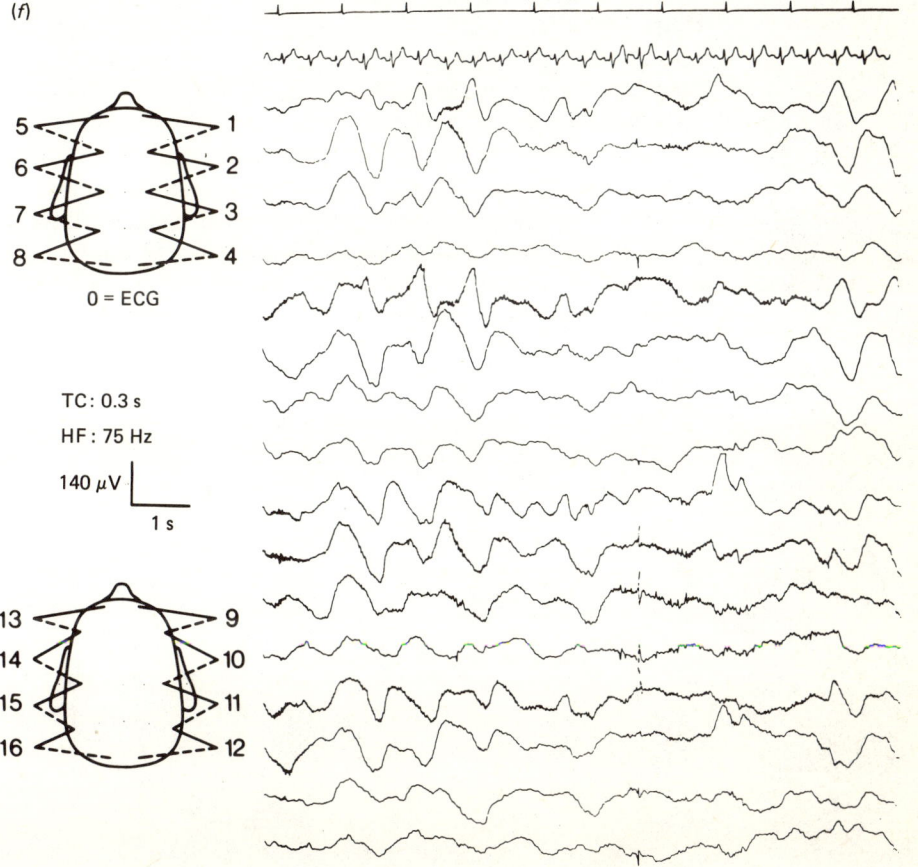

0 = ECG

TC: 0.3 s

HF: 75 Hz

140 μV

1 s

psychiatric manifestations. Such a seizure may begin with an 'aura' or warning which is actually the first stage of the seizure itself. The most common aura is a 'rising epigastric sensation', a strange and often indescribable feeling in the stomach which rises to involve the chest and neck. Other initial symptoms may include hallucinations of smell, taste, sound or vision, disordered perceptions, or emotional changes, for example a sudden irrational feeling of fear. After some seconds or even minutes the patient often suffers a loss of awareness which may be complete or partial, and he may stare into space for a period of some seconds. This stage is often followed by stereotyped simple motor activities such as licking or smacking of the lips, chewing and fumbling with the hands. These actions, known as *automatisms*, are not goal-directed; however, more complex automatic behaviour may be observed such as turning the pages of a book, stubbing out a cigarette or attempting to undress. If, as is sometimes the case, the automatisms are continuations of an activity which preceded the onset of a seizure, they may be difficult if not impossible to recognize. The patient may appear very restless and if restrained may be combative. This has led to a wide-spread and unjustified fear that epileptics are aggressive; in fact goal-directed assaultive or other dangerous behaviour is very rarely observed. The seizure which usually has a duration of several minutes is followed by gradual return to full orientation. The patient may remember nothing of the attack or perhaps only the initial aura. Such an

Fig. 2.19. Topographic representation of the body over the semato-sensory cortex (left) and motor cortex (right). After Penfield and Jasper (1943).

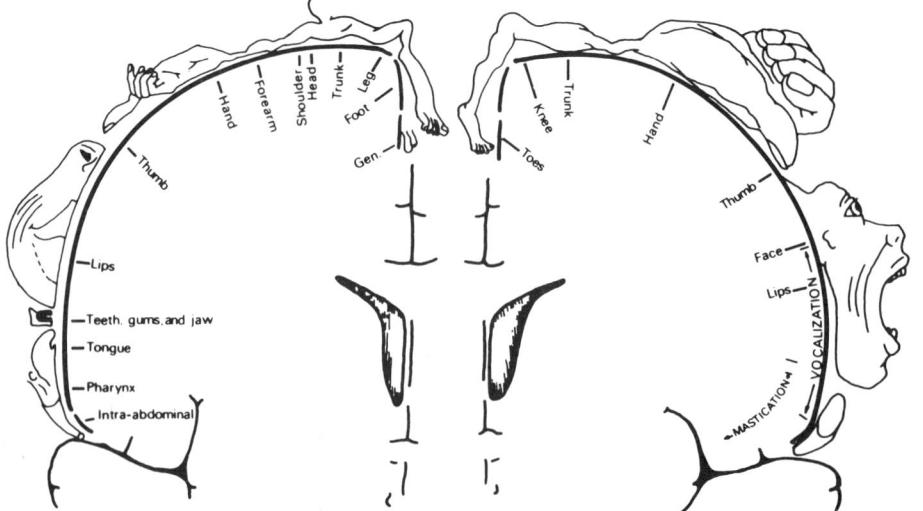

Fig. 2.20. Secondary generalization. The left frontal focus of spikes and spike-wave activity sometimes triggers a generalized discharge. Note that this consists of irregular, disorganized spike-wave unlike the rhythmic pattern seen in Fig. 2.17.

attack is termed a *partial seizure with complex symptomatology* and the most common site of origin is the temporal lobe, particularly from a scar in its antero-medial part (*mesial temporal sclerosis*). The ictal EEG usually shows highly rhythmic focal discharges confined to one temporal area, often maximal over the anterior temporal region and consisting typically of rhythmic spikes or other waveforms in alpha, theta or even beta frequency bands. Sometimes the initial EEG change is simply a reduction in amplitude of all ongoing activity. Partial seizures whether of elementary or complex type may exhibit the phenomenon of *secondary generalization*. The initially focal EEG disturbance spreads to become diffuse and possibly symmetrical and the clinical symptoms may also take on a generalized character such as a very prolonged absence attack or even a generalized convulsion (Fig. 2.20).

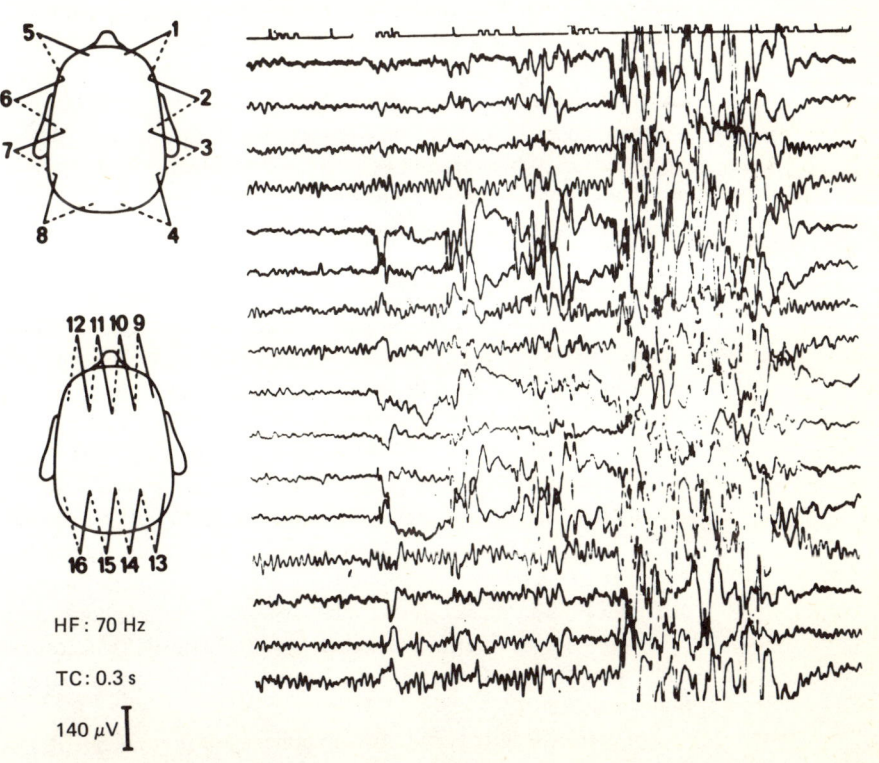

HF : 70 Hz

TC : 0.3 s

140 μV

1 s

Secondary generalization is an EEG phenomenon and must be distinguished from the type of epilepsy known as *secondary generalized epilepsy*. This is found in patients with diffuse brain damage and combines clinical features of both the primary generalized and partial epilepsies. Typically these patients suffer from multiple seizure types the most alarming of which is the *akinetic seizure*, characterized by the simultaneous and sudden occurrence of unconsciousness and a fall, the latter due to sudden loss of muscle tone. The patient often strikes his head and may have to wear a protective helmet in order to avoid severe head injury. Secondary generalized epilepsy usually results from severe brain damage suffered during intra-uterine life or at birth, and the patients often suffer from neurological handicap and mental subnormality. If the seizures commence in infancy they may take the form of *infantile spasms*, a type of attack in which the trunk is suddenly flexed and the arms thrown forwards (sometimes termed a *salaam attack*, due to a fancied resemblance to an Arabian gesture of greeting). Infantile spasms are often accompanied by a chaotic EEG pattern termed *hypsarhythmia*, characterized by high-voltage irregular delta activity and multi-focal spikes with no constant localization. In older children and adults the EEG of secondary generalized epilepsy shows diffuse slowing and disorganization of background activity, multiple foci of epileptiform activity and generalized discharges typically consisting of slow spike-wave activity (2/s or less).

Activation procedures, particularly hyperventilation and sleep, play an important role in the investigation of the epilepsies. Generalized spike-wave activity in patients with absence seizures can almost always be precipitated by hyperventilation. Other types of generalized and focal epileptiform discharges may either be brought out *de novo* or exaggerated during hyperventilation, although the effect on focal discharges is usually less marked. Intermittent photic stimulation elicits generalized spike-wave activity in some 5% of people with epilepsy, usually of generalized type. This reaction, termed a *photoconvulsive response*, is strongly supportive of a diagnosis of epilepsy, particularly if it continues after the stimulus has ceased. Short-lived or localized epileptiform discharges on photic stimulation are of less diagnostic significance and sometimes occur in relatives of people with epilepsy and even in normal children.

Epileptiform activity, whether in epilepsy or in non-epileptic disorders (see below) may often be activated by sleep. Focal discharges occur most readily in stages I and II and may also be present in REM. Generalized epileptiform activity is activated by deeper sleep and does not appear in REM. Recording after a night of sleep deprivation is a special case; sleep is readily achieved but does not seem to be the only factor responsible for EEG activation. Indeed, many patients show maximum activation during wakefulness and light drowsiness with a subsequent decline in paroxysms during deeper sleep. As pointed out above, epileptiform activity is not confined to people with epilepsy and it is found in 2–3% of large series of non-epileptic patients (Zivin and Ajmone Marsan, 1968). It is, however, more common in certain clinical groups: mental subnormality, biochemical disorders, cerebral palsy (neurological disability due to brain damage occurring before, during or shortly after birth, with or without mental subnormality). Epileptiform activity is particularly common in sufferers from migraine. About 30% exhibit temporal sharp waves and some authors estimate that as many as 10% have spike-wave discharges. In patients with cerebral tumours, with or without epilepsy, it is generally associated with slowly growing non-malignant processes which have a more favourable clinical outlook. In contrast, epileptiform activity caused by cerebral anoxia, for example after cardio-respiratory arrest, is an ominous sign, and such patients do not often survive. Among normal subjects from whom any with a history of neuropsychiatric disease have been excluded, epileptiform EEG activity is very rare (Robin, Tolan and Arnold, 1978).

2.2.4. Non-epileptic transients and periodic EEG patterns

Certain spiky EEG phenomena, particularly accompanying drowsiness and sleep, occur in normal subjects and must be clearly distinguished from those spiky waveforms associated with epilepsy. Fig. 2.21 shows rhythmic spikes which have the unusual feature of being surface-positive. These occur with a frequency of approximately 14 or 6/s and are seen in some 20% of records of drowsy healthy subjects in the second and third decades of life. Fourteen and 6/s positive spikes are sometimes misleadingly described as abnormalities on the grounds that they occur even more often in certain groups of patients. However, they are so common in health as to be of no clinical predictive value. A related phenomenon often seen in the same subjects is low-amplitude 6/s spike-wave activity or 'spike-wave phantom'. This too is of no clinical significance. A phenomenon less widely recognized which may be wrongly interpreted by the inexperienced as evidence of epilepsy consists of stereotyped bursts of very sharp spikes, sometimes followed by slow waves, maximal over the temporo-basal regions. These are seen only in sleep and have been variously named *short sharp spikes* (SSS) or *benign epileptiform transients of sleep* (BETS). They may be found in up to 40% of normal subjects and therefore have no clinical significance.

Triphasic waves resemble epileptiform discharges and occur typically in hepatic encephalopathy resulting from severe liver disease although they may also be seen in other acute diffuse cer-

Fig. 2.21. Positive spikes. (*a*) Both 14 and 6/s positive spikes are present in this tracing obtained during drowsiness from a healthy 22-year-old subject. Note the typical distribution, maximum in the posterior temporal regions. (*b*) Detail of spikes on channel 12.

(*a*)

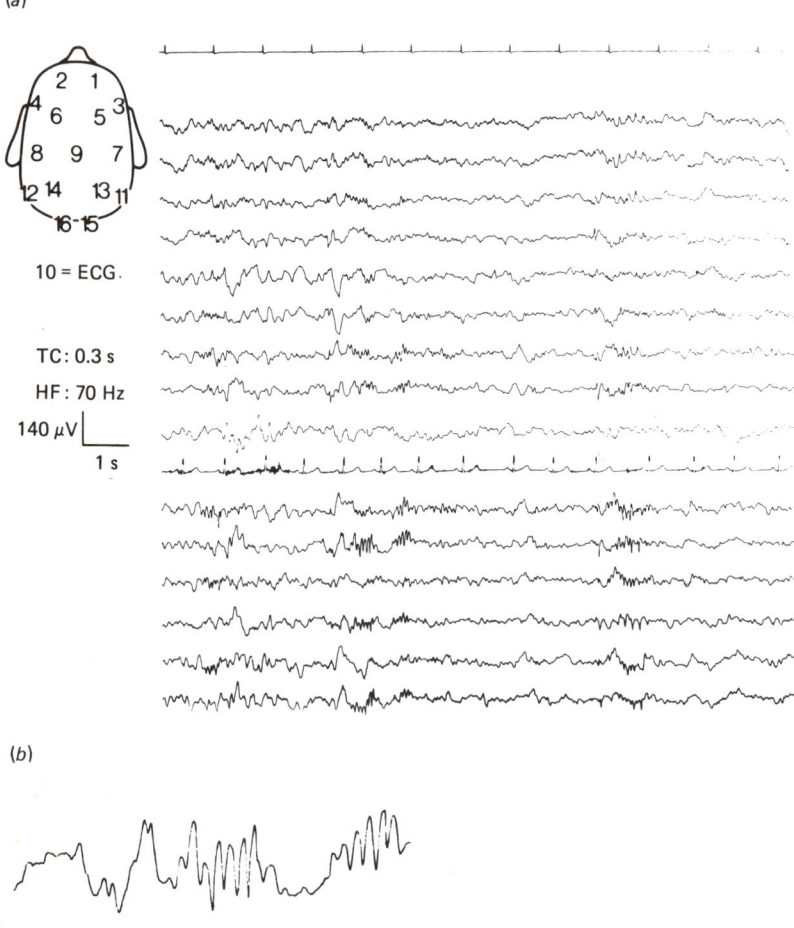

10 = ECG.

TC: 0.3 s
HF: 70 Hz
140 µV
1 s

(*b*)

250 ms

ebral disturbances. The waveform consists classically of a complex in the delta frequency band with three distinct phases but the number of phases may vary from patient to patient. They are of some technical interest as they arise from the front of the head and move posteriorly across the scalp (see Section 4.3).

Periodicity is a characteristic of various intermittent EEG patterns which occur at more or less regular intervals and often resemble epileptiform activity. This may be seen with certain unusual viral infections of the brain such as Creutzfeld-Jakob disease and herpes simplex encephalitis. In the former condition the discharges occur diffusely with a relatively high frequency and have a biphasic or triphasic waveform. In the latter the discharges are more complex and usually lateralized over one hemisphere, particularly in the temporal region. A particularly striking periodic pattern is seen in a rare viral infection of childhood called subacute sclerosing panencephalitis (SSPE). The earliest clinical manifestations are usually subtle changes in the personality and intellect. Increasing intellectual deterioration and neurological deficit follow, and toward the end of the illness jerky movements of the entire body appear regularly at intervals of several seconds. At this stage the EEG develops a pattern of generalized high-voltage polyphasic sharp and slow wave discharges of stereotyped waveform, occurring with a constant time relation to the jerks, but not necessarily synchronous with them (Fig. 2.22). This striking EEG picture may suggest the diagnosis even before it is suspected clinically.

Burst suppression, another periodic EEG pattern, consists of bursts of slow waves followed by intervals of nearly complete or total electrical silence. The repetition rate is variable, and the bursts less stereotyped than in the examples above. If a burst suppression pattern is present several hours after cerebral anoxia the prognosis is grave. It is also seen during deep anaesthesia or drug overdose, for example with barbiturates. In the latter case full recovery may occur if cerebral anoxia has not intervened. It has been postulated that burst suppression, and also periodicity in general, result from relative isolation of the cortex from the underlying white matter, a view supported by experimental studies.

Periodic lateralized epileptiform discharges (PLEDs) are unilateral periodic sharp waves repeating at intervals of 1–2 s. This pattern is most typically seen with acute cerebral lesions (infarction or haemorrhage) producing focal or generalized seizures which usually disappear after some days. However, PLEDs are seen in a wide variety of other conditions, acute or chronic, localized or diffuse, and are therefore not specific.

2.3. The uses and abuses of the EEG

As the EEG is complex and has engendered a scientific jargon which tends to impress the inexperienced, it seems to arouse the hope that it will aid neurological diagnosis in many situations, even those in which it has little value. Clinical decisions may be based on poorly formulated questions leading to inappropriate investigation, for example the request to exclude epilepsy on the basis of an interictal record. Unfortunately, many electroencephalographers co-operate in this misuse of the EEG and, apparently in a misguided attempt to be helpful, report every deviation from the most typical adult waking record as 'abnormal'. With some justification their colleagues conclude that all EEGs seem to be abnormal and therefore unreliable and unhelpful. Both over-, and under-evaluation lead to misuse of the EEG as a diagnostic tool; EEGs are recorded to answer unanswerable questions, and others are not ordered in situations where they could be most helpful. These remarks are highly relevant to the whole approach to EEG

Fig. 2.22. Stereotyped polyphasic complexes which occurred at intervals of about 15 s in a 7-year-old boy with subacute sclerosing panencephalitis. This EEG was recorded one month after an isolated episode of status epilepticus. At this time he was otherwise asymptomatic.

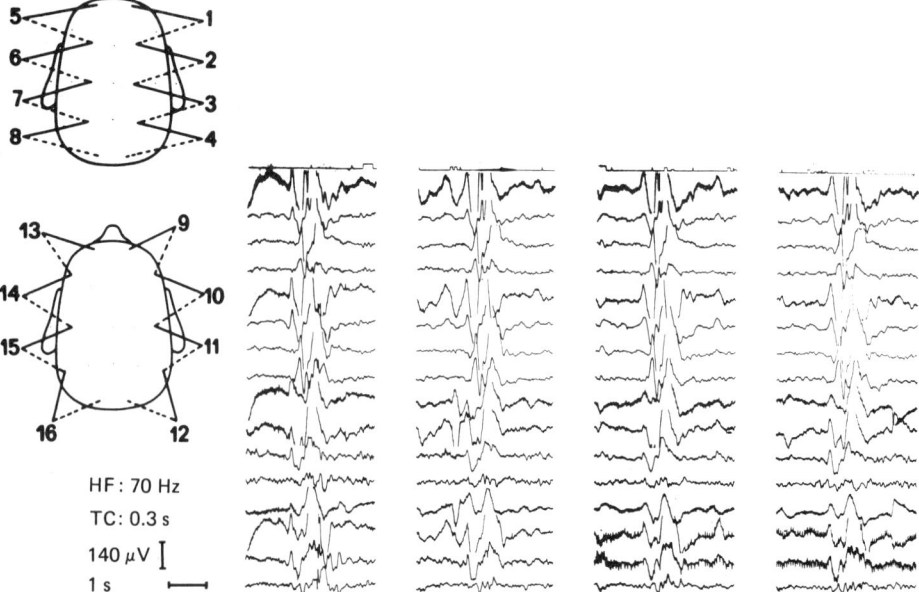

HF: 70 Hz

TC: 0.3 s

140 µV

1 s

recording; unnecessary investigations provide little motivation for careful technique, but EEG studies directed to solving worthwhile, clearly stated problems demand and justify the highest technological standards.

The reliable recognition of abnormalities in any investigation depends in the first instance on the presence of adequate data from normal subjects. Unfortunately, the earliest classical studies of the EEG in large numbers of normal subjects were based on youthful service personnel. Consequently there was a high incidence of maturational phenomena not present in older subjects which led to the conclusion that many normal people had 'abnormal EEGs'. It is of course illogical to describe findings which commonly occur in healthy people as abnormal. Recent studies using more appropriate criteria show that normal people have normal EEGs, and that an abnormal record in an apparently healthy volunteer usually indicates that he has, or has had in the past, a condition affecting the brain (Roubiček, Volavka and Matoušek, 1967; Robin et al., 1978; Binnie et al., 1978a). It must be emphasized that the converse is less likely to hold; that is, a normal EEG does not, with some exceptions, exclude the presence of a pathological process.

As should be apparent from the preceding sections, the EEG reflects structural abnormality only in so far as this affects activity of cortical neurones. It therefore cannot be equated with diagnostic techniques such as computerized transaxial tomography (CT-scan) or the cerebral angiogram which are used to investigate cerebral *structure*. Rather it complements these and, like neurological or psychological examination, is a means of assessing brain *function*. Until recently the EEG was one of the few and perhaps the most powerful non-invasive investigation of the brain which involved no discomfort or risk to the patient. In recent years the development of the CT-scan has changed this position. This special X-ray technique allows visualization of the brain itself without danger to the patient (Fig. 2.23), and has indeed revolutionized neurological diagnosis.

Despite the power of this new method, electroencephalography has held its position, for there remain many disorders which can be diagnosed by the EEG but not by the CT-scan, prominent examples of which are epilepsy and metabolic disorders. In the future many patients with suspected cerebral disease will require both investigations, the information from one complementing that from the other.

2.3.1. Epilepsy

The relationship of EEG phenomena to the types of epilepsies and seizures was discussed at length above. Obviously, the most convincing diagnostic data result from recording the EEG during a seizure. Unfortunately, this is rarely possible during routine EEG studies with the exception of absence attacks precipitated by hyperventilation. Nevertheless, interictal recordings can provide diagnostically valuable information in the majority of people with epilepsy. The probability of recording interictal epileptiform discharges depends on the frequency and circumstances of their occurrence, and therefore on the number, duration, and types of EEG recordings carried out. For example, repeated routine EEGs in a patient with infrequent epileptiform activity increases the chance of recording a discharge. In our laboratory a diagnostic EEG series including a waking record (of 40–60 min) with hyperventilation and photic stimulation, and recordings during drug-induced sleep and after sleep deprivation, yields diagnostically useful information in about 90% of people with epilepsy. In the remainder, it may be necessary to record the EEG under circumstances in which seizures or epileptiform activity are most likely to occur, for instance after reduction of medication or during the

Fig. 2.23. CT-scan. The symmetrical light coloured areas are the ventricles, the more irregular light-coloured region in the right centro-temporal region is a cerebral tumour.

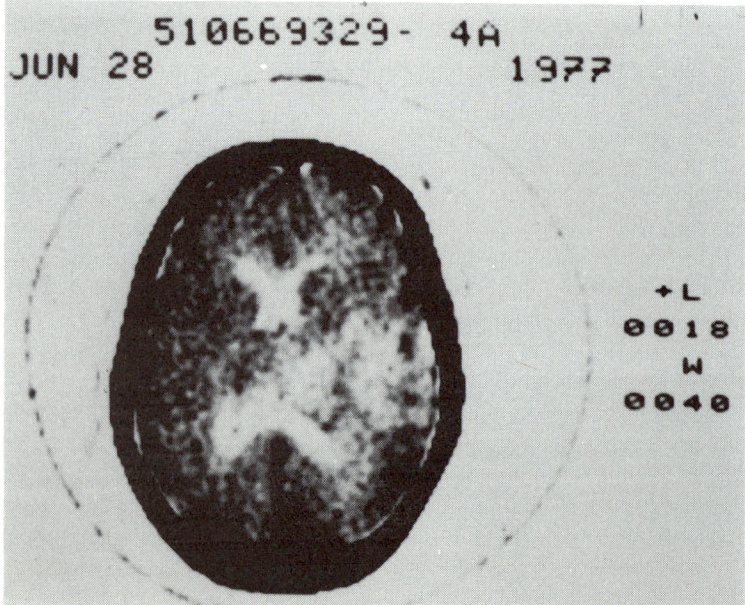

premenstrual phase in some women. Alternatively, prolonged recordings of many hours or days can be carried out by means of telemetry (see Section 9.3) until a seizure is registered. Attention should again be drawn to the dangers of excluding a diagnosis of epilepsy because of a normal EEG or interpreting normal EEG phenomena such as positive spikes or small sharp spikes during sleep as evidence of epilepsy.

2.3.2. Space-occupying lesions

The brain is completely surrounded by a bony encasement, the skull, and cushioned by the cerebrospinal fluid. While offering excellent protection, this arrangement can also be a disadvantage in the presence of expanding pathological processes such as tumours, intracerebral haematoma, or an abscess. As there is essentially no unused spaced within the skull, any process which itself occupies space will not only destroy cerebral tissue within its vicinity, but also produce local pressure effects and eventually a general increase in intracranial pressure. Both factors account for the often striking EEG changes accompanying *space-occupying lesions*.

Brain tumours may originate in the brain itself or its coverings (primary tumours) or may be spread from a primary location elsewhere in the body (secondary or metastatic tumours). The most common primary brain tumour is the glioma which in fact arises not from nerve cells but from the cells of the supporting tissue known as glia. *Gliomas* are commonly graded in terms of their rate of growth. The slowly growing glioma is graded I and may be present for many years before it is suspected. Grade IV gliomas are rapidly expanding tumours which often result in death within 6 to 12 months. The effects on the EEG depend to a large extent on the tumour's rate of growth and its location. Fast-growing tumours also infiltrate nerve fibre pathways destroying normal tissue. They may have a very rich blood supply, diverting blood from adjacent brain, and may themselves also suffer haemorrhage or infarction. These processes may produce marked EEG abnormalities, both local and generalized. Slow-growing tumours produce few EEG changes early in their course, although if they become large, the EEG abnormalities may be severe. The tumour's location is also an important factor; a process in the frontal lobe may attain considerable size before producing recognizable clinical symptoms or EEG changes, whereas a temporal location may declare its presence much earlier. The earliest

EEG disturbance may be low-voltage focal slowing in theta or delta ranges which becomes more prominent as the tumour increases in size. Focal EEG findings in the early stages of tumour growth are of great importance for they may lead to more definitive studies and timely operative intervention. In the case of advanced tumours which produce marked focal delta activity as well as diffuse abnormalities due to increased intracranial pressure, the EEG may only serve to confirm what was suspected clinically.

Of particular importance is the *meningioma*, a very slowly growing benign tumour of the dura which eventually compresses the underlying brain tissue. Early in its course the only clinical symptom may be epileptic attacks of partial type, with or without secondary generalization. The characteristic EEG pattern is focal theta activity with or without low-voltage delta waves and epileptiform discharges. Early diagnosis in these cases may make it possible to remove the entire tumour without resulting brain damage and neurological deficit (Fig. 2.24). In general the more slowly growing tumours are associated with clinical seizures and epileptiform activity in the EEG, whereas rapidly growing malignant tumours do not appear to allow sufficient time for the development of an epileptiform focus. These guidelines are not invariable, however, and other studies will be necessary in order to confirm a suspected EEG diagnosis. In summary, the EEG is an effective screening test for the early diagnosis of cerebral tumours and supplements the findings of other studies which may reveal the structure and precise location of the process.

Other pathological processes which occupy intracranial space may produce focal EEG findings similar to those of tumours; however, certain of them have rather characteristic patterns. For example, the untreated brain abscess, a localized purulent collection typically resulting from the spread of infection from the sinuses, mastoid bone or inner ear, may produce a prominent delta focus consisting of high-amplitude often triangular long-duration delta waves with destruction of background rhythms. Such patients are seriously ill with headache, nausea and vomiting, fever and neurological signs. This classical picture is not always present, however, and a partially treated abscess which has developed a firm fibrous capsule may produce a much less striking picture of focal slowing not unlike that of a slowly growing tumour.

The *subdural haematoma*, mentioned above, consists of an accumulation of blood between the dura and arachnoid resulting from tearing of the veins which bridge the subdural space. Head trauma some weeks or even months before the patient comes to clinical attention is usually the cause, although a history of head injury is not always obtained, particularly in the elderly. Headache is a nearly constant clinical feature and neurological findings may be sparse or absent. The progression of neurological deficit is insidious, but decompensation may occur rapidly with confusion, coma and death. Early diagnosis is essential for the operation is relatively simple and usually results in complete cure. The classical EEG findings of unilateral depression of cerebral activity have been described above; these are not always present and the EEG should never be used 'to exclude subdural haematoma'. In the majority of cases, however, the EEG is abnormal and often serves to draw attention to the serious pathology underlying apparently trivial symptoms, early in the course of the illness.

Space-occupying lesions of the posterior fossa: tumours or other space-occupying processes arising in the posterior fossa may originate in the cerebellum, brain stem, or cranial nerves. The *medulloblastoma*, for example, is a primary tumour of the cerebellar midline structures occurring in early life and producing headache, vomiting and unsteady gait. Other types of tumours may arise in a cerebellar hemisphere producing clumsiness of the limbs on the same side of the body. The EEG changes in these conditions are variable and non-specific. Early in the course of a tumour the EEG may be entirely normal; as growth occurs, slow waves, often rhythmic, appear in the posterior regions. Later, if cerebrospinal fluid pathways are blocked producing increased

Fig. 2.24. Left frontal meningioma: left-frontal delta and theta activity.

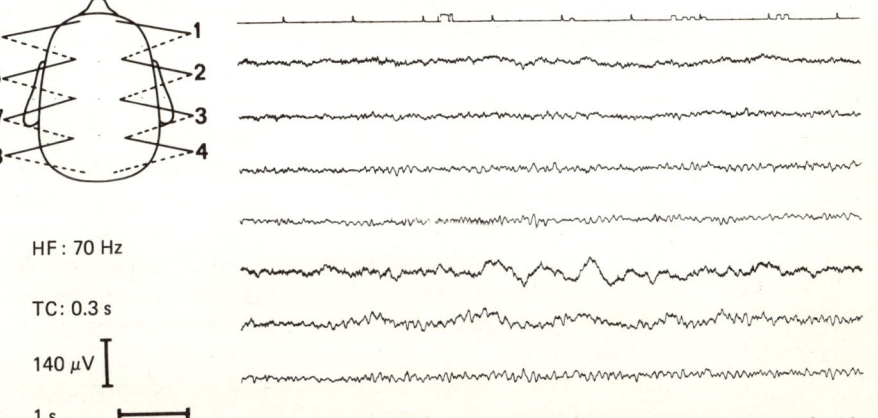

HF: 70 Hz

TC: 0.3 s

140 μV

1 s

intracranial pressure, FIRDA (q.v.) may be observed. Although the EEG is of limited value in the diagnosis of such lesions, a finding of FIRDA or excess posterior delta activity in a child complaining of headache without obvious or only subtle neurological signs can suggest the appropriate diagnosis.

A tumour of the VIIIth cranial nerve at the junction of the pons and medulla in the posterior fossa (the *acoustic neuroma*) produces a well-known syndrome with hearing loss and tinnitus on the affected side as well as the type of dizziness known as vertigo. The EEG is normal until the tumour enlarges and exerts pressure on the brain stem. At this point the EEG may record a rhythm at a distance similar to that of other posterior fossa lesions. 'Evoked responses' (see Chapter 12) may also be valuable for detecting pathology in the posterior cranial fossa.

Increased intracranial pressure (ICP): This is one of the most serious problems in neurology requiring prompt action by neurologists and neurosurgeons if the patient's life is to be saved. Increased ICP results when the cerebrospinal fluid pathways are interrupted, for example due to a blockage in the ventricular system, at the site of absorption of the cerebrospinal fluid, or at the base of the brain preventing return of cerebrospinal fluid to the site of absorption. (See Fig. 1.7.) The rising ICP produces expansion of the ventricular system and may force the brain stem through certain natural openings in the dura or skull (*herniation*). If the pressure is not immediately relieved, the patient will not survive. A cardinal neurological finding in increased ICP regardless of cause is papilloedema, swelling of the optic nerve head. Tumours of the posterior fossa produce an increase in pressure at an earlier stage than cerebral tumours, but in both cases the EEG findings are similar. The earliest sign is slowing of the posterior dominant frequency, with perhaps the appearance of some diffuse irregular slow waves. Later, FIRDA intervenes, although in the case of posterior fossa lesions the amplitude of the distant rhythms may be maximal over the occipital regions. This EEG finding requires prompt action and must be directly communicated to the referring physician.

An unusual condition producing increased intracranial pressure and papilloedema in the absence of demonstrable structural pathology is so-called pseudotumour cerebri (benign intracranial hypertension). The patients complain of headache but are alert and have no neurological deficit. The ventricles are not enlarged but on the contrary are small in size. Consequently the EEG in these cases is normal or shows only very mild abnormalities. The finding of a normal EEG in a young overweight woman with headache and papilloedema is highly suggestive of this diagnosis.

2.3.3. Cerebrovascular lesions

The brain requires for its survival a constant supply of glucose and oxygen provided by the cerebral circulation; consequently, interruption of the blood supply will result in death of cerebral tissue. Arteriosclerosis, a common degenerative condition of the cerebral vessels in later life, may occur locally in one vessel or involve the entire cerebral circulation. The resultant narrowing of the vasculature may be well tolerated for many years without evident neurological deficit. Eventually, an artery may be blocked by blood clot formation at a point which has been severely involved by the arteriosclerotic process (*thrombosis*). This results in death of tissue in the distribution of the affected cerebral vessel with resultant neurological deficit. Obstruction of small vessels may also result from *embolism*, which occurs when a fragment of blood clot becomes detached from a larger vessel and is impacted where the artery narrows. Such emboli arise most commonly from a diseased carotid artery at the site of an atherosclerotic plaque and may occur intermittently over many weeks or months. If the obstruction they produce is incomplete, episodes of transient neurological dysfunction may occur known as *transient ischaemic attacks*. In many cases the attacks are eliminated by surgery of the carotid artery or medical therapy. When one carotid artery is obstructed by an atheromatous plaque with clot formation, sufficient blood may be shunted from the other great vessels through the Circle of Willis to maintain the circulation on the involved side. Obstruction of any large vessel above the Circle of Willis usually leads to tissue destruction (*infarction*). The most commonly involved vessel is the middle cerebral artery which produces hemiparesis and a hemi-sensory defect, and a disturbance of speech (*dysphasia*) if the left hemisphere is involved. In the acute phase the EEG usually shows focal slowing in the frontal, temporal and parietal regions which increases if swelling in the involved area intervenes. Occlusion of the posterior cerebral artery produces a loss of half the field of vision (*hemianopia*) and less profound motor weakness, and the EEG shows disruption of the alpha rhythm on the affected side along with temporal-occipital slowing. Thus, broadly speaking, the EEG findings conform anatomically to the distribution of the involved cerebral vessels.

Haemorrhage within the brain usually arises in a setting of hypertension and is the result of sudden rupture of diseased small vessels, usually deep within one hemisphere. The haemorrhage causes severe local destruction of tissue, usually involving the main motor and sensory connections, producing paralysis and sensory loss on the opposite side of the body. It also acts as a space-occupying lesion. In fact, infarction and haemorrhage are inseparable: bleeding generally interferes with the blood supply of the surrounding brain and the destruction of tissue by an infarct also may lead to haemorrhage. In both cases the clinical picture is generally that of a stroke, with sudden onset of one-sided neurological deficit and possible loss of consciousness. Haemorrhage generally does more damage than infarction, is more likely to cause loss of consciousness and death and allows less complete recovery. EEG findings in the acute phase parallel the pathology: destruction of tissue leads to depression of normal activities, haemorrhage and swelling cause focal delta activity and generalized slowing due to raised pressure. If deep structures are involved FIRDA may appear.

In cases of acute vascular accidents, the EEG often serves only to support the clinical impression. However, it is not always possible to determine the anatomical location of the pathologic process on clinical grounds alone. A striking example is the occurrence of a stroke syndrome due to occlusion of small vessels in the pons or other white matter connections between the cerebrum and the brain stem (internal capsule). In these cases the clinical picture may be that of a profound hemiplegia whereas the EEG is entirely normal. The EEG also may be of particular value in following up a patient with an apparent vascular accident. Serial tracings which show progressive improvement serve to distinguish a vascular accident from a tumour, a problem which arises in patients in whom there is no adequate history.

Sometimes intracranial bleeding occurs from a small berry-like bulge (*aneurysm*) in the wall of an artery near the Circle of Willis. These aneurysms, which are usually of congenital origin, bleed outside the brain into the subarachnoid space and produce severe sudden headache. Blood may also spurt into the brain substance, producing destruction of tissue and spasm of the cerebral arteries. This combination of bleeding and vascular spasm is often fatal although in many cases the aneurysm can be treated surgically with successful results. As the spasm and site of bleeding depend upon the location of the aneurysm the EEG may be of some assistance in identifying the source of bleeding. *Angiomata*, malformations of cerebral blood vessels within the brain or sometimes on its surface, also give rise to subarachnoid haemorrhage. In these cases the bleeding is much less vigorous owing to the fact that it is venous and not arterial as in the case of aneurysms. Such malformations are therefore less life-threatening than aneurysms but are difficult to treat surgically unless they are relatively small and superficial. The EEG usually shows a prominent focus of high-voltage delta activity.

2.3.4. Infections

Infection of the meninges, *meningitis*, is generally associated with some cerebral involvement (*encephalitis*) and produces mild generalized EEG slowing. Acute viral encephalitis produces more profound EEG changes with generalized high-voltage delta activity sometimes in combination with periodic complexes of sharp and slow waves. Encephalitis due to the herpes simplex virus produces periodic stereotyped complexes which are particularly striking over the temporal lobes and indeed may be unilateral. In these cases the EEG gives an important clue as to the nature of the illness.

The *brain abscess* was discussed above but it should be added that early in the course of an abscess before the stage of purulence is reached, the clinical picture and the EEG findings may be difficult to distinguish from a viral encephalitis. Indeed, acute encephalitis may also be confused with other causes of impaired consciousness such as degenerative or metabolic processes. Since these illnesses have variable clinical courses including progressive improvement or deterioration, or gradual localization in a particular area of the brain, serial EEGs may be valuable in suggesting or supporting the correct diagnosis. Indeed, serial EEG changes sometimes occur before an alteration in the clinical picture is apparent. The more chronic forms of encephalitis often produce characteristic EEG patterns which may distinguish them from other, for instance degenerative, conditions producing similar symptoms.

2.3.5. Trauma

Head injuries which produce loss of consciousness are classified according to their severity. Commonly there is only brief loss of consciousness and no significant neurological sequelae (*concussion*) although headache and dizziness may persist for some time. In the post-concussional period the EEG usually shows no significant abnormality. More serious are the *contusion* (bruise) and *laceration*, an actual disruption of brain substance, often associated with a depressed skull fracture. In these conditions loss of consciousness may be prolonged and neurological signs are the rule. EEG changes are determined by a number of factors including the site and extent of brain damage, the state of consciousness, and the intracranial pressure. A combination of focal and diffuse EEG changes is commonly seen. A blow to the head may also produce damage to the opposite site of the brain (*contre-coup*) which may cause local depression of EEG activity. The main value of the EEG is for following the patient's progress and predicting outcome both in the acute phase and later. Paradoxically, a patient with neurological deficit who some months after a head injury shows an abnormal but improving EEG is more likely to exhibit further clinical recovery than one whose EEG is normal or static. A progressively resolving EEG abnormality following a head injury may be important for medico-legal purposes when there is uncertainty as to whether particular symptoms are a consequence of the trauma or due to a pre-existing condition.

The subdural haematoma has already been discussed. It is sometimes difficult on clinical grounds alone to differentiate between a cerebral contusion or laceration and a subdural haematoma. Indeed, these conditions may co-exist and complicate the diagnostic and therapeutic picture. The EEG may be of benefit if the classical signs of subdural haematoma are present; unfortunately this is often not the case. The CT-scan has altered clinical practice in these cases to a large extent although the supplementary information provided by the EEG is still of value.

2.3.6. Metabolic disorders

The proper functioning of nerve cells depends not only on an adequate supply of oxygen and glucose but also the constancy of the biochemical environment. Disturbance of blood electrolytes (e.g. sodium, potassium, chloride), due for instance to dehydration, or the accumulation of certain metabolic products if the kidneys or liver are diseased, produces a *toxic confusional state*. The result is diffuse cerebral dysfunction with increasing lethargy, confusion and eventual coma. While focal neurological signs are usually absent, this is not invariable; a patient may present the confusing picture of deepening lethargy and focal neurological dysfunction such as hemiparesis. If no history is available, a mistaken diagnosis of a cerebrovascular accident may be made. The EEG is a sensitive indicator in such conditions; indeed EEG changes may appear before there is any obvious clinical deterioration and provide a valuable early warning that urgent treatment is required to prevent the onset of coma (Fig. 2.11). The earliest EEG changes include slowing of the dominant rhythmic frequency and an increase in the diffuse slowing usually without focal features. As consciousness declines this slowing becomes more profound. An important feature may be the presence of triphasic transients which are seen in a variety of metabolic disorders but most characteristically in hepatic encephalopathy. Such a finding in a patient with stupor of unknown cause virtually confirms the true diagnosis.

2.3.7. Diffuse cerebral degenerations

Progressive, irreversible loss of mental function or *dementia* may occur in all stages of life. In childhood it may result from a number of rare genetic disorders whereas in later life the condition is unfortunately common although the cause is not known. Early signs of dementia include inability to concentrate and loss of memory, usually for recent events. Progressive deterioration of all mental functions occurs along with loss of emotional control and eventual helplessness. Focal neurological findings and even seizures may occur but these features are much less prominent than the cognitive dysfunction. The most common example in adult life is *Alzheimer's disease* which occurs not only in the elderly but sometimes in the prime of life. The EEG findings are very consistent with slowing of the alpha rhythm, bi-temporal slowing often in the theta range, loss of frontal beta activity and a marked reduction in amplitude with distortion of sleep spindles and K-complexes. As the degenerative process is not uniform, focal slow activity may also appear which should not be confused with that due to a tumour or treatable lesion.

2.3.8. Cerebral anoxia

Since the development over the past two decades of improved methods of resuscitation, cessation of respiration or of cardiac action no longer implies inevitable death. However, many patients remain unconscious after resuscitation, sometimes for years, and it is important to be able to predict the eventual outcome. Destruction of the cerebral cortex is incompatible with recovery of consciousness, and EEGs are often requested as an aid to the diagnosis of *brain death*. EEG findings suggesting an unfavourable outcome after resuscitation have been mentioned in previous sections and include: epileptiform activity, burst suppression, periodic transients, and generalized alpha activity in the presence of coma. Recovery of consciousness does not appear to have been reported in any properly documented case of isoelectric EEG persisting more than 6 hours after resuscitation and in the absence of intoxication, hypothermia or gross metabolic disturbance. The issue of brain death is a subject of continuing ethical and legal debate in which the electroencephalographer inevitably becomes involved. Criteria for establishing the diagnosis are not uniform and a central issue is whether or not these include cortical destruction, but it is likely that the EEG will continue to play an important medico-legal role. EEG recording under the circumstances of intensive care is technologically difficult (see Chapter 9).

2.3.9. The EEG in psychiatry

Hans Berger's hopes that the EEG would throw light upon the nature of mental disease have, alas, not been fulfilled. The EEG is certainly of great value for identifying patients whose apparent psychiatric disorders have an organic basis in cerebral degeneration, a toxic confusional state, intracranial space-occupying lesion, infection, or epilepsy. As an aid to identifying psychiatric disease the EEG is of minimal value. Statistical associations exist, for instance between immature EEGs and personality disorders or between unusually regular alpha activity and hysteria, but these associations are too weak to be of value either for predicting or excluding these conditions. It may nevertheless be hoped that the increasing use of EEG data processing in this area may in the future produce techniques of practical clinical worth.

2.3.10. Dynamic electro-physiological investigations

In Chapters 12 and 13 we mention various electrical responses of the cerebral cortex, brain stem, retina, inner ear and cranial muscles to sensory stimuli. In many areas, the recording of spontaneous EEG activity is giving way to the more dynamic *evoked response* techniques which form an electro-physiological extension of the traditional neurological examination.

2.3.11. Research applications

Electroencephalography has many uses for the scientific investigation of brain function in normal subjects. It forms an essential tool of sleep research and is sensitive to changes in attention and to a variety of metabolic factors. Combined with data processing to detect and quantify small changes, it is used to study alterations in human cerebral function in association, for instance, with psychological tasks, diurnal rhythms, the menstrual cycle, etc. It is claimed that certain centrally acting drugs produce EEG changes in normal subjects, specific to their pharmacological actions. If this is the case, EEG studies may be used to identify new substances as drugs of potential clinical value.

As means of detecting change in cerebral function the EEG also has a role in clinical research. It can, for instance, be used to determine the cerebral effects of a particular therapeutic or diagnostic technique and to study possible cerebral changes in the course of psychiatric disorders.

3. Electrodes

3.1. Introduction

The bioelectrical signals which make up the EEG are carried by ions in aqueous solution and have to be recorded by apparatus containing solid conductors; the electrodes constitute the interface between these two systems. When a metallic electrode is in contact with an electrolyte, atoms of the electrode become ionized and pass into solution and metallic ions from the electrolyte are discharged and attach themselves to the electrode. An equilibrium is established and an electrical double layer is set up, so there is a potential gradient between the electrode and the adjacent electrolyte. The electrical double layer has the properties of a source of e.m.f. together with a capacitance, in parallel with a resistance* (Geddes and Baker, 1967). The magnitude of the electrode potential is determined by the physico-chemical properties of both the electrode and the electrolyte. When two identical electrodes are immersed in a homogeneous electrolyte they will both assume the same potential with respect to the electrolyte and will therefore be equi-potential with each other. When dissimilar electrodes, for instance of different metals, are immersed in an electrolyte, the electrode potentials are unequal and a potential difference is established between the two electrodes; the electrodes and electrolyte together form a simple Voltaic cell. When a single channel of an EEG machine is connected to the head by a pair of electrodes, the circuit therefore incorporates the potentials, capacitances and resistances of both electrodes, all of which elements are variable (Fig. 3.1). In addition, due to random movement of molecules, electrical noise arises at the surface of the electrodes and this has an amplitude dependent on the material of which they are made.

3.2. Desirable characteristics of electrodes

3.2.1. Electrode impedance

In Fig. 3.1, it will be seen that the biological signal, E_s, is connected to the electrodes through the series and parallel impedances, R_s and R_p, of the surrounding tissues. R_p is generally much smaller than R_s, and the voltage available to the electrodes, E_{AB}, is therefore greatly attenuated; i.e. the EEG (E_{AB}) is considerably

---

* This model which is shown in the equivalent circuit of Fig. 3.1 is an approximation which holds for low-frequency signals such as the EEG. At higher frequencies series resistance and capacitance are more important and themselves vary inversely with the square root of frequency (Geddes, 1972).

smaller than the post-synaptic potentials (E_s) by which it is generated. There will be a further loss of signal E_{AB} unless the impedance of the external circuit is much greater than R_p. Moreover, the impedances of the electrodes and of the input of the EEG machine form a potential divider circuit such that E_{CD}, the signal available for amplification and display, is:

$$E_{CD} = E_{AB} \frac{R_i}{Z_1 + Z_2 + R_i}$$

where Z_1, Z_2 and R_i are the impedances of the two electrodes and of the input of the amplifier. Minimum signal loss will therefore be achieved if $(Z_1 + Z_2 + R_i) \gg R_p$ and $R_i \gg (Z_1 \text{ and } Z_2)$, i.e. the electrode impedances should be low and the input impedance very high.

In practice, with modern EEG machines and the types of electrodes generally used, the electrode impedances are extremely small compared with that of the input of the amplifier and well over 99% of the original signal is available for amplification. The only exception is provided by electrodes made of inert materials such as stainless steel (see Section 3.3.4) of which the conductance is largely capacitive; these electrodes conduct well at frequencies above about 1 Hz but exhibit a high impedance to very low frequency signals. They are therefore unsuitable for recording slow phenomena such as the CNV (see Section 12.3). A further effect of input impedance on electrode performance should be noted. The greater the current passing through the electrodes, the

Fig.3.1. Equivalent circuit of EEG generator, electrodes and recorder; for explanation see text.

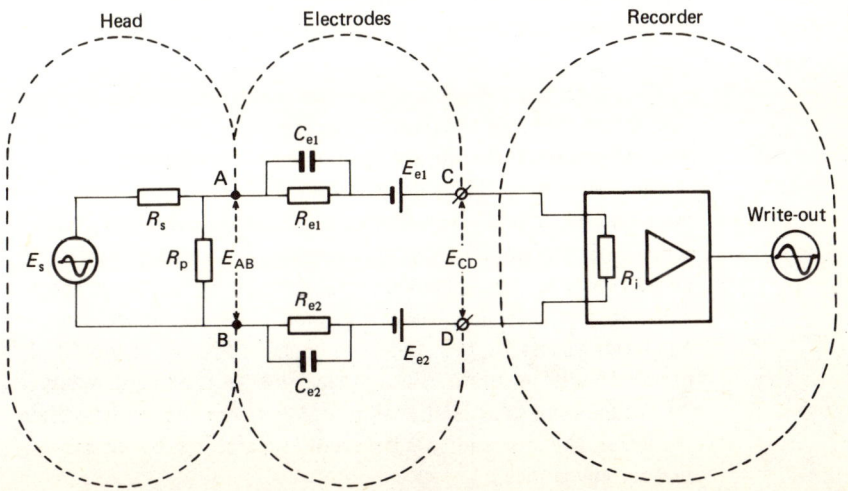

Head   Electrodes   Recorder

greater will be the frequency dependent phase distortion of the signals, due to the capacitance of the electrodes. This current is reduced by a high input impedance.

Electrode impedances should also be so far as possible stable. If the e.m.f. created in the input circuit by the electrode potentials is constant, it may produce a permanent offset in a DC recording system (which can if necessary be compensated by an externally applied potential) but will not produce AC signals which could be confused with or mask the EEG. However, if the resistance of this circuit also changes, there will be variations in the current, which will be recorded as spurious signals or artefacts. For instance, an e.m.f. at the electrodes of 100 mV will produce in an input circuit with a resistance of $2\,M\Omega$, a current of 5×10^{-8} A. A change in this resistance of only 0.2% (i.e. change of $4\,k\Omega$ in electrode resistance) will change this input current by 10^{-10} A. This is equivalent to the effect of a $200\,\mu V$ EEG signal in the same circuit.

So nearly as possible, electrode impedances should be equal. This is particularly important in connection with susceptibility to electrical interference which is dealt with more fully in Chapter 8. If a source of interference causes the subject to assume a potential difference with respect to the EEG machine, a current will flow through the electrodes and the input circuit of the machine to earth. Provided that the electrode impedances are equal this current will produce a common mode signal at the input and will not be registered (see Section 5.2.2). If the electrode impedances are unequal, however, differing currents will be produced in the two input leads and these will not be rejected but will appear as interference on the tracing.

The electrode impedance is determined largely by the area of contact and the material used. The stability depends on the method of attachment to the scalp and on the extent to which the subject moves. Although the three factors of magnitude, stability and equality of electrode impedance have been considered individually, in practice they are inseparable. Techniques which give a low electrode impedance will generally promote equality and stability; moreover if the impedances are low, minor inequalities or instabilities are less important. Finally, it should be noted that the absolute values of electrode impedances are less important than their relationship to input impedance; the higher the latter, the less readily is the recording affected by unsatisfactory electrodes.

3.2.2. Electrode potential

Unequal electrode potentials will produce a standing DC component at the input to the amplifiers. This will not ordinarily produce any major problem during AC recording except that it may, with some older types of machines, result in a reduced common mode discrimination ratio (Section 5.2.2.). For purposes of DC recording it may be necessary to 'back off' the electrode potentials by means of an external potential source and a potentiometer.

Of much greater practical importance than inequality of electrode potential is instability. The electrode potentials are typically some tens or hundreds of millivolts and a very small percentage change may produce a signal considerably larger than the EEG itself. The passage of current through an electrode system may change the physico-chemical characteristics of the electrodes and hence also their potentials. A rather gross analogy is provided by two iron electrodes immersed in a copper sulphate solution. Each will initially have the same potential with respect to the electrolyte and they will therefore be equipotential with each other. If a current is passed through the cell, copper ions will be discharged and deposited as metallic copper on the cathode. Thus the chemical composition of the latter is altered, the electrode potentials are no longer equal and an e.m.f. develops between the electrodes. An electrode/electrolyte system which can undergo such a change is described as 'polarizable' (arguably a misuse of the term). For the purposes of bioelectrical recording it is desirable to use a system such that the passage of charge will not readily change the physico-chemical characteristics of the electrodes, i.e. they should be non-polarizable, or 'reversible'. An example of a reversible system is provided by silver electrodes, coated with silver chloride, and immersed in sodium chloride solution. The passage of a current will cause more silver chloride to be deposited on the anode, whilst at the cathode silver ions are discharged, being deposited as silver atoms, and chloride ions pass into solution. The layer of chloride therefore becomes thicker on the anode and thinner on the cathode but, up to the point where the entire chloride layer on the cathode is exhausted, the physico-chemical nature of the electrodes remains essentially unchanged. Thus, unless a sustained DC potential is applied, the system is non-polarizable. The main extracellular electrolyte is indeed sodium chloride and the electrodes most commonly used for EEG recording are made of chlorided silver. Nevertheless they are not in practice entirely stable and careful preparation is necessary to minimize fluctuations in electrode potential.

Finally, electrode potentials should be as low as possible. The lower the e.m.f. in the circuit formed by scalp, electrodes and input of the EEG machine, the less marked will be the effect of fluctuations in electrode resistance. Tin/stannous chloride electrodes have a particularly low contact potential and produce satisfactory recordings even where mechanical scalp/electrode contacts are poor and the resistances very variable (Kado and Adey, 1968). Practical considerations have, however, prevented their routine clinical use.

3.2.3. Practicality

Electrodes should be easy to apply and to remove and should have a means of fixation which provides good mechanical stability and so far as possible constant contact resistance. For routine clinical EEG practice the electrodes must be securely attached so that they do not become displaced in restless sleep or during epileptic seizures. The method of fixation should not cause discomfort to the subject not least because a tense patient produces muscle artefact and is also unlikely to fall into natural sleep or drowsiness, which play an important role in diagnostic electroencephalography.

If it is intended to record from a moving subject, the electrodes and leads should be as light as possible and the insulation of the leads should not be of material which readily becomes electrostatically charged. Mechanical artefacts will be reduced if the electrical double layer is not in direct contact with the skin. This may be achieved by recessing the electrode in an insulating cup and bridging the gap with a conducting jelly.

E.m.f.s of hundreds of millivolts may be set up between dissimilar metals immersed in an electrolyte; consequently, connections between electrodes, clips, plugs and wires should be easily kept dry. The junction between the electrode and its lead is particularly liable to give arise to artefacts or to become corroded. A number of methods for protecting this joint have been employed: epoxy resin, varnish, silicone rubber and shrunk-on sleeving; none has proved wholly successful.

The electrode must be of a material which will not have a harmful effect on the underlying skin and is not easily corroded. For long-term depth recordings inert electrodes (gold or stainless steel) must be used: silver chloride is sufficiently soluble to be toxic when chronically implanted.

3.3. Electrode materials
3.3.1. Silver/silver chloride electrodes

In the preceding section a number of materials for the construction of electrodes have been mentioned. That most widely adopted for clinical EEG practice is silver/silver chloride. This material has been used in various forms, as compacted silver/silver chloride, chlorided silver wire or gauze in a plastic container, but most commonly as a solid silver electrode coated with chloride. Silver/silver chloride electrodes are reversible, have reasonably good stability and low noise level, have a low resistance and capacitive reactance, and with careful preparation have electrical potentials equal to within 0.5 mV (O'Connell *et al.*, 1960). The metal must be of at least 99.9% silver; this is a higher level of purity than that used for much jewellery. Low-grade silver contains copper as the main impurity which produces greenish marks on the scalp and sometimes ulceration. A suspect electrode should be immersed in 10% ammonia: a bluish colouration confirms the presence of copper.

Chloriding is sometimes carried out by chemical means but an electrolytic method is generally preferred. The technique usually recommended is the following: immerse the electrode in 5% saline together with a piece of scrap silver, connect the electrode to be chlorided to the positive pole of a 1.5 V dry cell or similar DC source and the piece of silver to the negative pole. Chloriding should be complete within 30 s. If the procedure is carried out in darkness the electrode will be covered by a white layer of silver chloride. In light, a photochemical reaction rapidly leads to the formation of a more stable allotropic form of silver chloride which gives the electrode a brown or deep purple colour. Slower chloriding appears to give a much more durable chloride layer and a reduced incidence of electrode artefact (Coles and Binnie, 1968; Roberts *et al.*, 1974). The electrodes are mounted in a specially constructed holder so that their surfaces are immersed in the saline but the electrode–wire junction is held clear of the electrolyte. The electrodes are connected in series–parallel with resistors of some tens of kilo-ohms (Fig. 3.2) so that the current through each channel is equal, constant and independent of the individual electrode resistances or potentials.

The period of chloriding should be at least one hour, but may preferably be extended to 24 hours. The total charge to be passed through each electrode should be about 1–2 C, that is a current of 0.25–0.5 mA per electrode will produce satisfactory chloriding within 1 hour.* To determine the total current to be passed through the apparatus this figure should be multiplied by the number of electrodes and divided by the number of hours over which it is intended to carry out the process. Chloriding reduces electrode impedance by increasing the capacitance, but excessive chloriding should be avoided; it gives high resistances and a thick deposit which rapidly flakes off.

If the surface of an electrode is not uniform, due for instance to defects in the chloride layer, a local current will be set up when

---

* There is a remarkable lack of agreement in the literature concerning the optimal charge. Estimates range from 0.048 C/cm² to 168 C/cm² (Geddes, 1972). 0.5 C/cm² appears to give the lowest impedance at EEG frequencies.

Fig. 3.2. System for slow chloriding of EEG electrodes. The electrodes are connected in series-parallel with 50 kΩ resistors (R_s), which ensure that the currents $I_1, I_2 \ldots I_n$ are virtually equal. An adjustable current source is connected in series with the electrodes, a silver plate cathode and a milli-amp meter used to monitor the chloriding current.

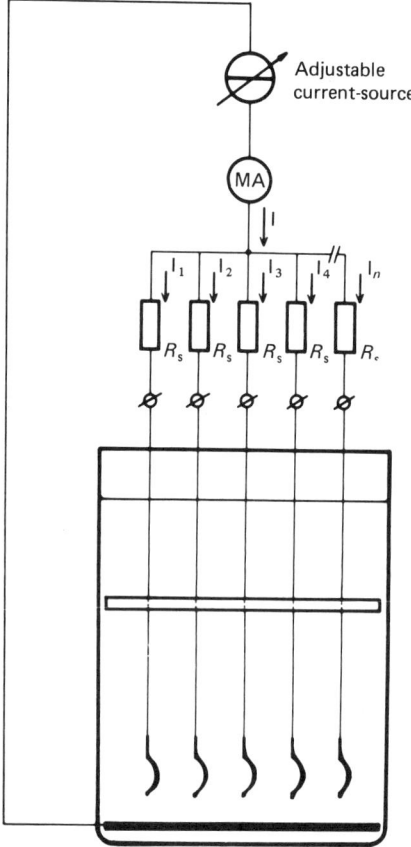

it is immersed in electrolyte. This causes 'self-chloriding' until the potential differences are eliminated. Thus, leaving the electrode in saline promotes the formation of a uniform chloride layer and hence a stable electrode potential. Similarly, if several electrodes are immersed in saline and connected together through their leads, the self-chloriding process will cause them to adopt equal potentials with respect to each other (Cooper, 1956). Apparatus is available commercially for electrode storage which also promotes self-chloriding, but note that silver chloride is soluble in concentrated saline solutions and, if the electrodes are stored for long periods in self-chloriding apparatus, it is important not to allow the electrolyte to become over-concentrated due to evaporation. Self-chloriding of newly prepared electrodes may be deliberately promoted by scratching away some of the chloride layer from that surface of the electrode which will not come in contact with the scalp and then immersing in saline for 15 min.

When old electrodes are re-chlorided they should be cleansed of fragments of paste or adhesive by means of acetone or alcohol. Remains of the old chloride layer may be stripped electrolytically: the electrode is immersed in a chloriding bath, but in this instance is made the cathode and a larger potential difference of the order of 9 V is applied. Alternatively ultra-sound may be used to remove both fragments of glue and the original chloride layer. A further refinement is to roughen the surface of the electrode by etching, so that the chloride will adhere more securely. For this purpose the same procedure is used as for chloriding but silver nitrate solution is substituted for sodium chloride. As silver nitrate is highly soluble, the surface of the cathode does not become coated with a layer of the salt but is simply eroded. Chemical etching is also possible by immersing for 20 min in an acidic solution of ferric chloride (conc. HCl 300 ml, $FeCl_3$ 300 g, distilled water 600 ml). This is corrosive and must not come in contact with clothing or skin.

It is important to keep apparatus used for chloriding scrupulously clean, and in particular to avoid contamination with other metals. Plugs, wires and clips must on no account be immersed in the electrolyte. Separate baths and indifferent electrodes should be reserved for chloriding, stripping and etching. Electrodes should never be cleaned with wire brushes, files, burrs or other metallic objects. If necessary plastic pot cleaners or scouring powder may be used.

3.3.2. Tin/stannous chloride electrodes

As mentioned above, chlorided tin electrodes have excellent recording characteristics, with a very low electrode potential and a lower noise level than chlorided silver. A serious practical difficulty is its marked toxicity and an elaborate method of construction is necessary to avoid direct contact with the skin. Practical details are provided by Kado and Adey (1968) but chlorided tin is rarely used for routine clinical practice.

3.3.3. Solder electrodes

A somewhat cavalier approach to electrode preparation was the use of solder. It is highly reactive and therefore gives a low contact resistance. Because of the low melting point of solder it was a simple matter to cast one's own electrodes in a wooden mould. However, the electrode potentials were high, unequal and unstable and solder has rightly fallen into disuse as a material for electrodes.

3.3.4. Inert electrodes

At the very low levels of e.m.f. involved in EEG recording there is no mechanism for transferring charge across the electrode/electrolyte interface if the electrode itself is made of a chemically inert material such as gold, platinum or stainless steel. Electrodes of these materials therefore have a very high ohmic resistance and conduct only by capacitative coupling to the underlying tissues. The capacitance will depend upon the area of the surface of contact. Inert electrodes generally take the form of wires or needles and the contact area may be a few square millimetres in the case of the scalp needle, but very much less for a depth electrode insulated up to its tip. The capacitive reactance of these electrodes increases with decreasing frequency. For scalp needles this is of little consequence within the range of frequencies encountered in routine clinical EEG practice (Zablow and Goldensohn, 1969), but they are not suitable for recording event-related slow potentials (see Section 12.3).

3.4. Types of electrodes
3.4.1. Stick-on cup or disc electrodes

Electrodes in the form of shallow cups or less commonly discs are widely used. They are 9–11 mm in diameter and made of chlorided silver. Many minor variations in form are encountered (Fig. 3.3): the lead may be soldered close to the edge of the electrode or attached to a short tail which makes the electrode easier to handle during application. A variant having similar characteristics is a plastic cup containing a coiled chlorided silver wire insert.

The electrode site is generally cleaned with alcohol or ether-meths, but some workers claim that, unless the skin is very dirty, omitting this step gives lower resistances and fewer artefacts. The electrode is positioned on the scalp and held in place by the technician's finger or by a special applicator (Fig. 3.4) and adhesive is applied around the edges, either directly from a tube or by means of a small paint brush. Collodion is generally used (14% nitrocellulose in solvent ether, 0.73 g/ml). The consistency is important, if too runny it will be spilled on the patient and if too stiff it is unworkable. The collodion is dried by means of a compressed air jet (which may be incorporated in the electrode applicator), an ordinary hairdryer, or simply by blowing upon it. This last method is the slowest and aesthetically least acceptable but may be appropriate when dealing with a frightened child easily scared by a compressed air gun. Rapid and secure electrode application is a knack which depends largely on applying just the right amount of collodion and spreading it dexterously around the edge of the electrode with a finger, producing a film which is thin enough to dry quickly but adequate to hold the electrode in place. It is good practice to position the electrodes so that all the leads run in the same direction, either towards the anticipated position of the headbox or towards the vertex. Further security may be achieved by covering the electrode with a small square of

Fig. 3.3. Cup or disc electrodes. (*a*) Conventional silver disc electrode with lead attached to short tail. (*b*) Silver cup electrode showing two variations: wire soldered close to the edge of the electrode and a detachable lead connected through a 1 mm plug. (*c*) Plastic cup electrode containing chlorided silver wire. (*d*) Disc electrode. (*e*) Two types of suction cup electrode: that on the left and centre is retained by applying to the skin, squeezing and releasing; that shown in section on the right is attached by a suction line to a vacuum pump.

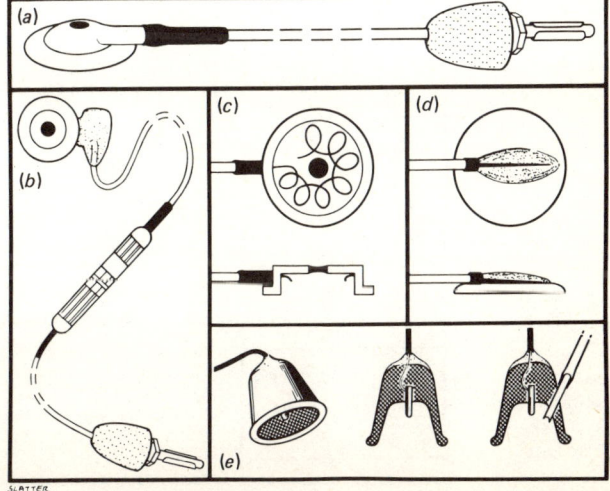

gauze soaked in collodion. Finally, electrode paste or jelly is inserted with a syringe and needle through a hole in the dome of the electrode. The needle has a blunt or, ideally, castellated end (Fig. 3.4) and by means of a rotating action it is used to abrade the outer layer of the scalp, helping to reduce contact resistance. Excessive abrasion is not only painful but leads to bleeding and severe, intractable artefacts. Sufficient paste should be injected to fill the cup and any excess should be wiped off. The resistance between a pair of electrodes should not exceed 5 kΩ and

Fig. 3.4. (*a*) Application of stick-on cup electrode. (1) Marking electrode sites. (2) Preparation of skin. (3) Use of special applicator which holds the electrode in place, a jet of compressed air used to dry the collodion is controlled by a valve operated between finger and thumb. (4) Spreading the collodion with the finger-tip; note that when not in use the tube of collodion is retained in a hole in the handle of the applicator. (5) Application of cup electrode using a paint brush and pot of collodion. (6) Abrading the skin after injecting electrode paste; note the rotary movement of the syringe between thumb and forefinger. (7) Needle with castellated end for injection of electrode paste and abrasion of skin. (8) For greater security a square of gauze may be stuck with collodion over the electrode.

(a)

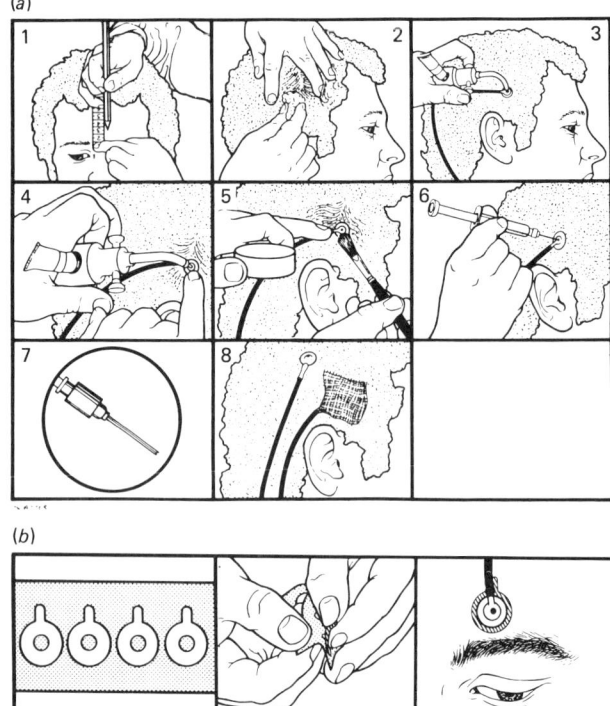

(b)

Fig. 3.4. (cont.)
(*b*) Application of cup electrode by means of double-sided sticky disc.

with good technique values of $2\,k\Omega$ can often be achieved. Cup
electrodes without a hole are also used, and the scalp must be
abraded and the jelly placed inside the electrode before it is applied. A convenient method of fixation is with a collodion-
soaked gauze square. A rubber tube is used to deliver compressed
air for drying the collodion, and at the same time to model the
gauze to the shape of the electrode. The internal diameter of the
tube should be slightly less than the width of the electrode.

To remove the electrodes the collodion should be dissolved
with acetone. Fragments of collodion are then dislodged by the
use of more acetone and a steel comb and the smallest remaining
particles with a fine comb of the type used for removing head-
lice. After use the electrodes should be scrubbed under running
cold water with a toothbrush, to remove remains of collodion
and jelly, and any in need of re-chloriding or with faulty elec-
trode-lead junctions should be set aside. Re-chloriding is necessary
after some 30 to 100 records, depending on the use made of the
electrodes and the method of preparation.

Solid disc electrodes are generally retained by means of a
pellet of bentonite paste which acts both as adhesive and conducting medium. Bentonite sometimes gives rise to skin reactions
(Clendenning and Auerbach, 1964) but the risk can be greatly
reduced if the preparation used is free of calcium (Appendix I).
Bentonite may also be used for cup electrodes, and this allows
more rapid application, which is of particular value when it is
necessary to obtain a record as rapidly as possible after an
epileptic seizure or cardiac arrest. Bentonite is suitable for many
routine purposes but is less secure than collodion and is not advised for sleep recordings, long-term tracings, or records from
restless subjects.

Over hairless skin, electrodes may be attached by means of
double-sided adhesive discs or (more securely and at lower cost)
by means of various paper or plastic tapes used for affixing
surgical dressings (Micropore, Leucopore, Blenderm, etc.).

Stick-on chlorided silver cup electrodes are by far the most
satisfactory for routine clinical and research applications. They
can be accurately placed and securely fixed and can give satisfactory recordings for periods of up to several days. After some
hours use the noise level increases, though not to an unacceptable value, but in this respect they do compare adversely with
stannous chloride (Kado and Adey, 1968).

3.4.2. Suction electrodes

Suction cup electrodes have been used particularly for electro-oculography but also sometimes for EEG recording from neonates. They consist of a rubber cup containing a chlorided silver core. They may be filled with jelly, and suction is achieved simply by squeezing them and releasing (Shackel, 1958). In a variant described by Cooper and Walter (1957), each electrode is attached by a suction line to a vacuum pump (Fig. 3.3).

3.4.3. Pressure contact or pad electrodes

These electrodes are constructed in many different forms but consist essentially of a piece of chlorided silver studding padded with sponge and gauze, supported by a plastic foot and retained by some form of cap of narrow rubber tubing or flat rubber bands (Fig. 3.5). The lead is attached by means of a banana plug or crocodile clip. Variants include tripods, consisting of three electrodes joined together, and simple silver clips attached to rubber strips. Tripods and systems where the electrode is located in a permanent hole in the rubber band are easy to use but do not allow any accuracy of positioning. Some skill is required to construct satisfactory headcaps and to adjust them to fit each individual.

The pads are soaked in saline before use. The application site is cleaned, as for stick-on electrodes, and a little electrode jelly is then rubbed into the scalp. This should be strictly limited to the region of contact, for the electrode will record the average activity over the whole area covered by jelly. Each electrode in turn is then positioned under the harness. This procedure is more difficult than might at first appear. Initially the cap is loose and the electrodes tend to fall out, but by the time the last electrode is applied it may have become too tight. Contact resistances should not exceed $10\,\mathrm{k}\Omega$ but will in general be higher than those obtained with stick-on electrodes. Lower contact resistance may be obtained by the cautious use of a battery powered burr or a sand-blasting nozzle (Shackel, 1959; Rémond and Torres, 1964). Within 20–30 min, or sooner if the recording environment is warm and dry, the saline on the electrodes begins to dry out. Sometimes it is possible to continue recording by applying more saline to the electrodes *in situ*. This is a difficult manoeuvre and if saline trickles down the scalp the electrodes will become short-circuited to each other. Within 30–40 min the chin strap of the headcap usually becomes uncomfortable, and recording must be terminated anyway.

When not in use, pad electrodes are stored in saline in a self-chloriding bath (Fig. 3.5). A grey discolouration of the pads indicates that re-chloriding is necessary. For this purpose the pads must be removed, but this type of electrode requires less frequent chloriding than discs.

It is claimed by those who use them that pad electrodes are

Fig. 3.5. (*a*) Pad electrodes. (1) Stages in construction of pad electrode. (2) The lead is connected by a plug or a crocodile clip. (3) Apparatus for storage and self-chloriding of pad electrodes. (*b*) Methods of attachment of pad electrodes. (1) Rubber head cap. (2) Electrodes in place. (3) Perforated rubber strips, may be more convenient for retaining pads on heads of unusual shape or in children. (4) Tripod electrodes, this method of attachment is simple but precludes accurate placement.

(*a*)

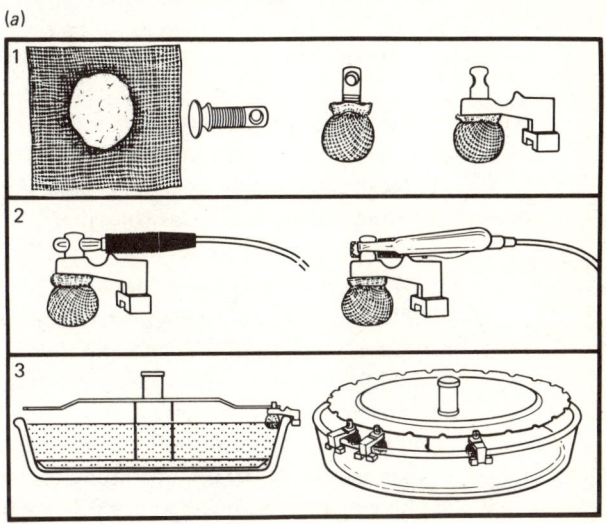

(*b*)

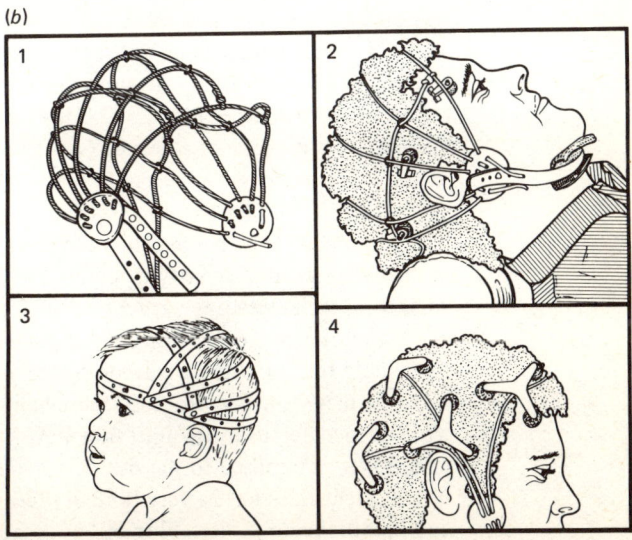

much easier and quicker to apply than stick-ons. This is probably true for trainee technicians, but in experienced hands pads are no faster to apply than discs. The disadvantages of pad electrodes are considerable. They give high contact resistances, are mechanically unstable and liable to artefact. They do not readily stay in place during seizures, sleep or in restless subjects. They are difficult to locate accurately and tend in any event to slide upwards towards to the crown of the head. The duration of recording is limited both by the drying out of the electrodes and by the discomfort of the headcap. The same discomfort also greatly reduces the likelihood of spontaneous sleep and indeed makes even drug-induced sleep recordings difficult to achieve. Despite the widespread use of pads in Europe we know no indication for their use, except in the occasional patient who strongly objects to having collodion in his or her hair.

3.4.4. Insertion scalp electrodes

Needle electrodes are commonly constructed of stainless steel, platinum or platinum with an iridium tip (Fig. 3.6). They can rapidly be applied and the sites of insertion can be accurately chosen. Nevertheless the effective recording location depends upon the orientation of the electrode after penetrating the skin (Tyner and Knott, 1976). The needles must be sterilized before use by a method adequate to destroy the virus of homologous serum jaundice (e.g. autoclave 20 min at 125 °C) which could be transmitted from one patient to another. The skin at the insertion site is first prepared with an antiseptic or alcohol and vigorous rubbing helps to divert the attention of the patient from the sensation when the needle is inserted. This causes suprisingly little discomfort but it is advisable to work from behind the patient, who may be worried by the sight of the approaching needle. The needle is thrust under the skin at an angle of 30° to the scalp and to a depth of at least 5 mm. The needles are self-retaining but occasionally greater security is required and can be achieved by anchoring each electrode with a tuft of hair soaked in collodion.

To remove the needle a pledget of cotton wool is pressed over the needle track and the electrode pulled straight out. Little bleeding may be expected. The technician must avoid all contact with the needles after use until they have been sterilized, otherwise he too is exposed to the risk of homologous serum jaundice. Needle electrodes have a very limited life span (15-20 recordings) and rapidly become bent, blunted, or detached from their leads.

They can be sharpened a few times on a fine oilstone.

Needle electrodes can be applied more rapidly than other types and are especially suitable for emergency records from deeply unconscious subjects. Though they are used in some departments for routine clinical EEGs they are susceptible to artefacts in restless patients, due either to abrupt changes in the physical properties of the electrode itself or to bleeding at the site of insertion. Needles are not acceptable for routine use in sleep recordings but, where it is essential to apply an extra electrode in a sleeping subject, this is virtually the only type that can be used without waking him. The effects of the high impedance to low frequencies have been noted above. The use of needle electrodes is absolutely contraindicated in patients with bleeding disorders or scalp infections.

A variant of the needle electrode is a wire hook which has been recommended for recordings of several days duration from neonates.

3.4.5. Electrodes for use in moving subjects

In an active subject the electrode surface may move relative to the skin; the electrical double layer is disturbed, electrode impedance and potential are altered, and artefacts result. Adequate recordings from moving subjects can be obtained with conventional cup electrodes, but where EEG telemetry is performed routinely special electrodes may be desirable. Many ingenious methods have been devised for reducing artefact in ECG recordings from subjects as varied as whales and astronauts (Geddes, 1972) and some may be applicable to EEGs. The electrode should be as light as possible, the most extreme instance of which is simply electrodeposition of silver into the skin itself (Edelberg, 1963). The electrode surface may be recessed so that it does not come in direct contact with the skin, the gap being bridged by electrode jelly. Recessed EEG electrodes include suction cups and the tin/

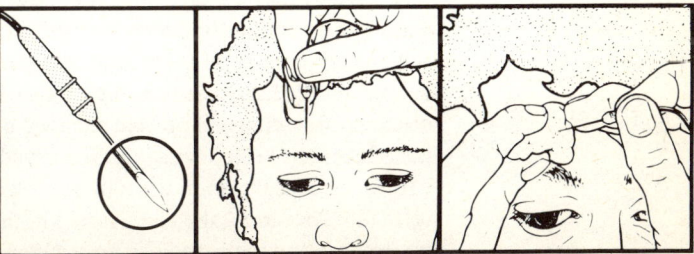

Fig. 3.6. The sub-dermal needle electrode, its insertion and removal.

stannous chloride electrodes of Kado and Adey (1968) but are quite large. The plastic cup with a silver wire insert is both re-cessed and light. Unfortunately, most types of recessed electrodes (with the exception of the chlorided tin variety) have a high im-pedance relative to their size.

3.4.6. Special purpose insertion electrodes

Recording from the undersurface of the brain, particularly from mesial temporal structures, is often crucial to the diagnosis of partial epilepsies. Activity from these basal regions may not reach the scalp but can be recorded with special insertion electrodes.

Sphenoidal electrodes

Jasper (1949) described the insertion under radiological control of a needle through the mouth to the region of the foramen ovale in order to record from mesial temporal structures. This method was superseded by a technique described by Jones (1951) and by Pampiglione and Kerridge (1956) for passing the electrode through the skin of the cheek below the zygoma and above the mandibular notch. The electrode may consist either of a 6 cm needle insulated with varnish or epoxy resin to within 2 mm of its tip or may be a flexible wire, itself inserted by means of a needle. As the needle electrode tends to produce spasm of the jaw muscles and hence artefact, the wire type is preferable and is moreover considerably less painful if recording from a conscious subject is required.

The wire electrode (Fig. 3.7) is of silver or stainless steel, in-sulated with varnish, and the tip is bared by scraping with a razor-blade or scalpel. The tip is bent back to form a hook. The wire may be passed up inside the needle with the hook exposed at the end; alternatively, the hook may be inserted in the pointed end of the needle and the wire carried back along the outside. The needle carrying the wire is inserted and then withdrawn, leaving the wire in place. When the needle has been removed the free end of the wire may be attached to the headbox by means of a lead bearing a crocodile clip. Alternatively, a 1 mm plug may be soldered to the end of the wire to provide a more reliable con-nection. In this case the wire must be carried up the outside, otherwise the plug will prevent removal of the needle. A special introducer has been devised by Townsend (1968) for inserting wire electrodes but even without this aid the technique is not difficult. The wires, already inserted in their needles or intro-ducers, must be sterilized before use by autoclaving, and sterile, preferably 'no-touch', technique should be employed for their insertion. The site of skin-penetration is a point 25 mm from the tragus of the ear along the line joining the incisura intertragica to the inferior margin of the ala nasae. This point should be identified by measurement and marked by means of an indelible dye or by lightly scratching the skin with a needle. One should then confirm by palpation that it lies over the space between the zygoma and the notch in the upper margin of the mandible. In edentulous patients this space may be obliterated when the jaws are closed, in which case dentures should be left in place during insertion of the electrode. The skin is cleaned with an antiseptic lotion and the needle inserted almost horizontally (ideally some 5° above the horizontal plane and 5° forwards from the coronal plane. At a depth of about 40 mm the needle will strike bone (the pterygoid plate of the sphenoid) and should then be withdrawn leaving the wire in place. On completion of the recording the wire should be gripped with a mosquito clamp flush with the surface of the skin and extracted with a sharp jerk. The distance from the clamp to the end of the wire should then be measured to confirm that it was indeed inserted to the appropriate depth.

Fig. 3.7. (*a*) Sphenoidal electrodes. (1) The Townsend introducer. (2) and (3) The sphenoidal wire inserted either through or on the outside of the needle (see text). (4) and (5) Removal of the needle leaving the hooked wire electrode in place. (*b*) Anatomical landmarks for insertion of sphenoidal electrodes (see text).

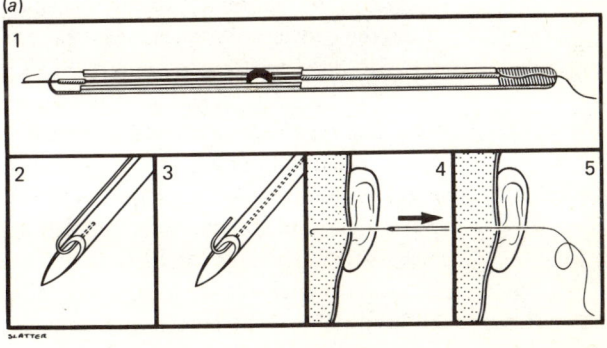

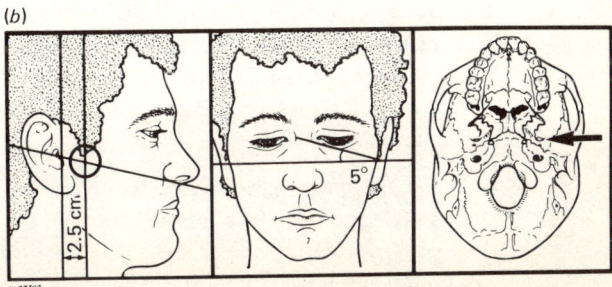

Regarding analgesia or anaesthesia there are some variations in practice. Infiltration of the skin with local anaesthetic serves no useful purpose, as this is no less uncomfortable than the insertion of the needle itself. In any event the main source of pain is abrasion of the periosteum on the pterygoid, or on the undersurface of temporal bone if the needle is angled too sharply upwards. Some skilled operators insert sphenoidal electrodes without any form of analgesia but this is distressing for the patient. Alternatively, as sphenoidal recording is often combined with sleep, one may insert the needle immediately after an intravenous injection of rapid acting barbiturate, as methohexitone. The present authors prefer to insert the electrode at leisure with a cooperative and conscious patient, and this may conveniently be achieved under light sedation (for instance intravenous neurolept-analgesia with droperidol and fentanil administered by an anaesthetist). The intravenous barbiturate is administered only after the commencement of recording to allow study of the early stages of drowsiness, during which information of diagnostic use is most often obtained.

The value of sphenoidal recording is debatable. Certainly a sphenoidal record combined with methohexitone-induced sleep provides information not readily obtained from waking EEGs using the conventional electrode locations of the 10–20 system (see Section 4.5) (Christodoulou, 1967). The amount of new information from sphenoidal recording is considerably less if sleep and night sleep deprivation records are routinely obtained and if low frontal or anterior temporal electrode placements are used, as described by Pampiglione (1956) and by Silverman (1960). Nevertheless, in patients with complex partial seizures and non-diagnostic wake and sleep EEGs, a 40% yield of useful information from sphenoidal recording has been claimed (Kristensen and Sindrup, 1978). The procedure is generally indicated only in patients being assessed for possible neurosurgical treatment of epilepsy, and if prolonged EEG telemetry is performed the wires may be left in place for several days (Ives *et al.*, 1977). Complications are uncommon but sometimes deep bleeding can occur if a small artery is penetrated, and the patient's face swells with alarming speed.

The nasopharyngeal electrode
An electrode may be inserted through the nose to rest against the posterior wall of the nasopharynx, recording from mesial temporal and basal frontal structures. The type of electrode currently

used consists of thin springy silver wire insulated with plastic sleeving and tipped with a small silver ball or with a bullet shaped head of the same external diameter as the sleeving (Fig. 3.8). The electrode should be disinfected in antiseptic solution to avoid the spread of nasal infections between patients, but strict sterile precautions are not necessary. It should be lubricated with glycerine or with catheter jelly (not with abrasive electrode jelly).

Nasopharyngeal recording should not be attempted in a patient with an upper respiratory infection, and should in any case be abandoned if repeated sneezing occurs. Although the electrodes are often inserted blindly, it is recommended that the nose first be inspected with the help of a nasal speculum or nasoscope. If the nasal septum is markedly deviated or the turbinates are swollen, difficulty may be anticipated, and one may decide to abandon the procedure. The patient should close his eyes and open his mouth. Two techniques for insertion are described. The first requires the electrode to be bent into a gently curving S (Fig. 3.8). The tip of the nose is pulled gently upwards and the electrode inserted in the nostril with the distal curve directed upwards. The electrode is then slid gently downwards and backwards along the floor of the nasal cavity below the conchae until the resistance of the posterior wall of the pharynx is met, at a depth of about 120 mm. The second method employs an electrode which is straight in its middle part; the distal curve extends only 4–5 cm and is directed downwards during insertion. When

Fig. 3.8. Nasopharyngeal electrodes. (1) The electrode. (2) and (3) The electrode tip may be fusiform or spherical. (4) The electrode in place.

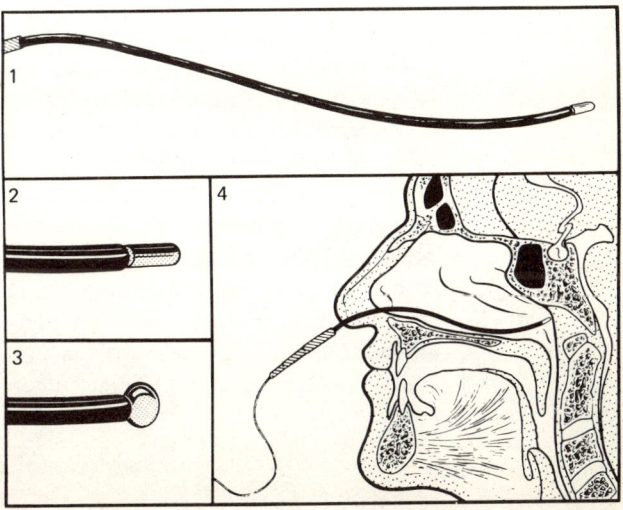

the posterior wall of the pharynx is reached the electrode tip is rotated laterally and upwards bringing the curve of the wire almost into the horizontal plane. Thus the tips are widely separated in the lateral parts of the nasopharynx and the proximal ends of the electrodes are crossed in front of the nose. The electrode is secured by taping its lead under slight tension to the opposite cheek. The sensation is mildly disagreeable but the procedure is generally well tolerated by adults and by cooperative children above the age of 10 years. A local anaesthetic ointment is sometimes substituted for the lubricating jelly but is rarely necessary.

Sometimes so much artefact is recorded, for instance from respiration or carotid pulsation, that no useful information can be obtained. It has been claimed that there is little advantage in using two electrodes as the tips are very close together, or indeed that the electrodes may become crossed at the back of the nose giving incorrect lateralisation of the activities recorded. The second technique described excludes both these possibilities and unilateral temporal discharges recorded at scalp electrodes may commonly be seen spreading to involve the ipsilateral but not the contralateral nasopharyngeal. On occasions focal paroxysmal discharges may be of maximum amplitude at one or other nasopharyngeal electrode but it is rare for any activity to be recorded which cannot be adequately demonstrated with a superficial anterior temporal placement.

The naso-ethmoidal electrode

An electrode similar to the nasopharyngeal may be inserted above the superior concha of the nose below the ethmoidal plate to record from the anterior fronto-basal region (Lehtinen and Bergström, 1970). Local anaesthesia and the use of a nasal decongestant are necessary. It is debatable whether this technique provides additional useful information.

The tympanic electrode

Arellano (1949) described a silver rod electrode tipped with sponge or cotton and inserted through the external auditory meatus to record from the eardrum. Before the electrode is inserted it is essential to check with an auroscope that the drum is intact. Contact with the eardrum at a depth of 50–60 mm produces a sudden but short-lasting pain. The technique is little used and its clinical value does not appear to be well documented.

3.5. Electrode jelly

Various different conducting pastes or jellies have been used to establish contact between the electrode and the skin. As the principal extracellular electrolyte is sodium chloride, isotonic (0.9%) saline is the obvious choice as the main constituent. Abrasives, such as pumice may be added to assist the removal of the outer layer of the skin, and gum tragacanth, glycerine or agar-agar to reduce evaporation. The use of calcium chloride appears to be associated with skin reactions and this is not included in some of the newer preparations.

For routine clinical recordings there is probably little to choose between the various commercial electrode jellies. For tracings of many hours duration possible skin irritation becomes an important consideration, as does the growth of micro-organisms, and a special formulation may be required. For instance, Day and Lippitt (1964) described a paste used for NASA space flights which produced no skin reaction after weeks of continuous use.

4. Derivation and montages

4.1. Introduction

When Hans Berger carried out his first recordings of his son's EEG he simply registered the potential difference between two electrodes, one on the front and one at the back of the head (Fig. 4.1*a*). The location of the electrical generators giving rise to the signals was for his purposes at that time immaterial. In 1935 Adrian and Yamagiwa demonstrated that the alpha rhythm was situated at the back of the head and the following year Grey Walter succeeded in locating cerebral tumours by means of the overlying delta focus. The method used for localizing focal EEG activity with the primitive apparatus available in those days was as follows. Two electrodes were used as fixed reference points and a third was used to explore the surface of the scalp. Each fixed electrode was connected to one of two channels and the exploring electrode was connected to both. Wiring was arranged so that an electrical potential at the exploring electrode which was negative with respect to the other two caused a downward deflection in the first channel and an upward deflection in the second. When the common electrode was positioned over a focus of delta activity the slow waves deflected the two channels in opposite directions, producing a 'phase reversal' (Fig. 4.1*b*).

In modern EEG practice with upwards of 20 electrodes and 8, 16, or more channels, techniques for demonstrating the topography of the EEG have become considerably more complex. There are certain underlying principles which may appear self-evident but their implications must nevertheless be clearly understood. The phenomenon to be studied consists of a complex electrical field distributed over the three-dimensional surface of the scalp and continuously changing as a function of time. The apparatus ordinarily used to display the EEG is a moving chart recorder: this shows the changes with time very adequately, but the distribution of the EEG must be deduced by combining the information provided by the individual recording channels, each of which registers the potential difference between its two input leads. The manner in which the electrodes are connected to these inputs is termed *derivation* and a particular pattern of electrodes and connections is a *montage*. Though our concern with locating cerebral electrical events may cause us to talk loosely of EEG activity at a particular site, it is in fact meaningless to speak of 'the electrical potential' at a particular point either on the scalp or indeed anywhere in the physical universe. **Only potential difference has any reality, and the differential amplifier of each**

Fig. 4.1. Early systems of EEG derivation. (*a*) A single channel registration as used in Berger's early studies; this cannot localize the activity recorded. (*b*) The use of an exploring electrode common to two channels allows localized phenomena to be detected by phase reversal.

(*a*)

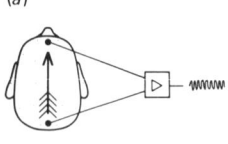

(*b*)

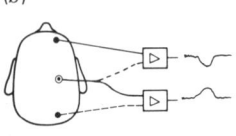

channel of the EEG machine registers the potential difference between its input leads. The concept of a localized EEG phenomenon
is, however, valid but only if it is conceived in terms of potential
difference. An EEG phenomenon may be regarded as localized if
it causes a restricted area of the scalp (or a minority group of
recording electrodes) to adopt a potential difference with respect
to the remainder of the scalp (or the the majority of the electrodes). This definition is of practical value, as such a potential
distribution commonly reflects a localized electrophysiological
event.

4.2. Methods of derivation

Various techniques are available for connecting combinations of
electrodes and recording channels in order to display the
topography of the EEG. The most obvious perhaps is to connect
one lead of each channel to a common reference point and to
display the potential difference between each of the recording
electrodes and this reference. This method is known as *common
reference derivation*. A similar approach is adopted by cartogra-
phers who show the height of features on their maps with
reference to a fixed datum, generally sea-level. A less obvious
method, but an obvious extension of Adrian's technique
mentioned above, is to connect electrodes in pairs to the channels
so as to display the potential difference between each electrode
and its neighbours. This method is called *bipolar derivation*. There
is no obvious analogy in conventional map-making practice, but
it is not difficult to imagine a plan intended for hikers, which
displayed local gradients rather than the overall topography of a
landscape. A third method, *source reference derivation*, has
recently been introduced but its definition will be postponed to a
later section (4.2.4). Another approach is to display the potential
differences between pairs of widely spaced electrodes; this has
no generally accepted name except possibly 'bipolar recording with
large inter-electrode distances'.

Though all methods of derivation present essentially the same
information, the displays produced are very different. Each
method is more suitable for the detecting and localization of some
types of activity than for others and no single method is satisfactory under all circumstances.

4.2.1. Common reference derivation

Fig. 4.2*a* is a contour map representing the potential distribution over the scalp at an instant in time corresponding to the peak of a spike. The potential distribution meets the criteria proposed above for a localized phenomenon. Electrode G and to a lesser extent electrodes, F, M, B, L, N and S are negative with respect to the others. The spike may therefore be considered to be electro-negative and focal at G, extending to adjacent electrodes particu-larly to F and M. The contour lines on the figure are spaced at $10\,\mu V$ intervals and the area to the right of them has been arbi-trarily designated zero; note that if a different site had been taken as the zero level, the position and shape of the contours would have been precisely the same.

In Fig. 4.2b the same spike is shown as it might appear in an EEG recording using electrode H (on the right ear) as the common reference. In connecting the electrodes to the recorder a certain

Fig. 4.2. Common reference derivation. The localized left fronto-temporal event (a), as displayed with a reference which is (b) unaffected, (c) minimally affected or (d) maximally affected by the phenomenon in question.

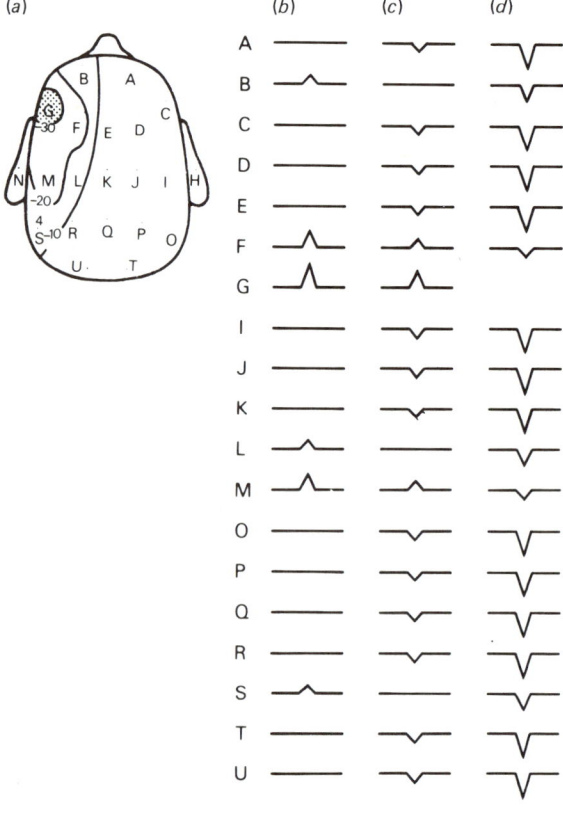

convention has been followed. The differential amplifier of each channel has two input leads designated '*I*' and '*II*' (or sometimes by the names of '*black*' and '*white*'). **When lead I of any channel is negative with respect to lead II, an upwards deflection is recorded on the chart; if lead II is negative with respect to lead I, it follows that the deflection will be downwards.** In some figures in this chapter, lead I will be shown diagrammatically as a solid line and lead II as a dashed line; in others each channel is shown by a numbered arrow pointing from the lead I to the lead II electrode. In common reference recording, the reference is always connected to lead II of every channel and the exploring electrodes to the leads I: any electrode which is negative with respect to the reference will therefore give an upward deflection. In the case of the spike in Fig. 4.2*b*, the affected electrodes are negative with respect to the reference, and therefore give rise to upwards deflections. The potential distribution is easily deduced from the display: the largest deflection occurs on the channel corresponding to electrode G and smaller deflections are seen on the channels derived from adjacent electrodes F and M. A few of the electrodes (B, L and S) are minimally affected and give rise to very small upward deflections. The spike is therefore seen to be focal at G. If this were the whole story, reading EEGs would be quite easy and the rest of this chapter would be superfluous.

Unfortunately, one cannot contrive that localized EEG phenomena always occur at a site on the head remote from the reference. Fig. 4.2*c* shows the display which would have resulted had electrode N been chosen as the reference.

The reference is now closer to the site of the focal spike and therefore affected by it to some extent. Electrodes G, F and M are still more negative than the reference N although the potential difference is less marked than in the first example. Consequently these electrodes continue to give up-going deflections which are lower in amplitude than when H was the reference. Because the reference is now $10\,\mu\text{V}$ negative with respect to the electrodes on the right of the head, and bearing in mind that the reference is connected to the leads II, it follows that the deflections in the channels from the right side will be down-going. Electrodes lying in the region at the same potential as the reference (B, L, S) record no potential difference; consequently channels recording from these electrodes show no deflection. The channel displaying the most prominent upward deflection (G) again indicates the location of the spike. The extent of its field is indicated not only by the channels giving smaller upward deflections but also, paradoxically, by those which show no deflection. The channels deflected downwards are connected to electrodes unaffected by the spike. This pattern is a consequence of the influence of the spike's electrical field on the reference.

An extreme case is shown in Fig. 4.2d. Here, the electrode G overlying the focal event, has been selected as the reference. Applying the reasoning followed above the result should be entirely predictable. G is still the most strongly negative but is now connected to all the leads II. According to the convention all channels will show a downward deflection. Note however that the largest deflections are recorded from those electrodes most different in potential from G. Electrodes F and M which are themselves affected by the spike give rise to much smaller deflections, being less different in potential from G. This pattern of display should be easily recognizable: if with common reference derivation all channels are deflected in the same direction, there is a localized event at the reference.

Though the displays illustrated in Fig. 4.2c and 4.2d are easily interpreted when there is a single isolated focal event, the picture becomes considerably more complex when there are two, possibly asynchronous, foci (Fig. 4.3).

Notwithstanding theoretical arguments about measurements of potential being relative and not absolute, the reader may feel intuitively that it should be possible to find a reference point unaffected by cerebral activity so that the condition shown in Fig. 4.2b always obtains. A reference located on some part of the head other than the scalp or even on another part of the body may seem an obvious solution. However, electrodes not located on the scalp do in fact record cerebral electrical activity: spikes from the orbital surface of the frontal lobe may for instance be strongly electro-negative at an electrode on the chin with respect to others over the scalp. It should also be noted that these locations tend to record EMG and ECG activity. A nose or chin electrode may be excellent for demonstrating widespread bilaterally synchronous activity over the convexity but any vertical eye movement will produce very large deflections in such a derivation and may obscure the EEG.

Because of the problems of artefact a scalp reference is often preferable to one elsewhere. It is possible to select a reference on the head which is inactive with respect to a particular EEG phenomenon of known distribution, but the problem is to find and localize the phenomenon in the first place. There are moreover a number of other difficulties. For instance, to record left temporal spikes, a right temporal reference could be ideal were it not for the fact that temporal spikes often occur bilaterally, possibly producing a confusing picture as shown in Fig. 4.3b. A reference at the vertex (Fig. 4.3a) will avoid this problem but may be unsuitable for a recording in which the patient is likely to become drowsy or sleep, owing to the presence of vertex sharp waves and K-complexes which will appear on all channels. Mention should also be made of a reference obtained by connecting two earlobe electrodes to each other. This offers no advantage over the use of one earlobe, and the considerable disadvantage that, though it records from both temporal lobes, the contribution from each side depends upon the ratio of the electrode resistances. Thus when activity is detected at a joined earlobe reference, it may not even be possible to determine from which side of the head it is coming.

Fig. 4.3. Common reference display of two focal events: (a) Unaffected reference. (b) Reference maximally involved by one of the two foci. (c) Complex display produced when the events are slightly asynchronous.

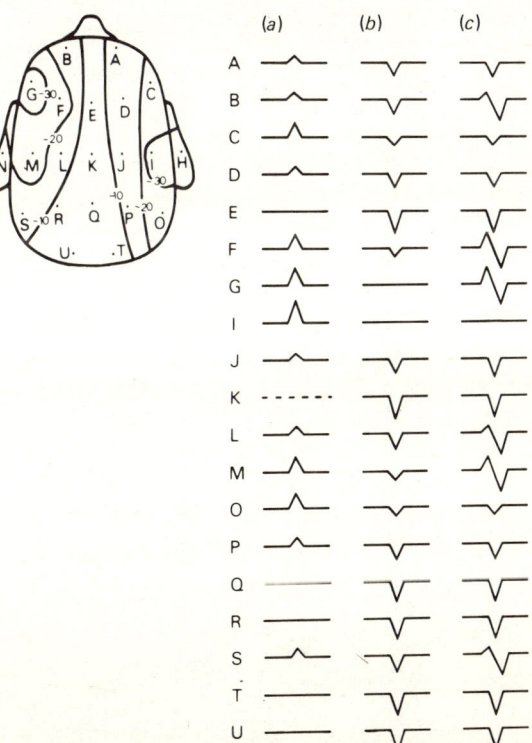

4.2.2. Common average reference derivation

Using common reference derivation it is not difficult with experience to determine whether a particular activity affects the
reference not at all, minimally, or maximally, that is to distinguish
the three conditions illustrated in Fig. 4.2b, c and d. There may
nevertheless be considerable advantages in ensuring that just one
of these conditions always obtains. The second type of display
(Fig. 4.2c), that seen when the reference is always slightly, but
not maximally, affected by any focal activity, may be achieved
by using an artificial reference obtained from the average of all
the electrodes in use, 'a common average reference'. Fig. 4.4
shows the same EEG phenomenon as in 4.2 recorded with this
reference. A property of the mean of a number of observations
is that the sum of differences from that average is always zero.

Fig. 4.4. Common aver-
age reference. The local-
ized event shown in
Fig 4.2 referred to the
average of all elec-
trodes in use. Note
simultaneous occur-
rence of upward and
downward deflections
with a sum of zero.

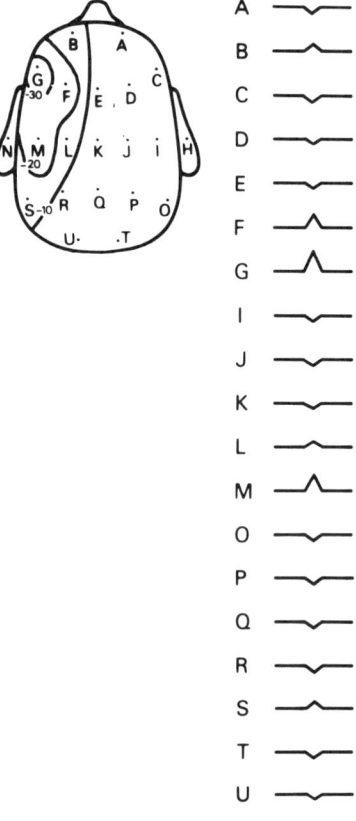

Fig. 4.5. Principle of common average reference. (a) Hypothetical potential distribution affecting only one of the electrodes in use. (b) The reference is derived by connecting all active electrodes through 1 or 2 MΩ resistors to a common point. (c) All electrodes are equipotential with respect to a remote inert reference with the exception of A which gives deflection equivalent to P (its potential with respect to the other electrodes). (d) When referred to the reference all unaffected electrodes are P/n positive with exception of A which gives a deflection equivalent to $P - P/n$.

Thus as Fig 4.4 shows, some channels exhibit upward deflections, others go downwards, but the sum of the deflections is zero. The display resembles that in Fig. 4.2c. The channel showing the most atypical deflection is again that recording from electrode G and there is thus little difficulty in identifying the localized event. The average lies between the extreme values of electrode G (which is most negative) and of the unaffected electrodes. Consequently, as the average is connected to the leads II, the channels from the right of the head give small downward deflections. In practice the average reference point is obtained by connecting each active electrode through a resistor of 1 or 2 MΩ to a common point (Fig. 4.5). Note that the maximum deflection is slightly less than that which would be obtained with a completely uninvolved reference as in Fig. 4.2b. If a localized phenomenon affects only one electrode, giving it a potential P with respect to all the others (arbitrarily designated zero), then the average reference has a potential P/n, where n is the number of electrodes contributing to the average. The deflection on the channel recording from the affected electrode will therefore be equivalent to $P - P/n$ (Fig. 4.5) and the unaffected electrodes give a small deflection P/n, of opposite polarity.

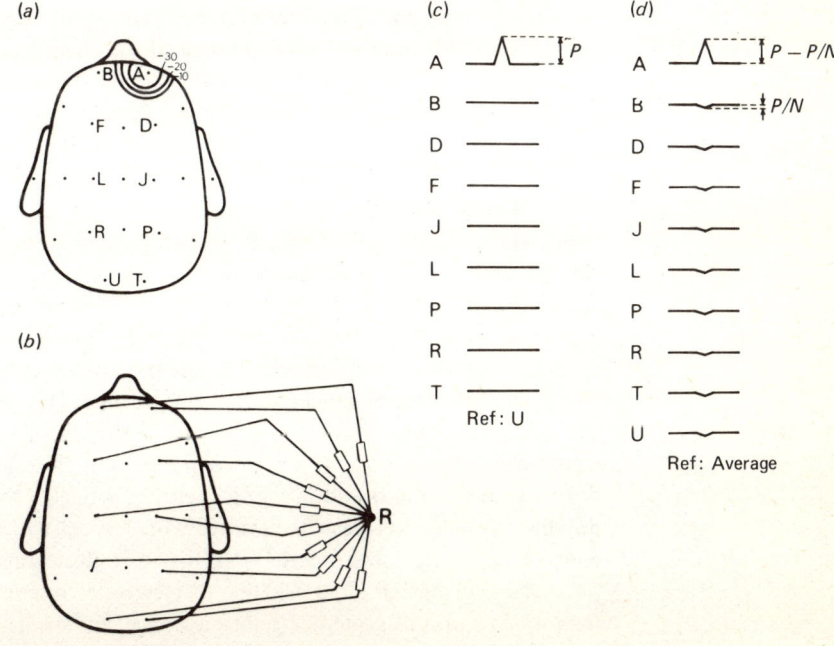

The rule that the instantaneous sum of upward and downward deflections is always zero will apply if the average is derived from all, and only, those electrodes attached to the leads I of the recorder. Some EEG machines have a fixed average reference derived from all the standard electrode placements with the omission, sometimes optional, of those electrodes particularly liable to record eye movement and muscle artefact. Others offer more choice and an average can be derived from all the electrodes on the front, the back, the right or the left of the head. Few if any standard machines offer the facility for deriving the average from the electrodes attached to the leads I whatever the montage, but this can generally be achieved by an inexpensive modification. If an electrode contributing to the average is not connected to lead I then activity, and particularly artefact, arising at that electrode will appear with identical amplitude and phase on all channels. Though one can readily recognize that this activity is coming from the reference, its source cannot be more precisely determined except by changing the montage to record from the other electrodes. Common average reference derivation can be particularly misleading when the number of recording channels is small and many of the electrodes contributing to the average are not connected to leads I. The problem is illustrated in Fig. 4.6: with 19 channels and an average derived from the 19 electrodes concerned, a bifrontal spike is easily identified; on an 8 channel machine and with an entirely reasonable choice of electrodes but the same average, the appearance is misleading and could suggest a surface-positive spike in the temporo-occipital regions.

4.2.3. Bipolar derivation

Mention has already been made of the use of bipolar derivation so that localized activity at an electrode common to two channels could be high-lighted by the phenomenon of phase reversal. To exploit this possibility, bipolar montages are composed of chains of electrodes all of which except the first and last are connected to the lead II of one channel and lead I of the next (Fig. 4.7). The EEG phenomenon previously illustrated in Figs. 4.2 and 4.4 causes electrode G to adopt a negative potential with respect to both its neighbours B and M; consequently channel 1 shows a downward deflection (lead II negative with respect to lead I) and channel 2 an upward deflection. Fig. 4.7c illustrates the potential distribution along the line of electrodes in another manner, as a plot of potential against distance, and displays

the potential differences between the electrodes which are
reflected in the deflections in Fig. 4.7*b*. Fig. 4.8 illustrates some
slightly more complex displays which may be obtained with a
single bipolar chain. If two electrodes are equally affected (Fig.
4.8*a*) the channel derived from them will show no deflection and
phase reversal will occur between the two adjacent channels.
One may infer that the focus lies between F and L but to prove it
one must apply an extra electrode. If the phenomenon maximally affects the last electrode in the chain (Fig. 4.8*b*) it is easily
recognized and gives rise to no phase reversal. When two electrodes at the end of the chain are equally affected (Fig. 4.8*c*)
the inexperienced observer may locate the phenomenon incorrectly
over the region of steepest potential gradient and not over the

Fig. 4.6. Misleading
display produced by
average reference deri-
vation using small
number of channels
(see text).

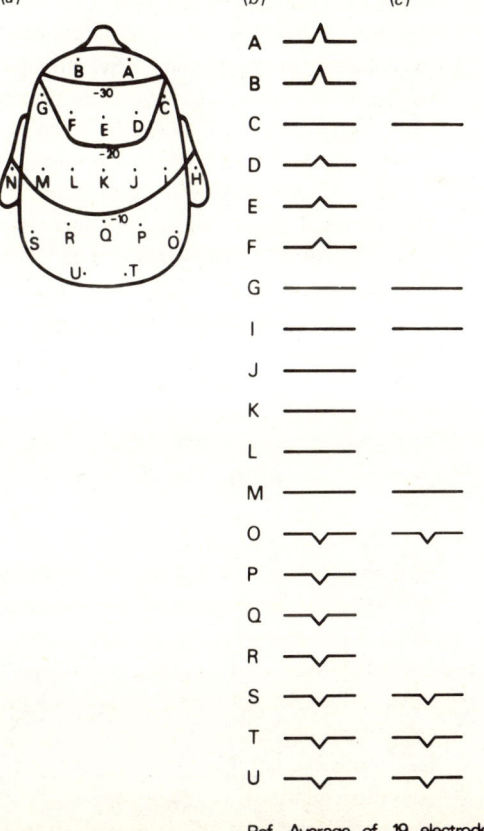

Ref: Average of 19 electrodes

potential maximum (i.e. between electrodes F and L and not over B and F).

The previous paragraph discusses only the localization of an EEG event with respect to a particular line of electrodes. It does not follow that because electrode L is the most affected of the chain B, F, L, R, U (Fig. 4.9), the phenomenon is in fact of maximum amplitude at L: a nearby electrode not included in the chain may be yet more strongly affected. One cannot claim to have located a focus by bipolar derivation unless the EEG event in question is shown to be of maximum amplitude at an electrode common to two bipolar chains mutually at right angles. Unless the electrode concerned is at the periphery of the scalp, it is essential to demonstrate simultaneous phase reversal at the common electrode in both chains (Fig. 4.9d).

Familiarity with EEG practice may lead one to accept the notion of bipolar recording somewhat uncritically. However the naive reader may reasonably enquire why it is necessary to go to such lengths to locate focal EEG phenomena by means of phase reversal when their distribution is already obvious on common reference derivation. The authors have been guilty of an oversimplification. It is not by chance that the preceding sections were illustrated with diagrams rather than examples of actual EEGs. Localization with common reference derivation depends largely on comparing the amplitudes of EEG phenomena in different channels. An unstable baseline of other activity of differing frequencies and possibly greater amplitude makes these comparisons difficult. An advantage of localization by bipolar derivation

Fig. 4.7. Principle of bipolar derivation.

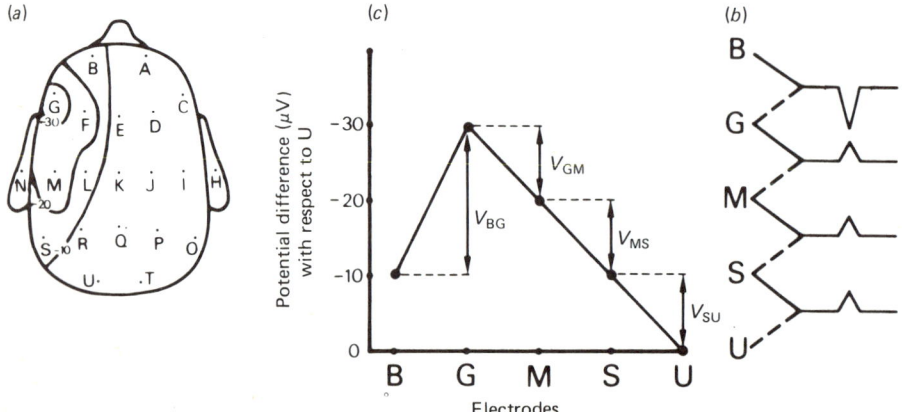

(a) (c) (b)

is that it depends only on comparing the directions, and not the amplitudes, of deflections in different channels.

4.2.4. Source reference derivation

Hjorth (1975) recently described an original method of derivation which, if it fulfils its early promise, may largely supersede the traditional methods. For a mathematical treatment of the under-

Fig. 4.8. Some more complex displays produced by bipolar derivation.

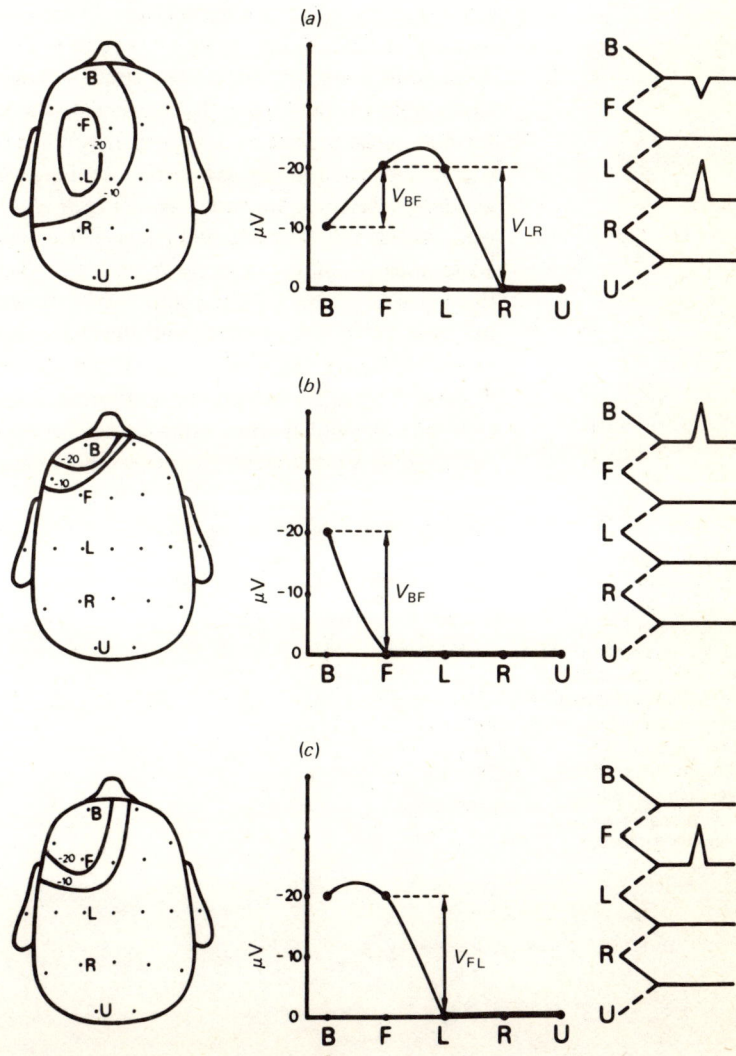

lying concepts the reader is referred to Hjorth (1975, 1979). The basic principle is that the activity recorded at each electrode arises partly from a local underlying electrical source and partly as a result of spread from other adjacent sources. It is possible to calculate the average potential gradient directed at each electrode from all the other electrodes and hence to estimate the activity at that site arising from all sources other than the primary local source. Thus recording between an electrode and its own local reference calculated in this manner should display only the activity uniquely arising under that electrode. In practice this requires an EEG machine with headbox pre-amplifiers and an operational amplifier circuit associated with each standard electrode input socket (Fig. 4.10) to calculate the source reference for that particular electrode. For a sharply localized EEG event, source derivation produces a display similar to that obtained with an ideal unaffected reference as in Fig. 4.2b, but without the need first to find a suitable reference. Thus, whilst sharing the advantages of common average reference derivation, it overcomes the practical defect of that method in that one does not see localized activities appearing with inverted phase on channels recording from unaffected electrodes. It also emphasizes focal features (Fig. 4.11) and has the additional advantage of avoiding the confusion which arises when discrete localized events spread and become superimposed on each other. With other methods

Fig. 4.9. Orthogonal bipolar chains. The potential distribution illustrated in (a) and (b) will not be correctly located by the use of the derivations shown in (c). Simultaneous phase reversal at the common electrode of two chains mutually at right angles (d) is necessary to locate the focus.

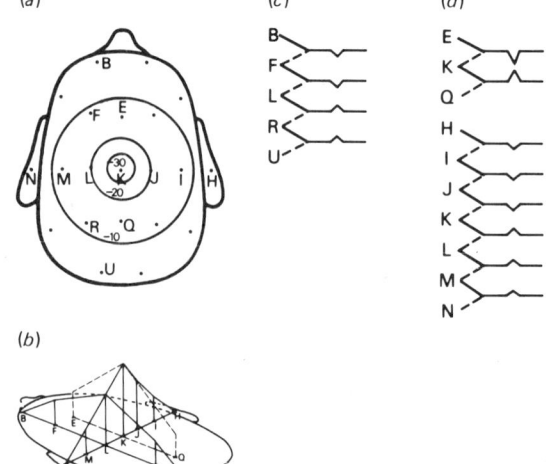

Fig. 4.10. Circuit for deriving source reference (after Hjorth, 1979). The source tracing Z_i at electrode i is obtained as shown by amplifying the potential difference between the signal Y_i recorded from i (with respect to an arbitrary reference) and an average of the signals Y_l, $Y_m \ldots Y_n$ at other electrodes. The contribution of each electrode to the average is weighted dependent upon its distance from i, the weighting factors being represented by the resistors b_{il}, $b_{im} \ldots b_{in}$.

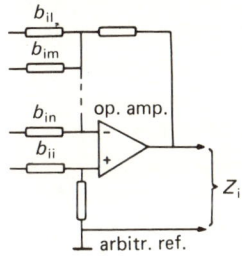

of derivation it may, for instance, be difficult to determine the waveform of an event in the midfrontal region in the presence of vertical eye movements. With source reference derivation the eye movement and the focal EEG event remain distinct and sharply localized. To exploit fully the advantages of this technique, one requires an EEG machine with sufficient channels to record from all standard electrodes simultaneously. It is then possible, contrary to all accepted practice, to perform the greater part of an EEG investigation using only one montage.

Source reference derivation suffers, however, from a number of theoretical deficiencies and there is not yet enough experience to determine whether these are likely to prove serious practical limitations. There is insufficient information from neighbouring electrodes to calculate accurately the source references for electrodes at the margin of the scalp. This may explain the apparently anomalous distribution of eye movement artefacts often registered by this method (Fig. 4.12). The source reference for a mid-line electrode cannot reliably be determined because the longitudinal fissure of the brain is not always in the mid-line and supposed mid-line electrodes often record predominantly from one hemisphere. A diffuse activity appearing on many channels in conventional reference recording will be seen only at the margins of the affected area with source reference (a feature shared by bipolar derivation, see Section 4.3). Attenuation, for instance due to a subdural haematoma, preventing registration both of local EEG activity and of components spreading from adjacent sources, may not be detected (a problem common to bipolar but not to other forms of reference recording).

4.2.5. Bipolar derivation with large inter-electrode distances
Recording from isolated pairs of widely spaced electrodes, which do not form chains, scarcely qualifies as another method of derivation. However it cannot readily be classified as a variant of any of the other techniques and does have some very specific applications which will be considered in the section on montages (4.6). The recording characteristics (see next section) are similar to those of common reference derivation because of the wide inter-electrode distance.

4.3. Recording characteristics of different methods of derivation
To explain the principle of the various methods of derivation we have chiefly considered focal EEG features. However, many

activities are diffusely distributed or produce electrical fields which do not satisfy the criteria for localized phenomena, as there is no minority group of electrodes adopting a potential difference with respect to the majority.

Figs. 4.13 to 4.16 illustrate the interaction between the methods of derivation and the topographic extent of an activity. In the extreme (and in practice very rare) case of a phenomenon localized to one electrode (Fig. 4.13), the maximum potential difference will be the same, whether measured with respect to an adjacent electrode of a bipolar chain or to a remote or source reference. Common average reference will give a marginally smaller deflection ($P - P/n$ – see Section 4.2.3). If the activity has a more diffuse distribution, however (Fig. 4.14), the method of derivation becomes much more important. The potential difference between an electrode and its neighbours is then small; the deflections on

Fig. 4.11. Source reference derivation. The potential distribution (*a*) is shown as displayed by common reference (*b*) or bipolar derivation (*c*). The principle of calculating the source reference value for electrode C from the potentials of its neighbours is indicated in (*d*). Approximate values of the source references for electrodes A to E are shown in (*e*) together with the display produced with such a source reference.

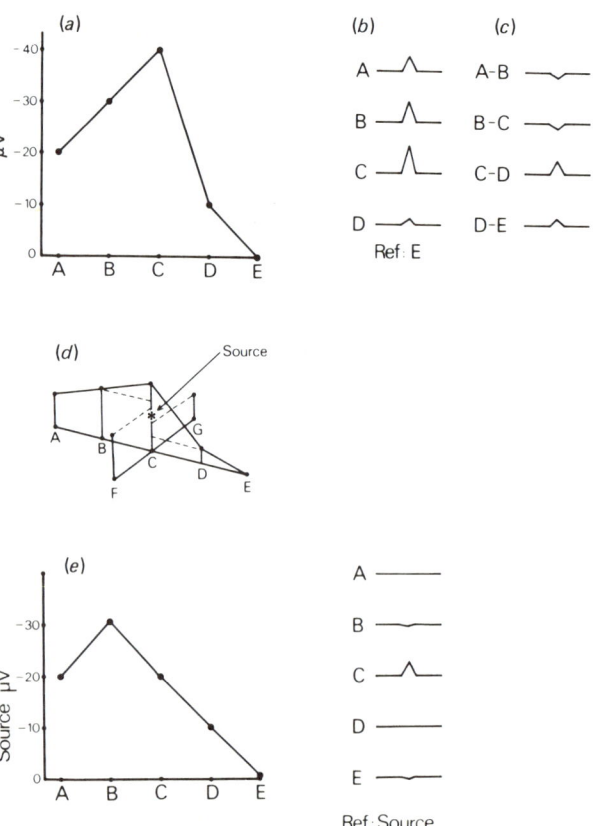

Fig. 4.12.(*a*) Comparison of average reference and source reference derivation. To obtain a similar amplitude tracing a higher sensitivity had to be used for source reference derivation. Note that the alpha activity seen in frontal leads with average reference recording (due to contamination of the reference – see Fig. 4.17) does not occur with source derivation. The right fronto-temporal spikes are marginally more prominent with source derivation (channels 14 and 19) than with common average reference (channels 3 and 8). When the patient becomes drowsy so that the 'frontal alpha activity' disappears (right-hand section) the advantages of one method over the other for displaying the focal abnormality appear minimal.

(*a*)

2 1
7 6 5 4 3
10 9 8
Ref: Ave
TC: 0.3 s
HF: 30 Hz
140 μV
1 s
11 = ECG
13 12
18 17 16 15 14
21 20 19
Ref: Source
TC: 0.3 s
HF: 70 Hz
100 μV
1 s

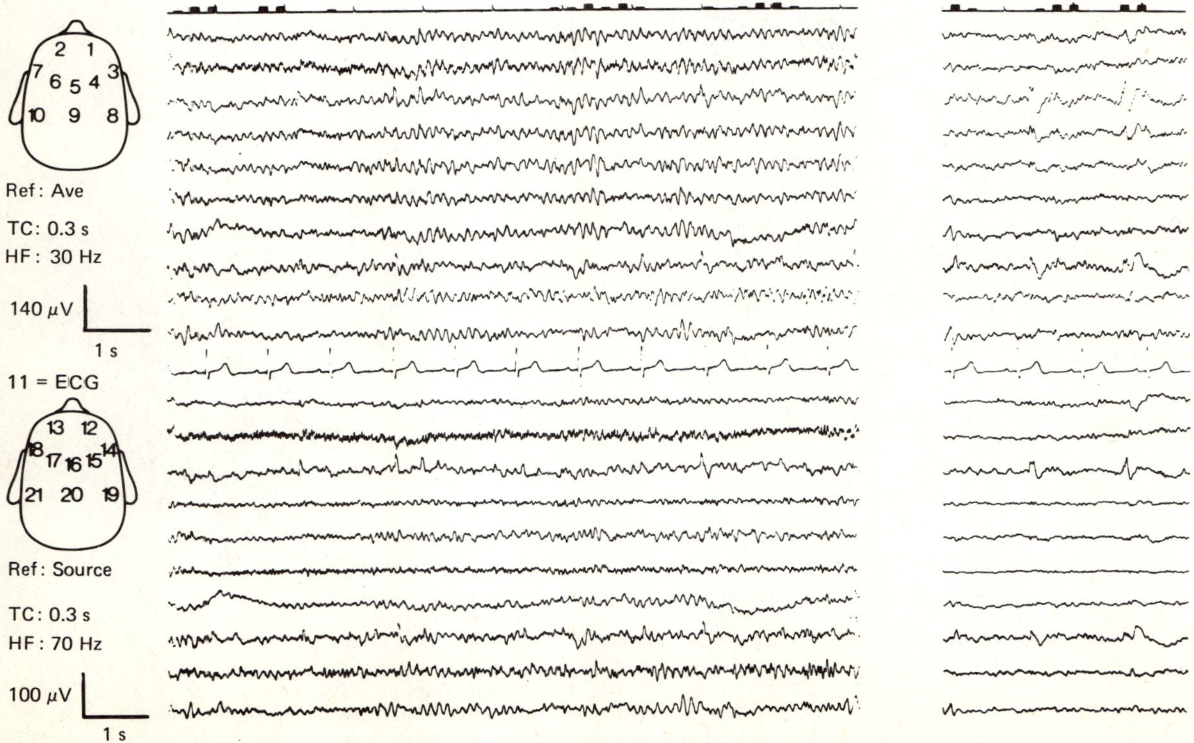

Fig. 4.12. (b) Comparison of average and source derivations. The apparent spread of the focal activity from the right superior frontal to pre- frontal regions (indicated by 'X' in channels 1 and 8) is less marked with source than with common average derivation and in this sense the source method may appear to give sharper localization. Note, however, that the down-going deflections marked '0' in channel 9 are most likely to be an artefact of source reference deri- vation due to the diffi- culty of computing an accurate source refer- ence for electrodes at the periphery of the scalp.

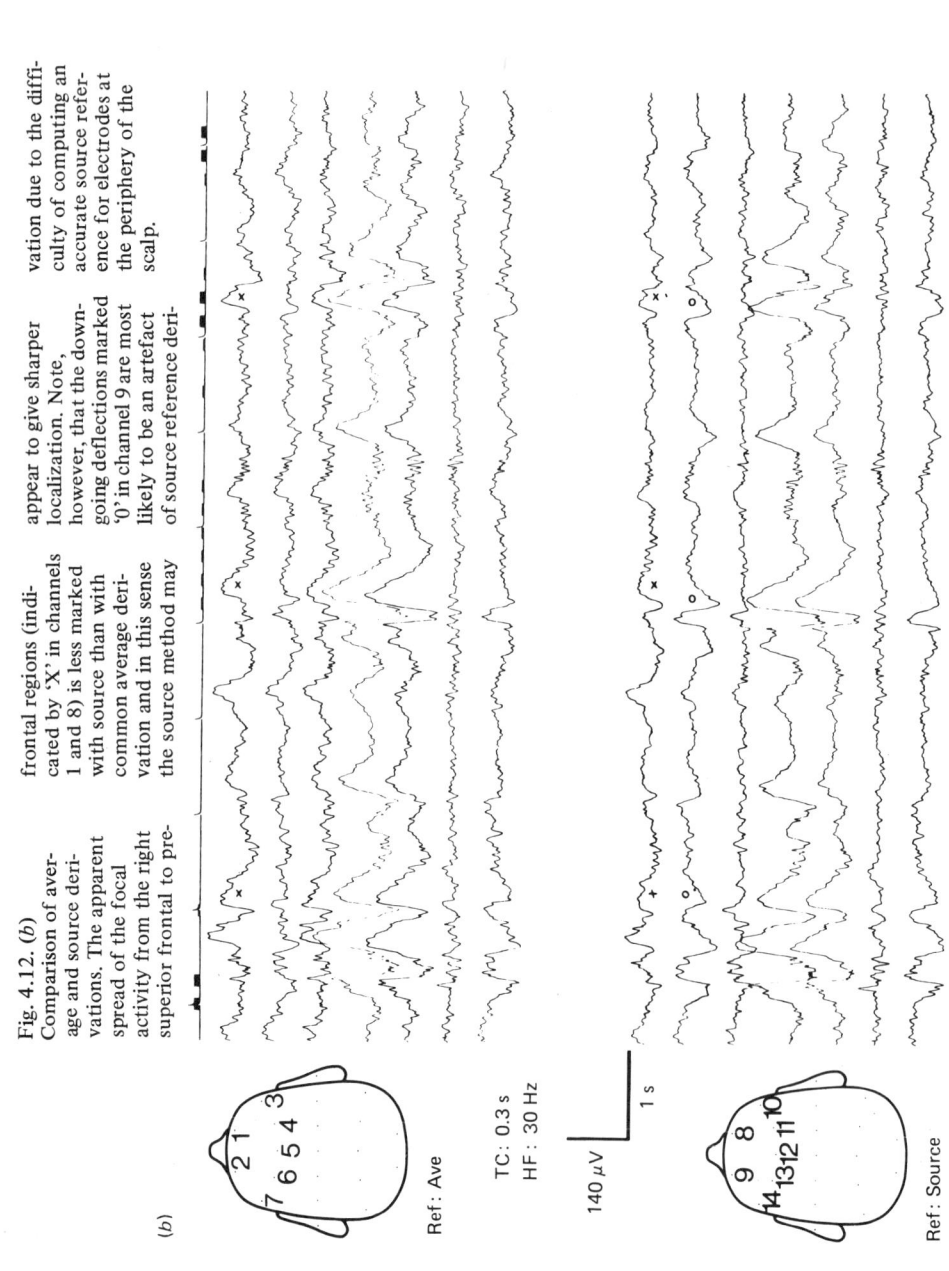

(b)

Ref: Ave

TC: 0.3 s
HF: 30 Hz

140 μV ⌐ 1 s

Ref: Source

bipolar recording are low and with source reference derivation they may be zero. By contrast, derivation to an unaffected reference gives an optimal display, indicating the amplitude, location and extent of the phenomenon. Common average reference is also satisfactory, for in the worst case, where half the electrodes are affected by the activity and the others not at all, the maximum amplitude recorded will be just half of that with an unaffected reference.

Interactions of derivation and topographic extent of an EEG phenomenon can also be considered simply in terms of inter-electrode distance. If the activity in question is diffuse, then the greater the separation of the pair of electrodes on a particular channel the greater also will be the amplitude of the write-out. In other words, there is an inverse relationship between inter-

Fig. 4.13. Sharply localized EEG event showing displays produced with bipolar, reference and average reference derivation.

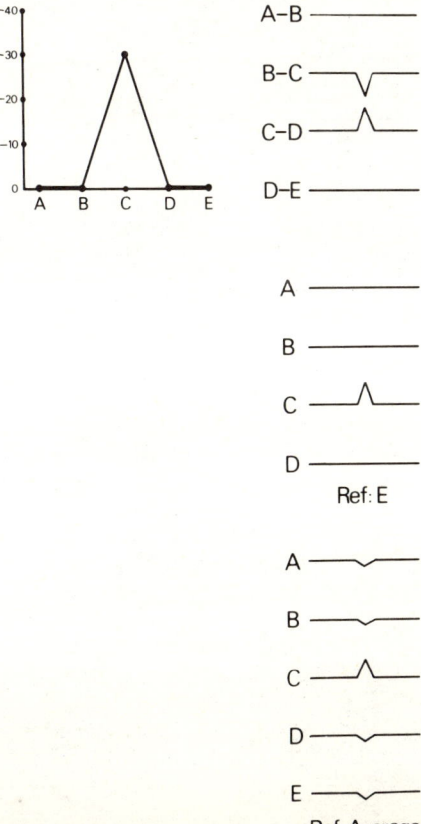

electrode distance and amplitude whether the derivation is bipolar or common reference. Slow components are often more wide-spread than faster background activities (Riehl, 1966); low-frequency activity will therefore be relatively attenuated with short inter-electrode distances, as in conventional bipolar record-ing, but will be more prominent with common reference, or bipolar derivation with large inter-electrode distances.

The question of displaying the topography of localized phenomena may also be considered from the standpoint of detecting regions where an activity is *not* present. This is of great clinical importance, as localized depression of normal activity is the most reliable EEG sign of discrete pathology. An absence of activity confined to one electrode (Fig. 4.15*a*) is virtually undetec-

Fig. 4.14. Diffuse EEG event showing displays produced with bipolar, common reference and average reference deri-vation.

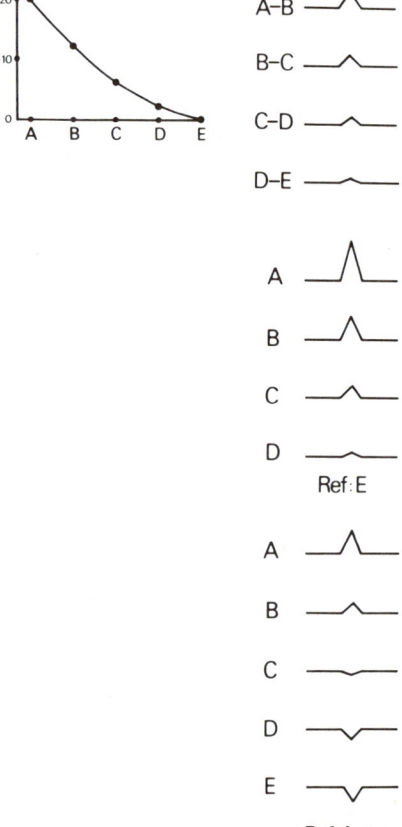

table by bipolar or source reference recording, though it may be suspected from the phase relations of channels displaying the difference between the inactive electrode and its neighbours. By contrast, common reference and average reference methods display it very adequately. When the attenuation extends to two electrodes it is seen on bipolar recording (Fig. 4.15b) but is still demonstrated rather inadequately by source reference derivation. Extrapolating from localized to more widespread absence of activity, one arrives at the condition in which an EEG component is present at half the electrodes on the head and absent at the others. Examples are provided by the alpha rhythm over the posterior half of the scalp, and less commonly, by a huge subdural collection of fluid suppressing all EEG activity on one

Fig. 4.15. Localized reduction of EEG activity. (a) Depression confined to one electrode is clearly displayed in common reference derivation but is likely to escape detection in a bipolar recording. In the event that there is common activity at the adjacent electrodes (D) and (P) phase reversal is produced in the derivations D-J and J-P which may draw attention to the presence of localized abnormality at J. (b) A more extensive area of reduced activity involving at least two electrodes is detectable also on bipolar derivation.

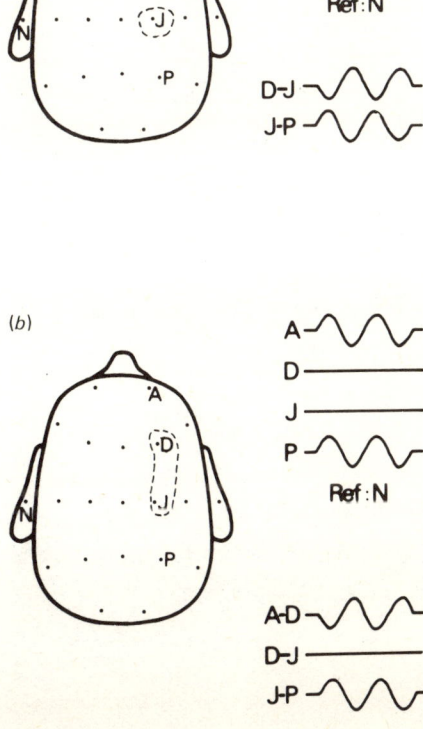

Fig. 4.16. Gross EEG asymmetry. (a) Total depression of EEG activity over the left hemisphere (shaded). (b) Bipolar derivation clearly demonstrates the absence of activity over the left hemisphere. (c) A reference in the electrically silent area also gives an easily interpreted display. (d) A reference in the area of normal activity presents a picture which on superficial examination is misleading and might lead to the impression that there was *right-sided* depression of activity particularly affecting electrodes I, J and P; the phase relations, however, indicate an active reference. (e) Common average reference derivation presents a grossly misleading picture; a clue to the true state of affairs is offered by the marked asymmetries in those regions where the faster activity (electrodes A and B) and the slower components (T and U) are of maximum amplitude; on other channels the phase reversal between the two sides of the head of activity of seemingly symmetrical amplitude is a further suspicious feature.

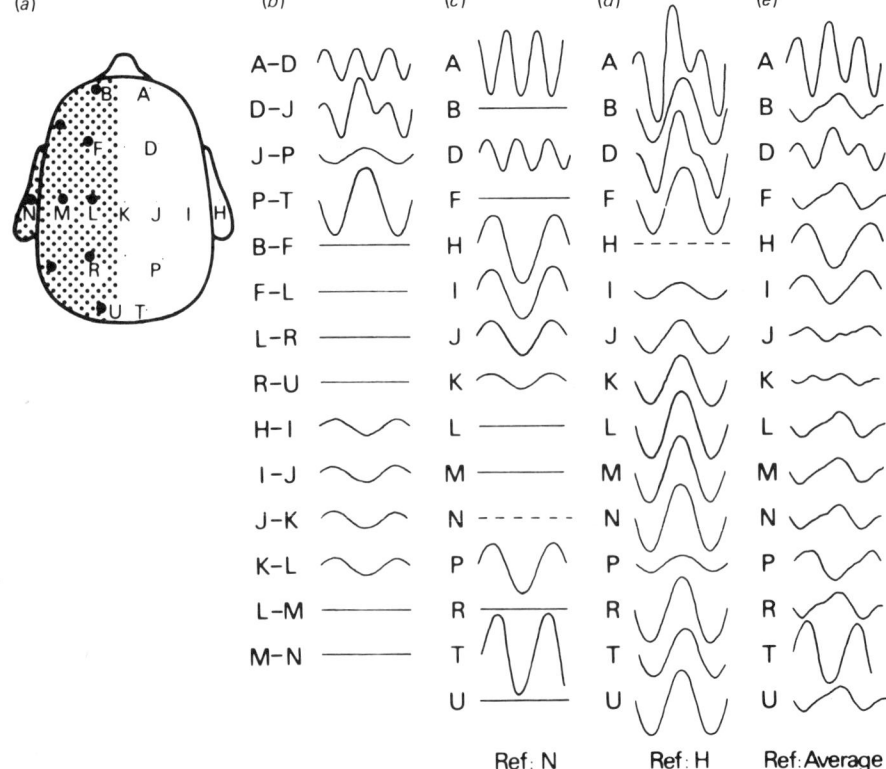

side. Bipolar derivation demonstrates this distribution very well
(Fig. 4.16b) although channels spanning the margins of the
affected region will register signals between the active and inactive
electrodes, leading the inexperienced to suppose the extent of
the phenomenon to be greater than it really is (e.g. Fig. 4.8c).
Source reference displays are satisfactory, as are common reference
(Fig. 4.16c), if the reference electrode is not located over the
active region. With an active reference (Fig. 4.16d), it may appear
that there is a greater EEG amplitude in the unaffected region.
Perhaps the worst case is common average reference (Fig. 4.16e)
which can show activities of equal amplitude and opposite phase
over the active and silent regions. In the case of the alpha rhythm
this effect is well known (Fig. 4.17) and presents no difficulty
(although one would not choose an average reference recording
to persuade a person unfamiliar with EEG that the alpha rhythm
arises at the back of the head). However, a patient with a large
unilateral subdural haematoma may appear to have a fairly
symmetrical EEG on common average reference recording.

Bipolar derivation can be equally misleading in respect to more
local asymmetries. Fig. 4.18a shows an asymmetrical alpha rhythm
recorded with bipolar derivation, apparently of higher amplitude
on the left than the right. From this bipolar display it is impossible
to predict what the pattern would be with an unaffected
reference. The bipolar derivation may correctly indicate that
there is more alpha activity on the left than the right (Fig. 4.18b).
However, the overall amounts of activity on the two sides, as
shown by reference derivation, do not necessarily parallel the
local potential differences shown by the bipolar recording (Fig.
4.18c and d). The apparently higher alpha amplitude on the left
may, for instance, result from attenuation of activity at one electrode, producing steep local potential gradients. If one asks
which of the two pictures is correct, the answer must be that
both are; however, from an interpretive standpoint, a gross
asymmetry in overall activity with respect to a reference electrode is more likely to be of importance than relatively minor
local differences in the gradient between one electrode and
another.

A common feature of paroxysmal discharges is that successive
waves, for instance the spike and the slow component of a spike-
wave complex, may be differently distributed (Fig. 4.19). Bipolar
recording correctly localizes the potential maxima of the spike
and slow wave at electrodes B and C respectively. However, on

some channels the waveform is distorted and scarcely recognizable. Reference methods of derivation, particularly source reference, give a clear representation of both waveform and distribution.

A similar but even more confusing effect is produced by a wave which, though focal at any instant, travels across the scalp reaching successive electrodes sequentially (for instance the tri-

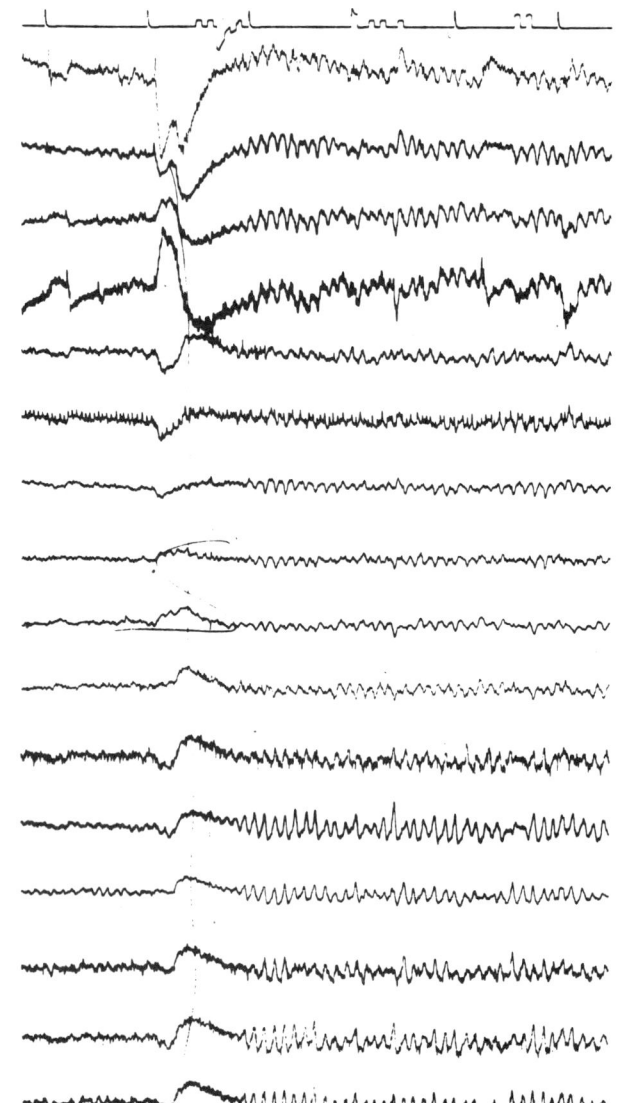

Fig. 4.17. 'Frontal alpha and occipital eye movements' on common average reference derivation. One would not choose this figure to persuade a sceptic that the alpha rhythm arose from the back of the head!

HF : 70 Hz

TC: 0.3 s

140 μV

1 s

phasic waves seen in hepatic coma). Only common reference derivation to an unaffected reference, possibly the chin or ear, indicates the true waveform. All other methods present a misleading picture, but in this respect common average reference recording is marginally the worst (Fig. 4.20).

4.4. Choice of method of derivation

All methods of derivation present essentially the same information. That is, given the results of common reference or common average reference recording, other methods of derivation and alternative montages using the same electrodes can be calculated:

Bipolar:

$V_{ab} = V_{ar} - V_{br} = V_{ao} - V_{bo}$
where V_{ab} is the potential difference between electrodes a and b; V_{ar}, V_{br} are the potential differences between electrodes a, b and the common reference electrode; V_{ao}, V_{bo} are the potential differences between a, b and the common average reference.

Common Average Reference:

$$V_{ao} = V_{ar} - \frac{1}{n}(V_{ar} + V_{br} \dots V_{nr})$$

where n is the number of electrodes averaged.

Fig. 4.18. Ambiguity of bipolar recording. (*a*) Asymmetrical bipolar display reflects only potential differences A-B and C-D. There is an infinite number of possible patterns of activity at these electrodes (with respect to a remote reference) which could produce this picture, for instance: (*b*), (*c*) and (*d*).

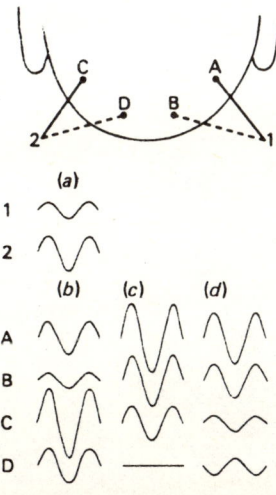

Source Reference:

$$V_{as} = V_{ar} \cdot W - V_{br} \cdot w_b - V_{cr} \cdot w_c \dots V_{nr} \cdot w_n$$

where V_{as} is the potential difference between electrode a and its corresponding source reference; w_b, $w_c \dots w_n$ are weighting factors related to the distance of electrode a from b, c $\dots n$; and $W = w_b + w_c \dots + w_n$.

Note that other derivations cannot reliably be calculated from bipolar recordings, and only with great difficulty (by solving simultaneous equations in n unknowns) from source reference. Skilled observers can predict the appearance of the bipolar derivations from common reference recordings and could indeed extract most of the information they require with this one type of derivation. This is certainly not true of the exclusive use of bipolar derivation. Nevertheless no single method will adequately display and detect every activity, whether focal or generalized, and also demonstrate local depression of activity and background asymmetries. If any dogmatic statement may be made about

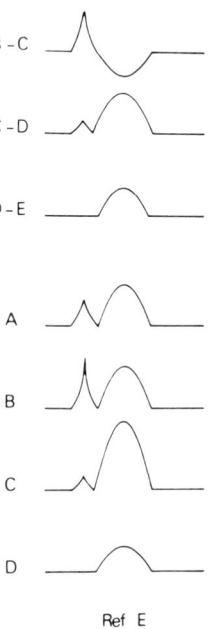

Fig. 4.19. Waveform distortion in bipolar derivation. A stylized spike-wave complex is shown, the spike being of maximal amplitude at B and the slow wave at C. Bipolar derivation correctly indicates the distribution but renders the waveform scarcely recognizable.

derivation it is that those who suppose that any single method is adequate for clinical EEG recording deceive themselves.

For routine purposes it is necessary to use at least two methods of derivation to obtain an overall picture of the EEG, and then to deploy the most appropriate techniques to investigate particular features of interest. One might for instance choose to commence the recording with montages composed of bipolar chains covering the head as widely as possible. If the number of channels is 16 or less, several such montages will be required. On a machine with 16 or more channels, but probably not on a smaller apparatus, it might equally be satisfactory to commence with a common

Fig. 4.20. A travelling wave. Only an inert reference (a) indicates the true waveform of this phenomenon.

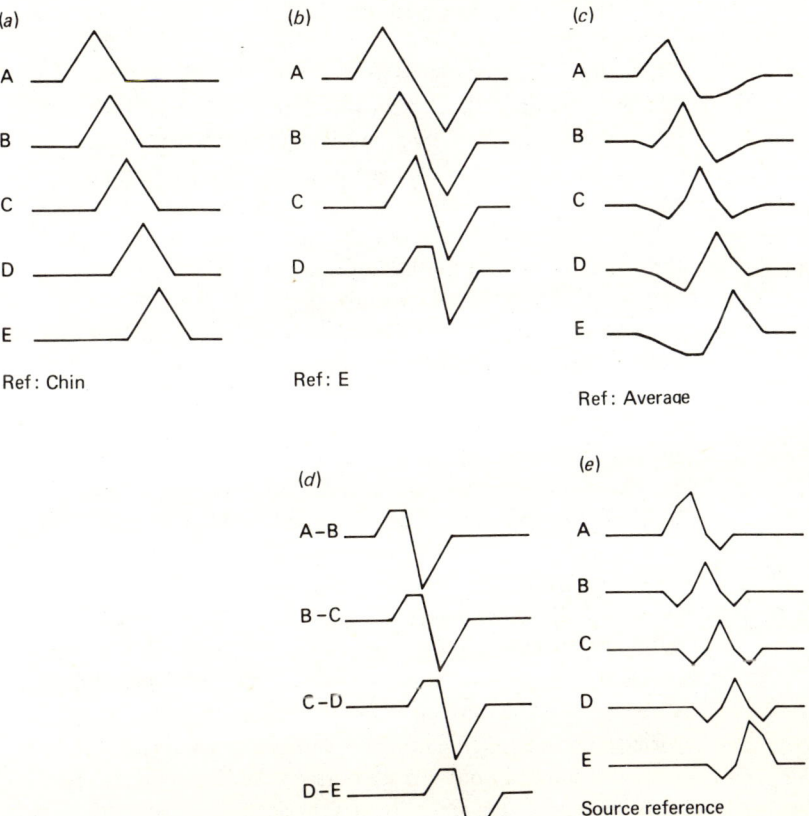

reference or source reference montage, again covering the head as widely as possible. During the investigation all regions of the head should be sampled both with reference and bipolar derivations. Further, because different physiological states, as waking, drowsiness and sleep, give totally different EEG patterns it is also desirable to use both bipolar and common reference derivation under each of these conditions.

4.4.1. Displaying background activity

The overall distribution of prominent background activities will be most obvious on bipolar recording. However, this must always be compared with the results of reference derivation, possibly using a midline reference electrode or common average reference, in order to detect localized attenuation (see previous section) and to detect and interpret asymmetries.

4.4.2. More localized phenomena

As demonstrated in the previous section, localized activities with an extensive potential field are registered at a higher amplitude in common reference or average reference derivations than with bipolar or source reference methods. Where the activity is also of low amplitude, which is often the case, it may be overlooked unless the appropriate method of derivation is used. Six and 14/s positive spikes are a good example: in bipolar derivations these may be suspected from their frequency and waveform and can almost always be detected with common average reference derivation. However an optimal display will be obtained only with derivation to a remote reference, usually the contralateral ear. Low-amplitude temporal sharp waves occurring in early drowsiness in patients with partial epilepsies may also have an extensive electrical field and similar considerations apply.

4.4.3. Localizing foci

Where there is a clearly defined stable focal feature almost any method of derivation will prove adequate to detect it. For precise localization it may be necessary to apply additional electrodes in the region of the disturbance.

Reliable localization by bipolar derivation requires the demonstration of simultaneous phase reversal at an electrode common to two bipolar chains mutually at right angles.

With common reference derivation it is desirable to find a reference point that is both unaffected by the phenomenon and free of other high-amplitude activities which make it difficult to compare the amplitudes of deflection in different channels. Ideally the reference should also be in the midline, otherwise unequal distances between the right- and left-sided electrodes and the reference will introduce apparent asymmetries. There is no site that consistently meets all these requirements. The main possibilities in the midline are the vertex, nose, chin, or possibly midfrontal or midoccipital placements. All of these under particular circumstances record unwanted high-amplitude activity (sleep phenomena at the vertex, eye movements at midfrontal, nose and chin placements, ECG and EMG artefact at nose and chin, and alpha rhythm in the midoccipital region). If the subject is relaxed and making few eye movements, nose or chin references may be excellent. The vertex is also very satisfactory in a waking subject and can also be used in sleep, provided the intepreter is sufficiently experienced to be able to distinguish vertex sharp waves and K-complexes (with their usual polarity inverted, as the vertex is connected to lead II) from other phenomena. A unilateral reference, for instance on the earlobe, may be suitable for demonstrating activity which is confined to the opposite hemisphere. Temporal epileptiform activity in particular is liable to occur bilaterally and may cause confusion as the ear reference picks up activity from the midtemporal region. Further the use of a unilateral reference will display background activity asymmetrically. A reference electrode over the mastoid process is less likely to be affected by temporal epileptiform discharges but is more susceptible to ECG and EMG artefacts. A popular method is to use two earlobe references, referring the right-sided electrodes to the left ear and vice versa. This reduces the likelihood of introducing spurious asymmetries but may cause a genuine asymmetry to be undetectable; it also solves none of the problems of bitemporal spikes or artefacts. It would be wrong to conclude from the above that common reference derivation is of little value. It is a powerful technique provided it is well understood by both the technologist and the electroencephalographer. When used without reflection, it will generally produce unsatisfactory results.

The most convenient routine methods for localizing clearly focal events are common average and source reference derivation, if only because they require least expenditure of thought and effort in selecting an appropriate montage or reference.

Where the focus is less consistent and has a more variable distribution different considerations apply. The appearances in bipolar derivation with multiple foci or a potential maximum of varying location can be extremely difficult to interpret and reference methods are generally preferable. In this application, source reference derivation is excellent, common reference is satisfactory if a suitable unaffected electrode can be found, and common average reference will succeed, provided the number of affected electrodes is not so great as to produce a highly unstable reference point.

For investigating an unstable focus a sometimes useful technique is deliberately to choose a reference at the expected site of the potential maximum (i.e. to attempt to achieve the condition d of Fig. 4.2). If one has been successful, all channels will be deflected in the same direction (Fig. 4.21a). If one has chosen incorrectly or the focus occasionally shifts to another electrode then one or more channels will show deflections out of phase with the others (Fig. 4.21b). This is a powerful technique of localization, which does not appear to be widely recognized nor to have any accepted name except perhaps '*active reference derivation*'. Its strength lies in the fact that it combines the advantages of common reference derivation with the use of phase relations in place of amplitude to achieve localization (which is of course the chief advantage of bipolar derivation, see Section 4.2.3 final paragraph).

If a transient focal event occurs only rarely, the opportunity to select an optimal montage for localization may not arise. The best chance of accurately localizing such events is offered by common reference or source reference derivation, unless one is in the unusual situation of using an EEG machine with so many channels (upwards of 32) that all bipolar linkages of adjacent standard electrodes can be displayed simultaneously.

Finally it should be noted that the choice of derivation may be determined not only by the EEG phenomena which have been found but also by predictions about what may happen. For instance one will not usually choose to use common reference or common average reference recording during hyperventilation, as movement artefacts may affect the reference and make the tracing unreadable. On the other hand, if a patient had an EEG abnormality in the past which was best displayed by reference derivation, and which is no longer present in the resting record one may deliberately choose to use reference recording for hyperventilation. Table 4.1 sets out the recording characteristics and the advantages and weaknesses of each method of derivation. It may also serve to emphasize once again the proposition that the competent technician or electroencephalographer must master and routinely use at least the three traditional methods of derivation.

4.5. Electrode placement

To determine the distribution of electrical activity over the scalp the positions of the electrodes must be known and, to ensure

Fig. 4.21. 'Active reference' derivation. (a) If a localized event is of maximal amplitude at the reference, G, it will produce in-phase deflections on all channels. (b) If the focus is in fact adjacent to the reference, at electrode F, the site of the focus is indicated by one channel deflected in the opposite direction from the others.

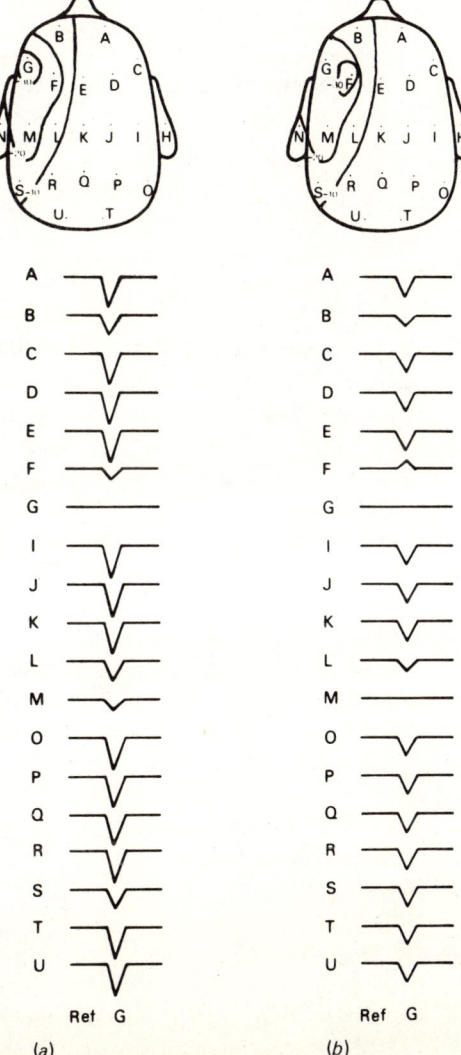

Table 4.1. *Properties of derivation methods*

	Method	
	Bipolar	Common reference
Principle	Displays local potential gradients between adjacent electrodes; localization by 'phase-reversal'	Displays potential difference between each electrode and common reference; localization by amplitude
Recording characteristics		
Discrete foci	Good detection and localization; special montage may be needed	Good detection and localization; may be difficult to select appropriate reference
Diffuse low-amplitude activity	Poor detection	Good detection and localization
General topography of background	Good display, extent of background activities exaggerated, slower components attenuated	Good display
Local reduction of activity	Poor detection	Good detection
Asymmetries	Unreliable, must be checked against a reference derivation	Good display
Waveform	Adequate for discrete stable focus, otherwise poor	Good display
Electrode and lead artefacts	Easily identified and located, affect few channels	Easily identified and located, affect all channels if at reference electrode
Common mode rejection	Good	Fair
Main uses	General display of background activity; locating stable foci	Displaying specific features, background asymmetries, local reduction of amplitude, diffuse activities, travelling waves; accurate display of location and wave form of focal activity

Common average reference	Source reference
Displays potential difference between each electrode and average of entire array; localization by amplitude and phase	Displays potential difference between each electrode and local weighted average; localization by amplitude
Good detection unless background amplitude is high; easy localization in 'routine' montages, false localization possible if too few channels	Good detection and localization, exaggerates focal character; requires at least 16 channels, not applicable to non-standard electrodes
Adequate detection and localization	Poor detection
Fair display, difficult for inexperienced interpreter	Good display, attenuates diffuse components
Fair detection	Poor detection
Good display, unless asymmetry gross – then misleading	Good display
Usually good; bad for widespread activities and 'travelling' waves	Fair to good
May be impossible to locate if number of channels is small; always affect all channels	Fairly easy to locate, affect several channels
Poor – unequal impedances on leads I and II	Fair
As for common reference, less reliable but more convenient for 'routine' use; excellent for preliminary screening of EEG	As for average reference, better display of focal features but less satisfactory than other reference methods for background activity

comparability between the findings in one patient and in another, a system of electrode placement must be employed which ensures so far as possible a constant relationship between the locations of the electrodes and underlying cerebral structures. In 1958 a committee of the International Federation of Societies for EEG and Clinical Neurophysiology (IFSECN) proposed an international system for electrode placement, the so-called '10–20 system' (Jasper, 1958). In a preamble to the report the committee listed the desirable characteristics of an electrode placement system which are set out below together with some additions which reflect widely held opinions:

(1) *'Position of electrodes should be determined by measurement from the standard landmarks on the scalp. Measurements should be proportional to skull size and shape, insofar as possible.'* The need for proportional measurements arises of course from the variability in size and shape of both normal and abnormal skulls. Absolute measurements from fixed bony landmarks would not result in consistent relationships between electrodes and underlying cerebral structures.

(2) *'Adequate coverage of all parts of the head should be provided with standard designated positions even though all would not be used in a given examination.'* It is debatable what precisely constitutes 'adequate coverage'; the 10–20 system itself covers only some three-quarters of the cerebral convexity and there is considerable variation in practice concerning the use of additional basal electrodes (Section 3.4.6).

(3) The electrode placements should be symmetrical about the sagittal plane or, more strictly, they should be symmetrically located with respect to the standard landmarks. Axial symmetry is important to EEG interpretation and asymmetry of the EEG often reflects cerebral abnormality. In fact most heads are asymmetrical: in a series of 20 normal subjects we found a mean difference in right and left antero-posterior circumferences greater than 1 cm and a mean difference of 6.5% in the distance from nasion to the right and left pre-auricular points. We are not aware of any studies relating the topography of the EEG to cerebral asymmetry in normal people but, as it is not possible to ensure equal inter-electrode distances on the two sides of the head, the most reasonable objective is to place right- and left-sided electrodes at homologous locations in relation to underlying brain.

(4) It is held that electrodes should be equally spaced along

antero-posterior and transverse axes of the head in order to ensure equal inter-electrode distances in bipolar chains. As indicated in the preceding paragraph, this ideal cannot usually be attained in transverse lines. Its importance in antero-posterior chains is also debatable; since the activity at the back of the head is different from that of the front, precise comparison of the amplitude in different channels along an antero-posterior chain would not seem very useful. Nevertheless, the general requirement for adequate coverage dictates that the electrodes should be as evenly spaced as possible.

(5) It should be reasonably easy to determine the sites and to apply and retain electrodes. Complex geometrical constructions over the surface of the scalp are almost certain to be inaccurate. Methods of electrode location based on the use of helmets, caps or elasticized bands have been used for research applications but rarely for routine clinical purposes (Rémond and Torres, 1964; Frost, 1973).

(6) *'Designations of positions should be in terms of brain areas (Frontal, Parietal, etc), rather than only in numbers so that communication would become more meaningful to the non-specialist.'*

(7) *'Anatomical studies should be carried out to determine the cortical areas most likely to be found beneath each of the standard electrode positions in the average subject.'* The committee reported that the relationships of the electrodes of the 10–20 system to underlying structures had been established anatomically. However, few such studies have been published concerning either the 10–20 or any other system.

Figure 4.22 is a schematic representation of the 10–20 system, a full description of which will be found in Appendix II. The system has been widely adopted since 1958. A survey of some 400 EEG laboratories in North America and Britain by Mavor *et al*. found a total of 20 different placement systems being used in 1965 but the majority of North American and European EEG departments now use either the 10–20 system or variants of it. Indeed, it could be argued that all users employ modifications of the system, for the original description assumes the unreal state of affairs shown in Fig. 4.22, namely that the four quadrants of the head between the inion, nasion and right and left pre-auricular points are equal in size. In fact not only are the two hemispheres unequal but commonly the ratio of the distances from the pre-auricular point to the nasion and to the inion is different on right and left. Every experienced technician using the 10–20 system recognizes this fact consciously or otherwise and modifies the system to overcome this difficulty. Unfortunately the use of ad hoc local variants negates the claim that the 10–20 system is an international standard which ensures uniformity between different departments. A number of other criticisms may be made. Coverage of the surface of the scalp and particularly of the temporal regions is inadequate and activity of clinical importance may therefore be missed. Wilson and Lloyd (1973) showed that posterior temporal slow activity is of maximal amplitude 2-3 cm below the posterior temporal electrode of the 10–20 system. There are no electrodes closely related to certain

Fig. 4.22. Stylized representation of the 10–20 system of electrode placement. (Reproduced with permission from Jasper, 1958.) Unfortunately, the head is not this shape!

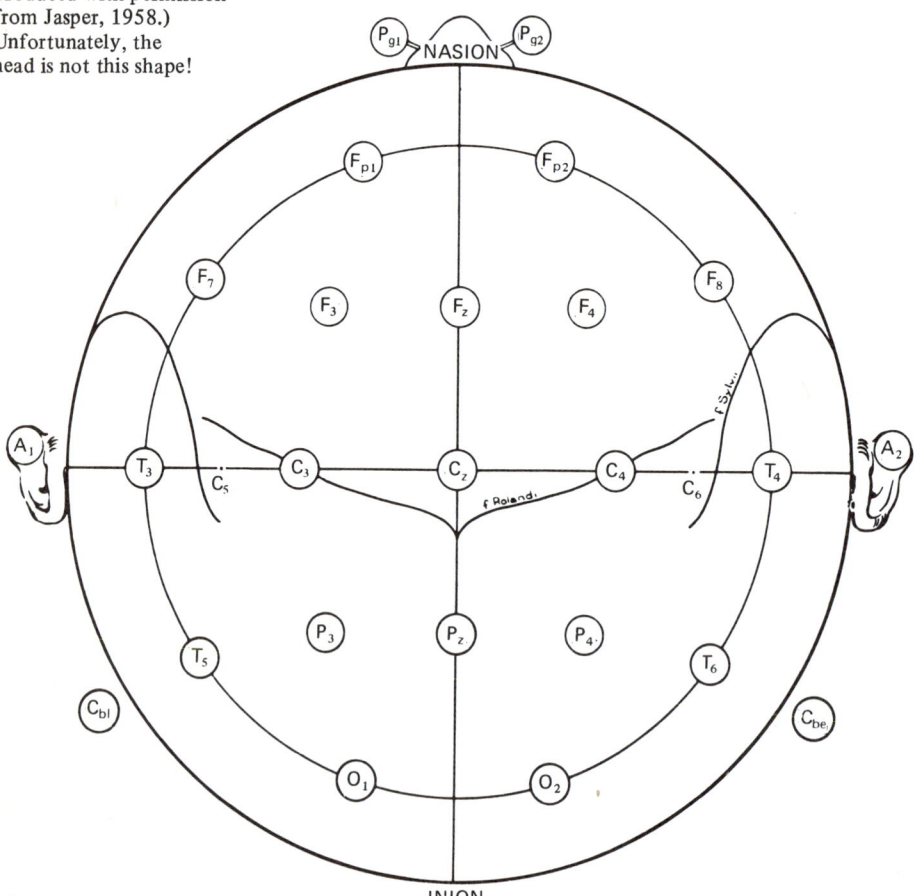

important anatomical sites such as the frontal, occipital and temporal poles. Silverman (1960) described an anterior temporal electrode which registered spikes of anterior or mesial temporal origin more satisfactorily than did the nearest electrodes (F_7 and F_8) of the 10—20 system. To the difficulties associated with pad electrodes (Section 3.4.3) may be added the fact that they do not readily stay in place at locations lower than the standard 10—20 placements.

Mention was made earlier of the fact that the relations of mid-line electrodes to underlying cerebral anatomy are uncertain due to the variable location of the attachment of the falx cerebri. Hess (1966) argued that it was therefore preferable to use no mid-line placements at all and proposed a symmetrical array of six antero-posterior lines without mid-line electrodes.

The introduction of the international 10—20 system was an important advance and has helped both to raise standards and improve communication between departments. However, it is not possible to follow the specification as published without modifications which are carried out on an ad hoc basis by most technicians. There is need for international agreement concerning the modifications required and yet there has been surprisingly little published criticism or discussion of the system in the two decades since it was introduced. Meanwhile, where optimal clinical practice appears to be more important than conformity with an international standard, one may need to consider other systems which provide more adequate coverage of the scalp and adapt better to individual variations in the shape of the head. One such system is described in Appendix II.

4.6. Montages

The combinations of electrodes connected to the channels of the EEG machine together constitute a montage. The design of montages follows from principles which have been set out in the sections on derivation. For instance, bipolar recording requires the use of consecutive chains of electrodes and, if the 10—20 system is used, this will generally result in lines of five electrodes linked to four channels (Fig. 4.23). Except for teaching purposes it is not customary to mix different methods of derivation in one montage except for monitoring variables other than the EEG. For instance a 16-channel bipolar pattern might consist of four chains of four channels (Fig. 4.23). On a 16-channel machine with a 17th reserve channel one might select a common reference

Fig. 4.23. 16-channel
bipolar montage com-
prising paired antero-
posterior parasaggital
and temporal lines.

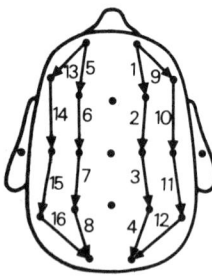

Fig. 4.23. 16-channel
bipolar montage com-
prising paired antero-
posterior parasaggital
and temporal lines.

Fig. 4.24. Common refer-
rence montage with 17th
reserve channel used to
monitor eye move-
ments.

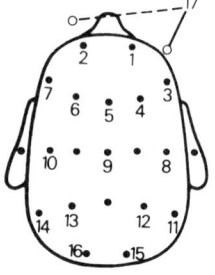

Fig. 4.25. 8-channel
bipolar montage for
investigating frontal
slow activity; channel
6 is used to monitor
the alpha rhythm.

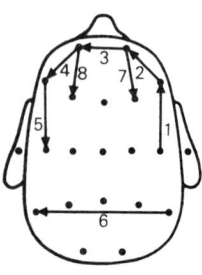

montage on 16 channels and use a transorbital bipolar linkage on
the 17th to monitor eye movement artefacts (Fig. 4.24). Often a
montage will be directed to some specific purpose, for example
obtaining a general view of the EEG, localizing temporal
paroxysmal activity, or monitoring responses to intermittent
photic stimulation. If the number of channels is so restricted that
the detailed examination of the activity of one region of the head
is incompatible with obtaining a general view, it may be important
to use one or two channels for monitoring other areas. For
instance, Fig. 4.25 shows an eight-channel montage intended
for examination of frontal slow activity with one post-central
channel allocated to monitoring the alpha rhythm, as changes in
vigilance have an important effect on certain types of frontal
slow waves. Where the number of recording channels is large, those
used to record physiological variables other than the EEG may
conveniently be employed to split up the montage in order to
enhance legibility (Fig. 4.26). The monitoring of other variables,
notably the ECG, is in any event good practice (see Chapters 8
and 9).

Most electroencephalographers have strong personal convictions
about the design of montages.* Some, for instance, favour
common reference montages in which homologous electrodes on
each side of the head are paired in order to facilitate recognition
of asymmetries (Fig. 4.27a). Others find reference montages based
on transverse or antero-posterior lines of electrodes easier to read
(Fig. 4.27b). Alternating between two bipolar chains so that
pairs of homologous right and left sided channels can more easily
be compared is a widespread practice which has little to commend
it; this renders phase reversals difficult to recognize (see Fig. 4.28)
and generally implies that the user is using bipolar derivation for a
purpose which would be better served by common reference
methods. An unorthodox use of bipolar derivation which may
however be useful is to record between homologous pairs of electrodes on right and left of the head in order to detect asymmetry.
If the activity is symmetrical with respect to both the amplitude
and phase, such a derivation will give a signal of low amplitude
whereas any difference in activity on the two sides will be high-
lighted (Fig. 4.29). Bipolar derivation with widely spaced electrodes (Fig. 4.30) is sometimes advocated on the grounds that the
wide inter-electrode distances give a better display of diffuse
activities. However, common reference methods have the same

*It should be understood that the illustrations of montages in this section
are intended as examples and *not* as recommendations.

advantage and permit much more reliable localization. In general the only useful application of bipolar montages with widely spaced electrodes is to record simultaneously from as many electrodes as possible on a machine with an inadequate number of channels. This may sometimes be appropriate during an activation procedure or in order quickly to check that the electrodes have been adequately applied and are not producing artefacts or interference.

The use of reference recording for various applications has been extensively discussed in previous sections. Note, however, that montage itself may influence the choice of reference. The amplitude of activity recorded is influenced by inter-electrode distance. Thus if a vertex reference is used, for instance, the activity recorded from the central, mid-frontal, and mid-parietal electrodes will appear lower in amplitude than that from the temporal regions. Such a display may be entirely acceptable, provided the implications of inter-electrode distance are understood. For an application where it is not acceptable one may prefer to use a chin or nose reference, for instance, or to refer the electrodes over each hemisphere to the contralateral ear.

Fig. 4.26. 24-channel montage. Note use of three polygraphic channels to separate the EEG channels into conveniently recognizable groups.

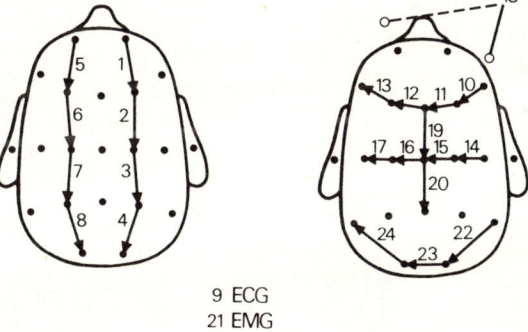

9 ECG
21 EMG

Fig. 4.27. A common reference montage showing two alternative sequences of channels, both having certain advantages.

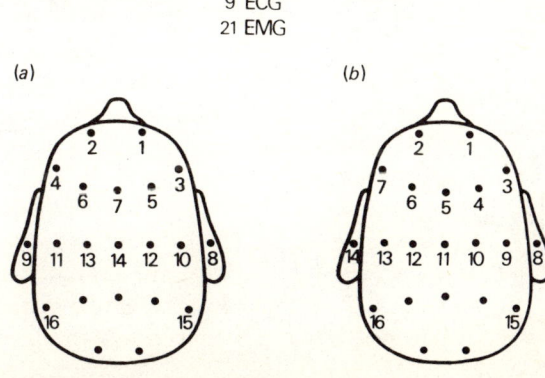

Fig. 4.28. Alternating homologous bipolar derivations. A phase reversal adjacent to a pair of equipotential electrodes (a) becomes separated by three intervening channels when an alternating montage is used (b). In a real EEG where other activities are superimposed upon the localized event the use of montage (b) is likely to cause the phase reversal to be overlooked.

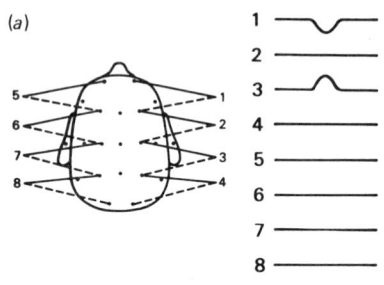

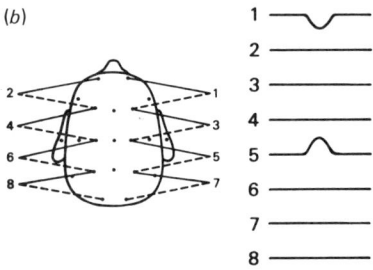

Fig. 4.29. The use of derivations spanning homologous right- and left-sided electrodes. (a) Channel 3 highlights the asymmetry of the spikes which is not apparent in the anteroposterior derivations 1 and 2. An extension of this principle would lead to the montage shown in (b); note that this montage would be virtually useless for any other purpose than that of detecting slight asymmetries.

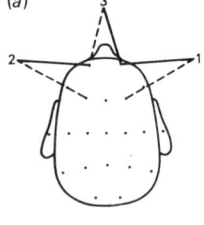

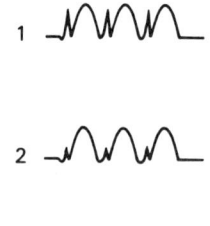

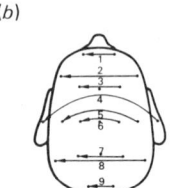

Fig. 4.30. Bipolar mont-
age with wide inter-
electrode distances.

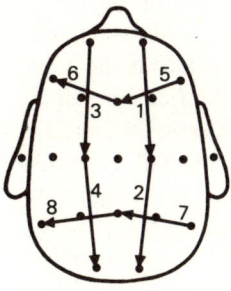

Fig. 4.31. (*a*) A common
reference montage
which is useful for
studying localized
temporal phenomena
but which violates
conventions concerning
the right-left sequence
of channels.
(*b*) Another montage
which may be useful
for recording from naso-
pharyngeal electrodes
but which also violates
the convention of chan-
nel sequence.

The committee on methods of clinical examination in EEG of the IFSECN (Jasper, 1958) also made recommendations concerning the design of montages. They suggested that bipolar recording should always include montages with linked serial pairs in straight antero-posterior and transverse lines. Traces from the right side should take precedence over those from the left and a transverse sequence should read from right to left. Adherence to such a convention makes for greater legibility, particularly if it is also followed when non-standard montages are devised. Obviously flexibility is necessary and for some purposes it may be desirable to use a montage which is symmetrical about the mid-line, even though this violates the convention of a right to left sequence (Fig. 4.31*a*). Similarly, one may sometimes wish to use a montage which incorporates a continuous ring of electrodes, again violating the conventions on right-left and antero-posterior order (Fig. 4.31*b*).

In conclusion, the intelligent use of montages depends upon a good understanding of derivation. Even for the registration of an apparently normal EEG in routine clinical practice it is necessary to use both bipolar and reference methods. On the other hand, if the EEG machine has 16 or more channels no useful purpose is served by the ritual use of a large number of different montages. Complicated and unusual montages intended to highlight particular details in the EEG often render other features unreadable. If 16 or more channels are available it is advisable to use only five or six simple montages routinely (perhaps two common average reference and three bipolar) but always to be ready to select appropriate and if necessary non-standard montages, possibly incorporating additional electrodes, as the situation demands.

(*b*)

(*a*)

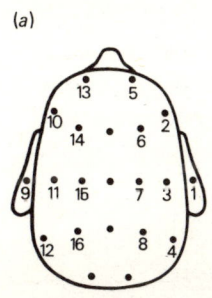

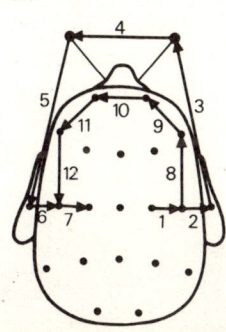

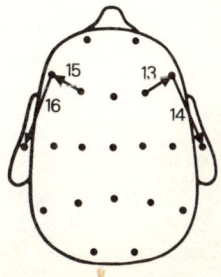

5. Recording systems

5.1. Introduction
The EEG is technically a difficult signal to record. It is of much lower voltage than the ECG with which it is commonly, and wrongly, compared, and indeed sometimes it is necessary to record EEG signals of an amplitude similar to that of the background electrical noise produced by the random movement of electrons. Secondly, it is a slow signal and falls outside the bandwidth of the amplifiers used for audio and radio frequency applications. Until recent years the desirable specification for an EEG machine for routine clinical use could not be met with the available technology. Lately, there have been a number of important innovations in design which will probably render any but the most general remarks about EEG machines rapidly out of date. For some particular research or monitoring applications, single channel EEG recorders with unorthodox forms of display may be required. However, commercial electroencephalographs for routine diagnostic use have 8 to 20 channels (or sometimes more) and a write-out, usually in ink, on a moving paper chart. The maximum available recording sensitivity is generally of the order of 1 μV per mm; that is, when the maximum gain of the system is selected an input signal of 1 μV gives a deflection of 1 mm on the chart.

The general layout of an EEG machine is shown in Fig. 5.1. The basic structure and function of an EEG machine are discussed in this chapter but consideration of the practicalities of its use and the effects of control settings on performance is deferred to Chapter 6.

5.2. Input circuits

5.2.1. Electrode connections
The electrode leads are plugged into a *headbox* which in turn is connected to the EEG machine by a screened multiway input cable. Sockets corresponding to each electrode site are usually labelled and arranged according to the 10–20 system on a panel engraved with a stylized outline of the head. For most routine

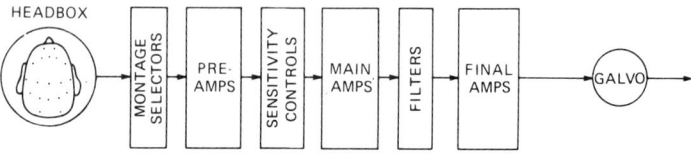

Fig. 5.1. Block diagram of EEG machine.

applications a minimum of 26 microvolt level sockets is a reasonable requirement and there should also be a number of sockets
equipped with switched attenuators for recording higher amplitude signals such as ECG. Some headboxes incorporate other
features such as a meter for testing electrode resistances, pre-
amplifiers (see following sections), and a means of earthing sockets
not being used during the investigation. A headbox may weigh
1 or 2 kg, but miniaturized headboxes are available which may
be attached to the patient, thus permitting additional freedom of
movement during recording. If the cable is detachable from the
EEG machine it allows more flexibility in that a patient may be
fully prepared for an EEG study while the machine itself is still
in use.

Within the EEG machine the electrodes are connected to the
inputs of the amplifiers by means of *selector switches*. In the
most modern recorders these switches are solid state and controlled by a microprocessor, but in traditional machines gold or
silver contacts are used and the switches so designed that the
surfaces slide over one another with a wiping action which helps
to remove any deposits of oxide. Mechanical switching of signals
as small as the EEG often presents difficulties and switch faults
are a recurring problem on machines with conventional mechanical switches. Often these can be reduced by treatment with
special cleaning fluids, subject to the manufacturer's recommendations. The provision of amplifiers in the headbox (see below)
also helps to provide a solution, as the signals to be switched are
then some tens of millivolts. Commonly, the electrode input leads
are AC coupled before the selector switches. This helps to eliminate standing potentials, which would overload the amplifiers when
different electrodes were selected. There may also be an automatic anti-blocking system which short-circuits the inputs to the
pre-amplifiers every time the selector switches are operated. On
all but the simplest machines intended only for emergency recordings, there is a choice between the use of preset montages and
manual selection of patterns of channels and electrodes. Ideally it
should be possible to use a combination of these facilities, that is
to select a preset montage and then change the connections on
some individual channels. On EEG machines with only eight
channels, it is necessary in the course of a routine record to use
many different montages and a minimum of ten preset patterns is
desirable. On a machine with more channels, the value of large
numbers of preset (as opposed to manually selected) montages is

debatable (see Section 4.6). A '*sindex*' switch may be provided to interchange connections to right and left sides of the head as an aid to checking asymmetries and detecting faults in the EEG machine.

The circuitry used to generate the average reference or source references is associated with the input stages of the machine, and indeed the resistors of the AC coupling circuits used to reduce standing potentials on the selector switch contacts may also serve to form the average.

5.2.2. Pre-amplifiers
It may be taken for granted that an amplifier amplifies the signal applied across its two input leads, but in most simple amplifiers only one of these two leads is regarded as active and the other is an indifferent reference point which is connected to earth, to the chassis and to the zero volts line of the power supply. If such

Fig. 5.2. (*a*) Simple or single-ended amplifiers: only one lead of each amplifier is considered active and the other is connected to earth; any signal between the patient and earth will appear across the input of each channel. (*b*) Differential amplifiers: each channel registers the potential difference between two active leads; an interference signal between patient and earth should be of identical phase and amplitude on both active leads and is not therefore amplified.

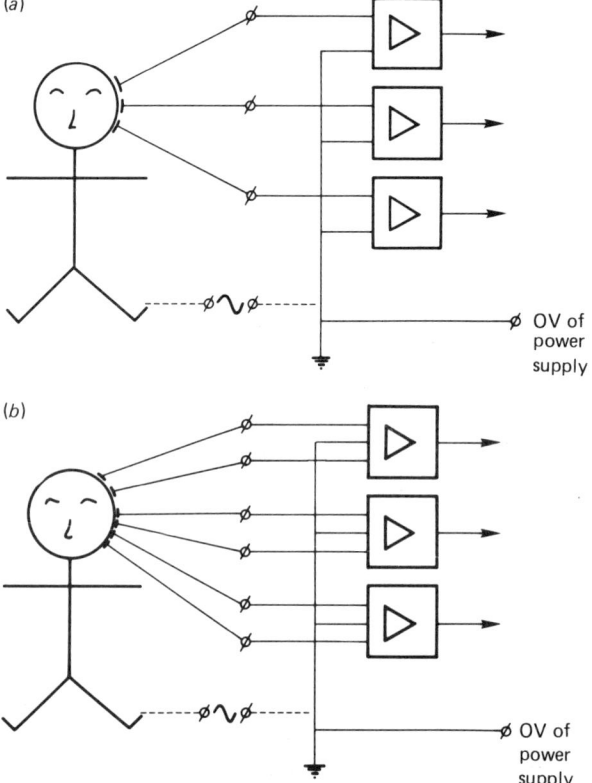

'single-ended' amplifiers were used for a multi-channel system such as an EEG machine, each channel would have to record between one active electrode and a common reference point (see Section 4.2.1.). Moreover such a system would not only record electrical signals arising on the head but also differences in potential between the patient and the EEG machine (Fig. 5.2a). Such potential differences do in fact commonly arise, due to electrical interference from the environment (see Section 8.1.) and are often of much higher voltage than the EEG signals. The solution lies in the use of a *differential amplifier* which registers the signal between two input leads and rejects any potentials which are common to these two leads with respect to earth (Fig. 5.2b). To maintain adequate rejection of these so-called 'common mode' signals on the valve EEG machines of 15 years ago, it was necessary for the technician to understand and to be able to adjust the differential amplifiers. Modern EEG pre-amplifiers consist of integrated circuits on chips which cannot be serviced by the user. An elementary account of the electronic principles of the differential amplifier would therefore serve little practical purpose here, but can be found in some older texts on EEG technology (Walter and Parr, 1963; Margerison, Binnie and Venables, 1967; Margerison, St John-Loe and Binnie, 1967). The effectiveness of discrimination against common mode signals is expressed by the *common mode rejection ratio*. This is the ratio between the magnitude of a common, equal, potential change on both input leads with respect to earth and the magnitude of the potential difference between the input leads with respect to each other, which will produce an identical output from the amplifier. A value of at least 10 000 may be expected of any modern machine, although if a suppressor amplifier is used (Section 5.9.) a ratio as low as 1000 to 1 may be acceptable. To maintain common mode rejection and also to reduce susceptibility to other forms of interference arising at the electrodes themselves, it is necessary that the input impedance (the impedance between the two input leads of each channel) should be high (Section 3.1.).

Paradoxically, there is a current trend in designing EEG machines for the first amplifier stage to consist, not of differential amplifiers located in the machine itself, but of simple amplifiers situated in the headbox or even in the electrodes themselves. It is possible to achieve rejection of common mode interference with such a system, but there is essentially one *single-ended* amplifier associated with each electrode and only within the EEG machine itself, after the selector switches, does one find the traditional arrangement of an array of channels each registering the potential difference between a pair of electrodes. Such systems have a number of advantages.

The outputs of the headbox pre-amplifiers have a lower impedance than the electrodes themselves; therefore there is less liability to interference during transmission via the input cable to the recorder (see Chapter 8). Further, pre-amplification close to the head ensures that the wanted signal will be large relative to any interfering potentials picked up during transmission to the EEG machine. Artefacts from selector switches are also less troublesome. Finally, it is possible after amplification in the headbox to transmit the EEG as optical, radio or infrared signals. This provides isolation of the patient from the recorder in the interests of electrical safety, and may also permit transmission of the EEG to a recorder situated some tens of metres from the patient.

5.3. Main amplifiers

5.3.1. Types of amplifiers

The total gain required in an EEG machine depends upon the sensitivity of the write-out system and different types of galvanometers give a full scale deflection at from 1 to 30 V. However, the primary purpose of amplification is not to increase the voltage but rather to provide sufficient power to drive the write-out

Fig. 5.3. (a) Principle of the chopper amplifier: the EEG signal (above) is 'chopped' into short sections which are alternately phase inverted, producing a signal of higher frequency and narrow bandwidth. (b) Amplitude modulation: the amplitude of a sinusoidal 'carrier' is modulated so that its envelope represents the original EEG waveform.

(a)

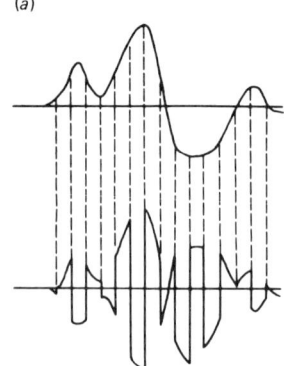

(b)

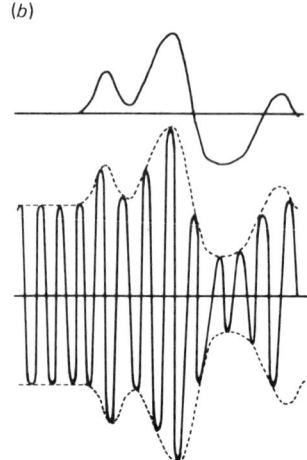

system. The early commercial EEG machines used AC amplification, as successive amplifier stages had to be coupled through
resistance-capacitance networks (Walter and Parr, 1963), which
imposed a lower frequency limit of about 0.5 Hz. Subsequently a
variety of DC recorders appeared. These used 'chopper' or carrier
amplifiers, which translated the low-frequency information in the
EEG (if necessary down to DC) into a signal of a much higher and
constant frequency (Fig. 5.3). This audio frequency signal could
more easily be amplified and the amplifier itself could be tuned
to reject interference at other frequencies. Finally, after amplification the chopped or modulated signal was converted back to
the original EEG waveform to be written out. Nowadays inexpensive high-gain DC amplifiers are readily available as integrated
circuits and the low-frequency response is determined not by
design considerations but by the requirements of the user. DC
recording is little used, however, and presents practical difficulties
due to standing potentials at the electrodes and thermal instability
of the amplifiers.

5.3.2. Gain or sensitivity controls

Each channel ordinarily has at least two gain controls. One is
stepped, generally at intervals of $\sqrt{2}$ to allow a sensitivity to be
selected appropriate to the amplitude of the signals. The second
(*channel equalization control*) is continuously variable and is used
for setting up the sensitivity of each channel to correspond to the
nominal values shown on the stepped gain control. There is
usually a master stepped gain control which allows sensitivity of
all channels to be changed simultaneously. Problems arise from
the interaction between the master and individual stepped controls. One solution is to have no master control but rather a
mechanical arrangement for optionally linking the switches of
individual channels. Another and less convenient arrangement
consists of a master control calibrated in units of sensitivity
(μV/mm) and individual controls calibrated in multiplication
factors (0.5, 1, 2, 4, etc.). To determine the sensitivity of any
channel one multiplies the master gain setting by the factor
selected. Another solution is to provide an illuminated display
which indicates the product of the master and individual settings.
Sensitivity settings from at least 1 μV/mm to 100 μV/mm should
be available and other, lower sensitivities may be required for
polygraphy (see below).

5.3.3. Filters

Fig. 5.4 shows the basic frequency response characteristics of the amplifiers and write-out systems of two EEG machines. It should be noted that the frequency has been plotted on a logarithmic scale and the apparently steep fall-off in high-frequency response in fact occurs over a range of several hundred hertz. The two machines differ in two respects: one (Fig. 5.4a) has DC amplifiers and there is therefore no attenuation of low frequencies, the other (Fig. 5.4b) has a write-out system using jet galvanometers (see Section 5.4.) and responds to much higher frequencies than do other machines. Both characteristics show a peak due to galvanometer resonance (see next section).

Filters are provided to modify the basic frequency characteristic of the machine, limiting sensitivity either to high or low frequencies and thus reducing the amount of certain unwanted

Fig. 5.4. Characteristics of EEG machines. (a) A pen recorder with DC recording facilities: note the peak of sensitivity due to pen resonance at 70 Hz and the rapid decline of sensitivity above 100 Hz.
(b) Machine without DC recording facilities but incorporating jet galvanometer: note the decline in sensitivity at frequencies below 0.2 Hz (determined by the longest time constant setting available) and the marked sensitivity to frequencies up to and beyond 1 kHz. The increase in sensitivity between 200 and 800 Hz is due to galvanometer resonance.

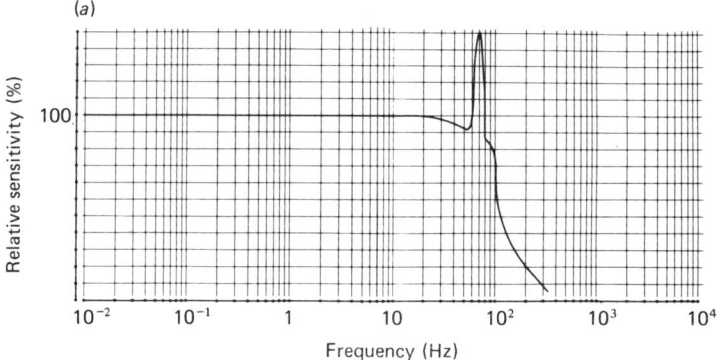

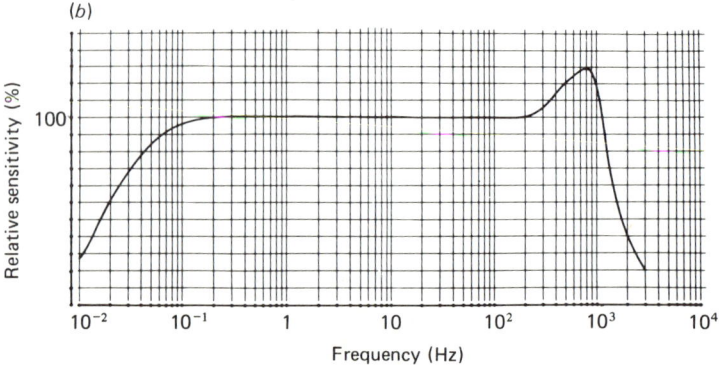

activities in the write-out. The use of filters is discussed in Chapter 6.

High-frequency (low-pass) filters are used in particular to reduce high-frequency electrical noise, mains interference, and muscle artefact. Several different settings are available which are generally specified by the frequency at which the sensitivity is reduced by 3 dB (i.e. to 70.7%). Typical values would be 15 Hz, 30 Hz, 70 Hz and no filter. The effects of these settings on sensitivity and on sine-waves of various frequencies are shown in Fig. 5.5. The filter itself generally consists of a simple capacitance and resistance network (Fig. 5.5c) which gives a very gradual fall-off in sensitivity.* For instance, as the figure indicates, the so-called 15 Hz filter still lets through 15% of a 100 Hz signal. For some applications filters with a much steeper cut-off are desirable, notably to prevent aliasing when an EEG machine is connected to a digital computer (see Section 13.1.). Special 'notch filters' may also be provided to give a very sharp reduction in sensitivity at mains frequency (Fig. 5.5d). It should be noted that the actual frequency characteristic of an EEG machine as measured from the paper chart is determined by a combination of the filter setting and the basic characteristics of the amplifier and write-out system, particularly the latter. For example, if the pens resonate at 70 Hz (see Fig. 5.4) and then show a marked fall-off in sensitivity at higher frequencies, the actual performance may be very different from that suggested by curves such as those in Fig. 5.5a, which show only the characteristics of the filters themselves.

Low-frequency (high-pass) filters by contrast, limit the low-frequency response of the system. As shown in Fig. 5.6 they attenuate low-frequency signals and could also be described by specifying the 3 dB attenuation points. However, their effects are most dramatically seen when a square-wave calibration signal is applied to the machine: this decays exponentially and the time taken to fall to 37% of the initial value is known as the *time constant*. By tradition, low-frequency filters on EEG machines are specified by the time constant values, which are related to the

---

* The relative sensitivity at any frequency is $\dfrac{2}{1 + 2\pi fRC} \times 100\%$ where f is the frequency in Hz, R the resistance in ohms and C the capacitance in farads. For a filter with a -3 dB point at fo Hz, the product RC is $1/2\pi fo$ ohm-farads. From this information the attenuation of any of the filters at a given frequency can be calculated.

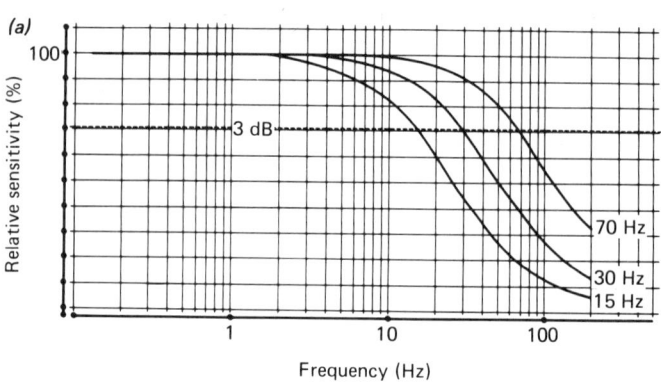

Fig. 5.5. High-frequency (low-pass) filters. (*a*) Characteristic at three typical filter settings, these are specified by the frequencies at which the sensitivity is reduced by 3 dB. (*b*) Response at three different filter settings to sine wave inputs of various frequencies. (*c*) The low-pass filter consists of a simple resistance-capacitance network. (*d*) Characteristic of 50 Hz Notch filter.

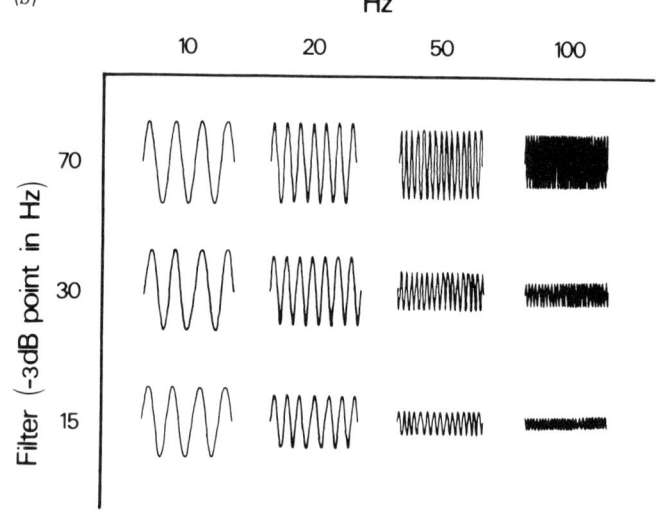

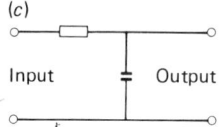

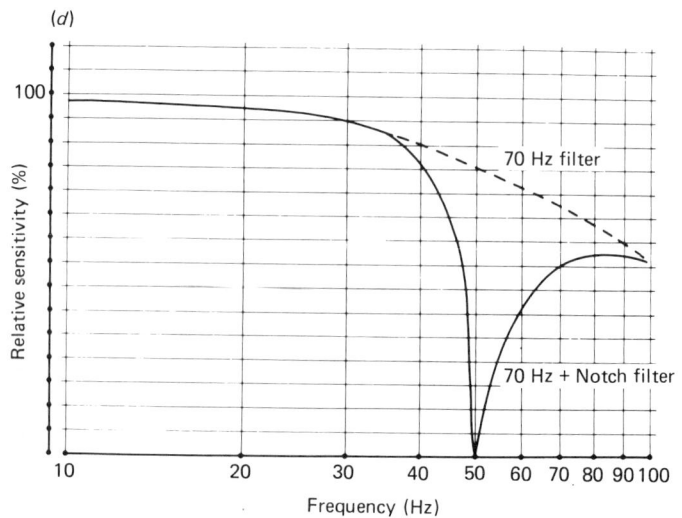

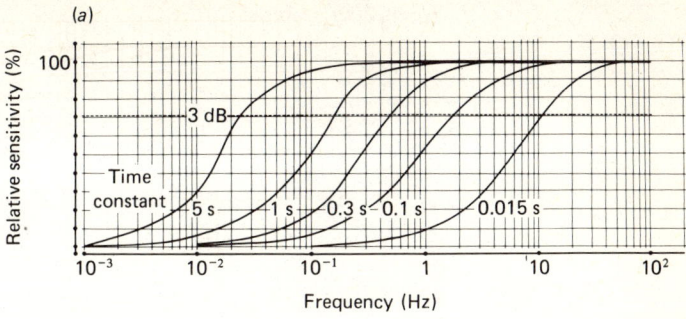

Fig. 5.6. High-pass (low-frequency) filters or time constants. (a) Characteristics at various typical time constants. (b) Responses to various sinusoidal or square wave inputs at different time constant settings. (c) The high-pass filter consists of a simple resistance-capacitance network. (d) The log of the frequency at which 3 dB attenuation occurs is inversely proportional to the log time constant.

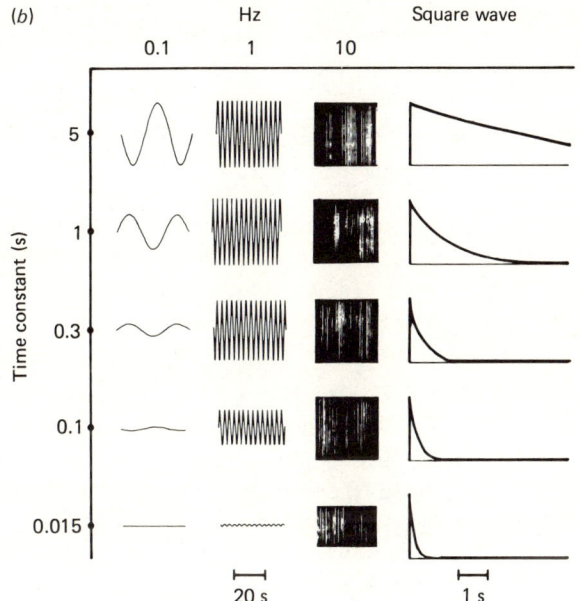

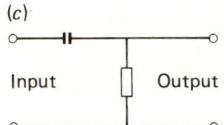

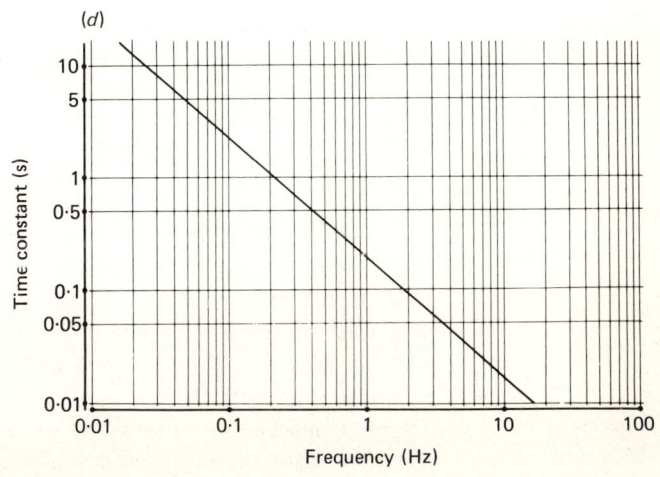

minus 3 dB cut-off frequency by the expression $f = 1/2\pi T$ (where f is the frequency in Hz at which 3 dB attenuation occurs and T is the time constant in seconds). Typical values for time constants would be 5, 1, 0.3, 0.1 and 0.015 s which correspond to cut-off frequencies of 0.03 Hz, 0.16 Hz, 0.53 Hz, 1.6 Hz and 10.6 Hz. Their effects can be illustrated by a family of frequency characteristics (Fig. 5.6a) or by a figure relating cut-off frequency to time constant (Fig. 5.6d). The time constant circuit consists of a simple resistance-capacitance network (Fig. 5.6c), although the actual values exhibited by the machine are also influenced by various resistive and capacitative elements in the headbox, cable and input circuits.

On all but the simplest machines HF and time constants are selectable both by master switches and by independent controls on each channel. In contrast to the sensitivity switches, these controls do not normally interact and the individual filter switches over-ride the master controls.

5.3.4. Outputs

Apart from providing signals used to drive the write-out system, the EEG amplifiers may also have additional outputs for connecting to tape-recorders or computers. These are generally analogue but on some modern machines may be digital (see Section 13.1.). They should if possible conform to certain international standards to ensure that they are suitable for connecting to data acquisition apparatus without the need for pre-processing by amplifiers, attenuators, etc. As the pen-writers themselves differ slightly one from another, when the machine has been correctly calibrated by use of the channel equalization controls, the amplifiers on different channels will have unequal gains. Computer or tape-recorder outputs must therefore have their own continuously variable sensitivity controls which are independent of those used to adjust each amplifier to the corresponding galvanometer (Fig. 5.7).

5.3.5. Other features of amplifiers

After the filter switches, the EEG machine is directly coupled and DC offsets may arise in the amplifiers. The final amplifier stage of each channel is therefore provided with an electrical centering control to correct for DC level (see also Section 6.2.). Sometimes, if the EEG machine is being used to write out signals from a data processing system one may use centering controls deliberately to offset a channel, for instance if the output consists exclusively of pulses all of the same polarity arising from a zero base-line.

Electrical noise is inevitable and arises both from the random thermal movements of electrons and the fact that a constant current is not in fact continuous but is made up of discrete units of charge. Noise covers a wide frequency band but within the usual recording limits of an EEG machine (for instance 0.5–70 Hz) should not exceed 2 μV peak-to-peak. Manufacturers often express noise levels not as peak but as root mean square values, which are substantially lower.

In the older types of EEG machines sudden overload by large signals charges the capacitances linking the different amplifier stages, producing 'blocking' of the system for some seconds. With modern design this is a much less serious problem and additionally the selector switches are often equipped with anti-blocking devices and a manual de-block control may also be provided.

5.4. Write-out systems

Each channel is equipped with a galvanometer or pen-motor. Usually this consists of a coil mounted in the field of a permanent magnet. When a current is passed through the coil, this rotates through an angle determined by the magnitude of the current and the recoil of a spring which tends to restore the galvanometer to its initial position. On some machines, mostly of older design, the coil is stationary and it is the magnet that rotates. Over a certain limited range of excursion the angle of rotation is proportional to the applied current. When the current changes, the galvanometer must move: work must be done to overcome its inertia and bring

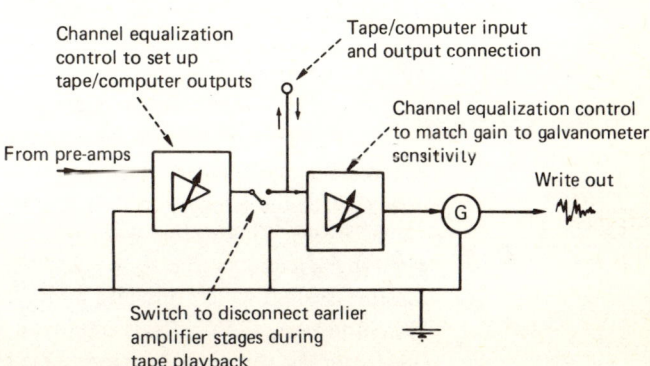

Fig. 5.7. Input/output facilities for connecting the EEG machine to a tape-recorder or computer. Electrical equalization of the channels is independent of the adjustment required to compensate for mechanical differences between galvanometers.

Channel equalization control to set up tape/computer outputs

Tape/computer input and output connection

Channel equalization control to match gain to galvanometer sensitivity

From pre-amps

Write out

Switch to disconnect earlier amplifier stages during tape playback it into motion, and energy must then be dissipated by 'damping' to stop it when it has reached its new position. The more rapidly the signal changes, the faster the galvanometer must move, and the requirements both for power and for damping increase. These factors impose a limit on the frequency response of a write-out system and, at best, the sensitivity of pen-writers declines rapidly above 100 Hz. Moreover the system may show a greatly heightened sensitivity to signals at its resonance frequency (see Fig. 5.4). A partial solution to the problem is provided by a very small moving iron galvanometer which writes with an ink jet in place of a pen. This has very low inertia and readily achieves a high angular acceleration in response to rapidly changing signals with the expenditure of little energy. It also requires little damping to dissipate its angular momentum. Jet galvanometers can be constructed with an almost linear frequency characteristic up to 1000 Hz (Fig. 5.4b). The implications of frequency response and damping of the galvanometer for the overall performance of the system are further considered in Chapter 6.

Fig. 5.8. Arc distortion of pen galvanometer. (a) Amplitude distortion. (b) Distortion in amplitude and time axes. Note that both are determined by the amplitude of deflection.

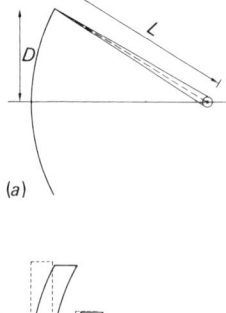

(a)

(b)

As a conventional pen galvanometer rotates about a vertical axis, the tip moves in an arc, distorting the write-out (Fig. 5.8). Though it may be hoped that the angular deflection is proportional to the applied signal, the vertical deflection from the base-line clearly is not. There is an amplitude error of $D^3/6L^2$ (where D is the vertical deflection and L the distance of the writing tip from the axis of rotation. Thus the greater the deflection the more the amplitude falls short of the correct value. In practice pen recorders are not usually capable of a pen deflection greater than 20 mm in either direction, and within this range the response is fairly linear. It can further be improved by modifications of the amplifier. Arc distortion also produces an error along the time axis equal to $D^2/2SL$ (where S is the paper speed). Jet galvanometers move about a horizontal axis and therefore give a rectilinear write-out with no distortion along the time axis. There is, however, a different form of arc distortion; in contrast to the pen-writer, the jet exhibits an increasing sensitivity as the deflection becomes greater. For aerodynamic reasons the stream of ink actually moves more slowly when the angular velocity of the galvanometer increases (Sima, 1966). This causes a distortion which is apparent only when high-frequency signals are displayed at a high paper speed. Another system which provides a rectilinear write-out avoiding distortion along the time axis employs a stylus which presses the chart against a carbon ribbon over a knife edge.

5.5. Paper drive and time marker

The paper must be drawn past the write-out system at constant speed. Usually it is gripped between a roller driven by a servo-controlled motor and an idling capstan which provides counter pressure. Few paper drives are entirely satisfactory; if the driving capstan is narrow the paper may slip, if it is wider or if two wheels are used without differential gearing, the paper may veer from side to side. This is especially likely to occur when the chart is not quite straight, as is often the case if supplies of paper are stored against a wall in a damp environment. A choice of paper speeds is provided and for most routine purposes 30 mm/s is appropriate. To investigate high-frequency components, including suspected mains frequency interference, a speed of 60 mm/s or more may be required. For longer registrations of a fairly conventional nature, for instance waiting for a patient to fall asleep, a paper speed of 15 mm/s may be used and for some applications, such as obtaining a compressed display of an entire night's sleep recording, much lower paper speeds are desirable. Selection of speeds may be achieved electronically or by means of gearing.

As a further check on paper speed an extra galvanometer is provided to write out a pulse on the edge of the chart at intervals of 1 s and possibly smaller pulses at 200 ms intervals. There may be advantages in having time markers running synchronously on both margins of the chart, as this enables one to line up events on different channels even if a faulty paper transport is causing the chart to slew from side to side.

Facilities may also be provided on the time marking channels for recording a pulse to mark various events (signalled by the technician pressing a button) and possibly to write out codes indicating control settings, warning that the sindex switch is in use, etc.

The paper should be visible and accessible for annotation by the technician for some 600 mm after leaving the pens. A receptacle is provided into which the paper falls from the recording table but unfortunately few manufacturers have yet produced a machine on which a continuous Z-folded chart falls tidily back into its natural folds.

5.6. Calibration facilities

All EEG machines have some means of injecting a square-wave signal for test purposes and in some cases other wave forms are also available. Usually the calibration signal is applied at the selector switches of each channel. This may, however, present

difficulties on those machines having headbox amplifiers, as a
signal injected at the selectors will not test the pre-amplifiers.
Moreover, since there is no fixed combination of pre- and main-
amplifiers associated with each channel, even if calibration is
carried out from the electrode sockets, it needs in theory to be
repeated for each new montage. Calibration signals of various
amplitudes should be available, sufficient at least to allow a
deflection of 10 mm to be obtained at any of the settings of the
stepped sensitivity controls. As will be shown in Section 6.2., a
great deal of information about machine performance can be
obtained from the response to the square-wave calibration pulse.
Some manufacturers also provide the means of injecting a calibration signal in series with the EEG when the machine is in use.
This is not suitable for accurate calibration but does give a rough
check on sensitivity which is useful, for instance, if the EEG
appears to be asymmetrical.

Facilities are also provided for testing electrode resistance.
Commonly this is carried out by means of a micro-ammeter and a
DC source of about 1.5 V which can be connected in series with
any pair of electrodes. This has the disadvantage both that it may
cause polarization of the electrodes and that impedance at EEG
frequencies is of greater interest than DC resistance. Some
machines therefore have the means of measuring impedance with
an applied test-signal of 10 Hz, which also avoids polarization.
The result may be displayed on a meter or written out on the
chart as a sine wave with an amplitude proportional to the impedance at the electrode tested. For this purpose the circuit is
generally completed through all the other electrodes on the head,
or a large proportion of them. Alternatively there may be a head
outline with an array of light emitting diodes (l.e.d.'s) which flash
when the corresponding electrode exceeds a preset value of impedance. As high impedances require one to adjust the electrodes
it is helpful for such a display to be provided on the headbox
where it can be seen by the technician when working by the
patient. Some modern machines have facilities for checking electrode resistance whilst the EEG is being recorded.

5.7. Polygraphic facilities

As will be indicated in Chapters 8 and 9 it is often desirable to record a variety of other signals simultaneously with the EEG. Some
of these are of greater amplitude, requiring a lower recording
sensitivity. Others are monitored by means of special transducers

with their own amplifiers. Appropriate inputs for signals of 1 mV to 1 V are therefore required either at the headbox or on the console of the machine itself. Amplifiers for use with polygraphic transducers are often provided by the manufacturer as optional modules which can be built into the mainframe.

5.8. Power supplies

Some of the older machines were extremely sensitive to fluctuations in mains voltage and required special stabilized and filtered power supplies. Modern apparatus is very tolerant of fluctuations in the mains and only exceptionally, perhaps in remote country districts, are special facilities necessary. However in many hospital environments, the earth connections of the sockets outlets may be inadequate and in the case of a portable machine it may be advantageous to have complete independence of local mains supplies by the provision of a rechargeable battery-pack.

5.9. Suppressor amplifiers

It will be shown in Chapter 8 that sensitivity to certain types of electrical interference may be minimized if the body of the patient can be maintained equipotential with the chassis of the EEG machine. Ordinarily this is achieved by connecting him through an 'earth electrode' to an earthing point on the machine. Nevertheless the lowest contact resistance which can consistently be obtained with the EEG electrodes is about 3 kΩ. Some manufacturers have therefore devised a more effective method of reducing the potential difference between the patient and the machine. The potential difference between a sensing electrode on the head and machine earth is applied to the input of a *suppressor amplifier*. This amplifies the signal some 50 times and reverses its polarity. The output is then fed back to the

Fig. 5.9. The suppressor amplifier: the potential difference between a sensing electrode on the patient and earth is amplified, phase inverted and fed back to the subject.

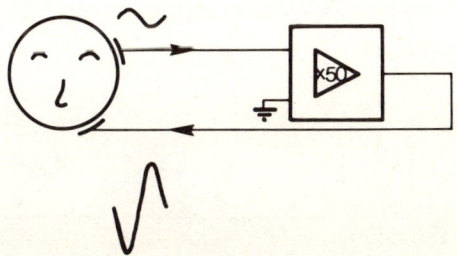

patient through another electrode, thus tending to cancel out
the original potential difference detected between the patient
and the machine (Fig. 5.9). This feed-back system thus helps to
keep the patient equipotential with the EEG machine. Such
systems are generally very effective and reduce the need for a
high common mode rejection ratio.

5.10. Electrical safety

It does not seem to be widely realized (even by engineers if they
have no experience of bio-medical applications) that the safety
requirements for the EEG machines are very much more stringent
than those which apply to domestic or industrial electrical apparatus. The body is normally protected from the effects of external
electrical potentials by the high resistance of the skin (some
hundred $k\Omega$ or more). When a patient is connected to an EEG
machine, steps are deliberately taken to obtain a good contact
between electrodes and the body and the resistance between the
patient and the chassis of the machine may be of the order of
$1 k\Omega$. As the internal resistance of the body is low, it follows that
the current which may be produced by a given applied potential
may be a hundred times greater than under normal circumstances.
A current of only 500 μA passed through the heart is sufficient to
produce ventricular fibrillation in dogs. This is of the same order
as the current which might be expected if a potential difference
of only 1 V was connected across a pair of EEG electrodes care-

Fig. 5.10. Earth-leak
current through patient
from a machine with a
faulty earth connection.

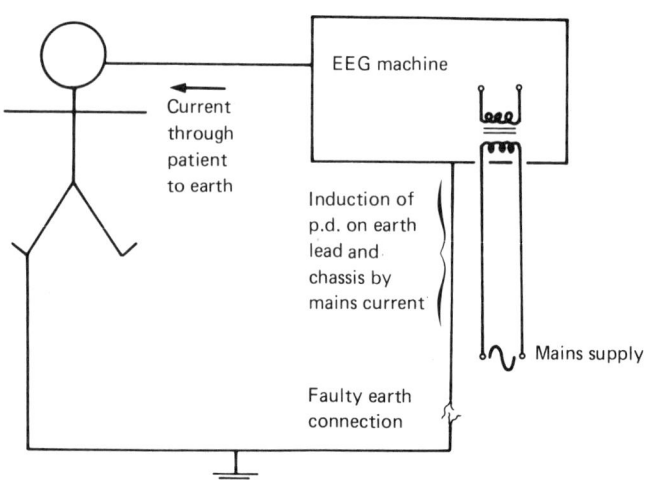

fully applied one on each arm. An important measure in defining standards of electrical safety for bio-medical equipment is the earth-leak current which could pass through the patient's body if the machine's own earth connection was broken (Fig. 5.10). In recent years a maximum earth-leak current of 100 μA has been regarded as acceptable but new international standards are currently in preparation which will undoubtedly be more stringent. Both the earth connections and earth-leak currents of new apparatus should be checked on delivery and re-checked at regular intervals in the course of routine maintenance.

As a general principle, design should ensure that at least two independent faults must exist before a hazard arises. Though the EEG machine may itself conform to accepted safety standards, it may cease to do so when connected to an extra long mains extension lead or to tape-recorders, computers and other apparatus not intended for bio-medical applications. Users of computers in electroencephalography have often been particularly lax in overlooking safety considerations. Though heroic attempts may be made to modify the power supply of a computer in order to meet safety regulations, every addition to the system, a new teleprinter for example, may necessitate fresh remedial action. The wisest policy is to avoid modifications of the EEG machine and to be sure that it is electrically isolated from all other apparatus. This may be achieved by making the necessary connections through 'optical couplers'. A better approach which has been adopted by the manufacturers of some modern machines is to provide isolation between headbox pre-amplifiers and the rest of the system, so that the patient is 'floating' with respect to earth. Even this does not provide absolute safety, as currents can flow between various items of equipment without involving ground and, in any case, the patient may become earthed by touching a grounded bedframe or water-pipe. For specifications of electrical safety the reader should refer to regulations of the appropriate authorities in his own country or of the International Electrotechnical Commission (1973). Useful reviews are provided by: Compes (1977), Miller (1977) and Strong (1973).

Responsibility for patient safety is shared by the manufacturers of equipment, the installer (supplier or local electronics department) and the user.

The *manufacturer* should:

(1) supply a clear manual in the language of the country of operation;

(2) certify compliance with international and national safety regulations;

(3) provide a detailed schedule for testing and installation;

(4) avoid other hazards not foreseen in the regulations. For instance in the last 10 years at least three manufacturers have supplied machines with which it is possible to pass a dangerous current through the patient by plugging the headbox lead into a matching socket intended for a tape-recorder output.

The *installer* should:

(1) check earth, signal connections and earth-leak current;

(2) comply with the manufacturer's instructions;

(3) ensure that connections to non-standard equipment or other modifications do not violate safety regulations;

(4) provide the user with documentation of all modifications and certify completion of safety tests.

The *user* must ensure:

(1) operation by trained personnel;

(2) that no unauthorized modifications are carried out;

(3) routine safety checks by qualified persons;

(4) documentation of all accidents and performance of safety tests before the apparatus is re-used.

6. Recording the EEG

6.1. Preliminaries

A successful EEG recording requires advance preparation. Even the making of an appointment involves informed decisions regarding the date, time, location and apparatus for the investigation. The implications should not need to be spelled out in detail but, by way of example, many departments choose to perform drug-induced sleep recordings after lunch, in the quietest recording suite and on the machine with the most channels. Alternatively, a record after nocturnal sleep deprivation requires similar recording facilities but will ordinarily be arranged for early in the morning. The availability of staff must be taken into account: for example if an unco-operative patient is expected two technicians may need to be allocated; if a patient has established a good relationship with a particular technician further investigations should if possible be carried out by the same person. For drug-induced sleep recordings in out-patients it is necessary to arrange transport and an escort home, and for an EEG after sleep deprivation similar arrangements must be made for the journeys both to and from the department. Time can be saved by sending out-patients a pre-paid postcard to confirm that they will keep the appointment. At the same time printed instructions should be sent giving details of any necessary preparations (washing the hair, fasting, continuing or discontinuing medication), together possibly with a pamphlet explaining in lay terms what the investigation involves. A freshly washed head is not in fact ideal for satisfactory electrode application but is preferable to a scalp encrusted with scurf, which gives high contact resistances. The use of hair oil and particularly of lacquer before the investigation should be discouraged and women should be warned against investing in an expensive coiffure prior to an EEG. Fasting is necessary only before those investigations involving drug administration (see Chapter 7). Existing medication should in all cases be continued unless otherwise instructed by the referring physician, for instance in order to observe the effects of drug withdrawal on the EEG.

Departments differ in the amount of information which they require with the EEG referral. One school of thought claims that EEGs should be recorded and reported 'blind', without reference to the clinical picture, and that interpretation should be left to the referring physician. It is not a view which we share. The recording procedure itself and the sequence of possible further

EEG investigations should be adapted to the clinical problem. Moreover, a descriptive report is an inadequate vehicle for communicating information about an EEG, and the majority of users of EEG services have insufficient knowledge of the subject to make a reliable clinical interpretation of a factual EEG report. It is difficult to find an efficient and acceptable method of obtaining clinical data from the referring physician. An over-detailed request form may not be completed but leaving the user to decide what to write often produces inadequate or irrelevant information. There is no uniformity of practice. Some departments offer a simple multiple choice, for instance 'reason for EEG: episodic phenomena – headache – neurological deficit – other'. Others require the referring clinician to answer a large number of questions, few of which will be applicable to any particular patient. Fig. 6.1 shows an example of a form which has been gradually evolved in several British departments over a period of some 20 years. This usually elicits the necessary information from the inexperienced, and a sophisticated user merely ignores the irrelevant questions and states his problem as concisely as possible.

In general the following information is required:

(1) *Administrative details*, including address and telephone number, hospital record number, and the name of the referring physician, who may need to be contacted for clinical discussion or to receive an urgent report.

(2) *Brief history* with approximate dates. Referring doctors do not always consider the relevance of the timing of historical events to interpretation of the EEG. The EEG findings to be expected in a patient with a life-long hemiparesis are for example very different from those in someone who has only recently suffered an acute hemiparesis.

(3) *Findings on examination*.

(4) Any history of *epileptic seizures* or other significant *disease of the central nervous system* even if these are not the reason for the present referral.

(5) *Age* and the presence of possible *mental subnormality* or *psychiatric disturbance* provide the department with advance warning of a potentially difficult patient.

(6) All current and recent *medication*, not only drugs pre-scribed for the condition under investigation.

(7) *Recent events which may alter the EEG*, for example a carotid angiogram, a head injury or an episode of status

Fig. 6.1. EEG request
form.

DEPARTMENT OF CLINICAL NEUROPHYSIOLOGY

This is a permanent record—Please Complete Legibly   E.E.G. No.............................

SURNAME (Mr./Mrs./Miss ....NAMES..AGE............SEX......

PATIENT'S ADDRESS (If appt. to be sent) ....

....Phone No. ....

HOSPITAL ....WARD/O.P.D. ....HOSPITAL No. ....CONSULTANT ....

PROBLEM: Provisional diagnosis and reason for referral ....

....

....

Main Symptoms (with dates if possible) ....

....

If seizures or other attacks occur, specify: Age of Onset.................................... Frequency...........................

Last Occurence ....Describe Attack ....

....

....

Main Sign...

....

RESULTS OF OTHER INVESTIGATIONS (Including Biochemical)..

....

MEDICATION (Drug Regime to be FULLY Stated) ....

....

PREVIOUS HISTORY (Infantile Convulsions, Head Injuries and Sequelae, Psychiatric Disorders, etc.)..........................

....

....

HAS THE PATIENT RECENTLY HAD: E.C.T., Lumbar Puncture, Anæsthesia, Neuroradiology, or any disturbance of consciousness not
mentioned above? ....

....

FAMILY HISTORY (Epilepsy, Other Neurological, Psychiatric, Systemic, etc.)..

....

REMARKS (E.E.G.s elsewhere, etc.) ....

....NEXT O.P. APPOINTMENT ....

Signature... Date...

epilepticus, or even a recent metabolic disorder such as hyponatraemia.

(8) The above may still not indicate why an EEG has been requested at the present time, and the referring physician should be asked to state the *clinical problem*.

With this information the technician will be able to individualize the EEG investigation to the patient and his problem. It may be useful for the medical and technical staff to discuss each study before it is carried out, for instance at the start of the working day. This provides not only an opportunity for technician-training about clinical matters, but also helps to improve the quality of the individual EEG recording. One can for instance discuss the appropriate procedures to be followed in the light of the clinical referral or past EEG findings, allocate work on the basis of the abilities and interests of individual technicians and arrange for extra help if an unco-operative patient is expected.

6.2. Calibration checks

Although, with improving electronic and mechanical design, EEG machines are becoming increasingly reliable, all are to some extent unstable and their recording characteristics should be regularly checked. Many machines require a warm-up period of at least one hour before reasonable stability is achieved and either they should be kept permanently switched on (subject to the approval of the hospital fire officer) or arrangements should be made for them to be turned on an hour before the first appointment. The following checks should be carried out at the commencement of each working day to be sure that the machine is correctly set up before the arrival of the first patient, and they should be briefly repeated at the beginning and end of every tracing. The detailed procedure and the sequence of tests will depend upon the particular machine.

6.2.1. Adequacy of paper and ink supplies

6.2.2. Zero-setting of meter

This is used for electrode resistance measurement (and also on some older machines for checking power supplies).

6.2.3. Voltage of batteries

These are used only in some very old machines and in certain portable equipment.

6.2.4. Adequacy of inkflow

On some machines the pens readily become blocked overnight and particularly over the course of the weekend, and it is often necessary to clear or replace blocked pens. This problem seems to have become very prevalent in recent years with the increasing use of very fine sapphire-tipped pens, which in other respects give a greatly improved performance.

6.2.5. Trace thickness

Some machines, particularly those using jet galvanometers, have a facility for injecting a low-amplitude high-frequency signal to increase the trace thickness. Opinions differ as to the optimal line thickness for legibility but if adjustable it should be equalized on all channels.

6.2.6. Pen or jet alignment

The pen tips must be correctly aligned at right angles to the direction of movement of the chart. Malalignment may result in misinterpretation of the time relations between channels of high frequency components, notably spikes.

Fig. 6.2. Test for alignment of (a) pens or (b) jets. These tracings were produced by the following procedure: at settings of calibration and sensitivity which will produce a maximal pen deflection, start paper transport, disengage paper drive, depress calibrate button, briefly re-engage drive to advance paper about 1 cm, release calibrate button, again advance paper 1 cm, depress and release calibrate button, re-engage paper drive. Performed this way the test checks not only alignment but also mechanical centering, dynamic range, and possible skewed mounting of jet galvanometers (Section 6.2.7 b and d). Note that in (b) channel 2 is out of alignment and the galvanometer on channel 4 is mounted skew.

(a)

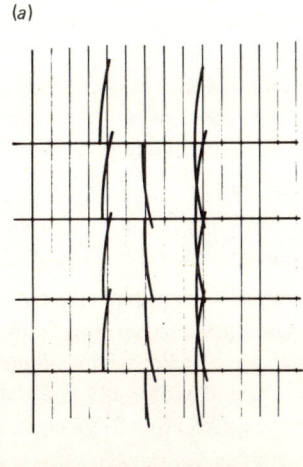

(b)

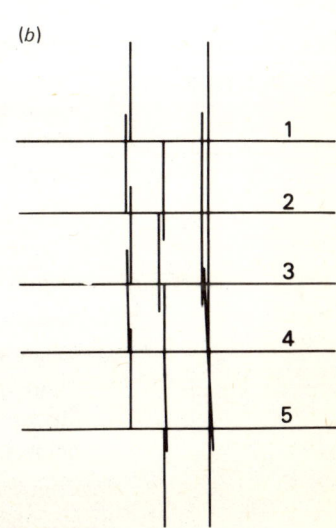

Test: A square-wave test signal is injected on all channels and alignment checked against a ruler or the vertical rulings on the paper (Fig. 6.2).

Adjustment: Pen alignment should be set up to within half a millimetre. On some machines fine adjustment is possible by means of a screw, on others it can be achieved only by bending the pens, a manoeuvre which frequently interferes with either inkflow or damping.

6.2.7. Centering

Each recording channel has a limited range of excursion about its zero-position, and, as the limits of this dynamic range are approached, the amplitude responses may become increasingly non-linear. Moreover, pen-writers are subject to arc-distortion which both alters waveform and displaces the tracing along the time axis. To minimize the distortion of waveform and of time relations and to ensure that large excursions both upwards and downwards can be reproduced, centering must be correctly adjusted:

(*a*) The amplifiers must be electrically centered, that is with zero input signal (e.g. with the machine switched to calibrate), the output from each amplifier should have a value of zero.

Test: Methods of checking vary for different machines but there is usually some means either of disconnecting the galvanometer from the final amplifier or for switching the final amplifier off. If this is not possible, one must turn off the mains switch of the machine, advance the paper a few centimetres by hand to mark the true zero positions of the pens, and then switch on again. Should these manoeuvres produce a sustained displacement of the pen on the paper, the system is not electrically centered (Fig. 6.3).

(*b*) Galvanometers should be mechanically centered so that with zero input signal they adopt the mid-point of their range of maximum excursion.

Test: Galvanometer-centering may be checked by injecting a square-wave calibration signal slightly in excess of the maximum dynamic range of the system. This will produce a distorted flat-topped write-out, and deflections above and below the zero position should be equal (Fig. 6.4).

(*c*) Centering of the pen on the galvanometer-spindle is checked by eye: the pen should lie parallel with the direction of movement of the paper.

Fig. 6.3. Electrical centering. The brief deflections represent the true zero positions of the galvanometers; thus channels 2, 3 and 4 respectively show large, small and minimal errors of centering.

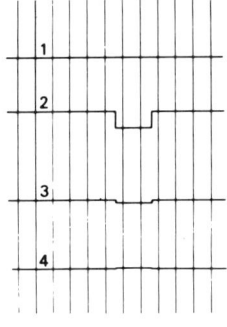

(*d*) Jet galvanometers rotate about a horizontal axis and, if they are mounted skew, their excursion will not be at right angles to the direction of motion of the paper.

Test: Stop the paper drive and inject a square-wave test signal (Fig. 6.2). This test can be combined with that for alignment.

It should be noted that the purpose of adjusting centering is to optimize the performance of the recording channels and not simply to produce traces which are equally spaced on the paper. Indeed if the galvanometers are unevenly mounted, which is often the case, the tracings will not be equally spaced when the system is correctly centered.

Adjustment: On most machines a control is provided to adjust electrical centering. Some manufacturers suppose their apparatus to be so stable that the centering control need be accessible only to a service engineer with a screwdriver; in some cases their confidence is justified, but often it is not! Mechanical centering of galvanometers can rarely be adjusted on modern equipment. An off-centre galvanometer is usually defective and should be replaced. There is often a tightening screw which can be released to allow centering of the pen on its spindle.

Fig. 6.4. Checking range of pen deflection as a test of mechanical centering. If the electrical centering is correct, the galvanometer on channel 4 is probably faulty.

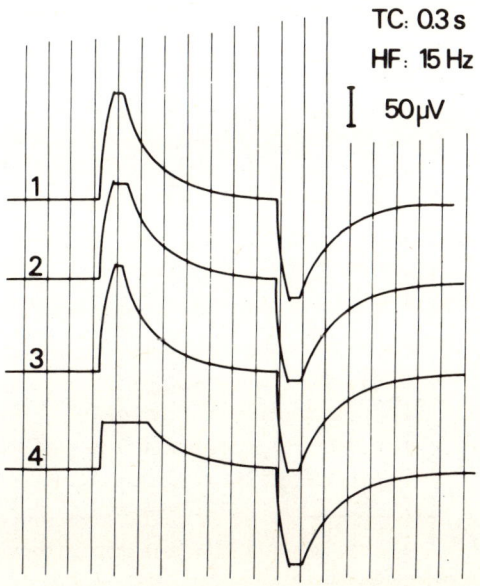

TC: 0.3 s

HF: 15 Hz

I 50 μV

6.2.8. Damping of write-out system

Because of the inertia of the moving parts, galvanometers always introduce some distortion of the signals. For instance when a square-wave is applied they both lag slightly behind the signal on the one hand, and tend to overshoot on the other. Attempts by the designer to improve one of these deficiences will tend to aggravate the other: for instance if overshoot of the pen is reduced by increased 'damping', the acceleration of the system will be reduced and its response to high-frequency signals impaired (Fig. 6.5). On the older types of pen-recorders it is necessary to accept slight underdamping, for instance a 5% overshoot when a square-wave signal is applied, in order to obtain an adequate high-frequency response. However, modern amplifiers incorporate frequency compensation, providing in some cases an almost linear high-frequency response up to 100 Hz without the need for underdamping. Jet galvanometers are underdamped but this is apparent only when very high-frequency signals are applied, for instance a square-wave at a high-frequency filter setting of 700 Hz.

Test: With the high-frequency filter switched out and the paper speed set to at least 30 mm/s, inject a square-wave test signal to give a trace excursion of at least one centimetre. On machines without frequency compensation a 5% overshoot should be produced. On more modern apparatus *critical*

Fig. 6.5. Damping: (1) underdamping, (2) 5% overshoot, probably the optimal condition on the older types of recorders, (3) critical damping (4) overdamping.

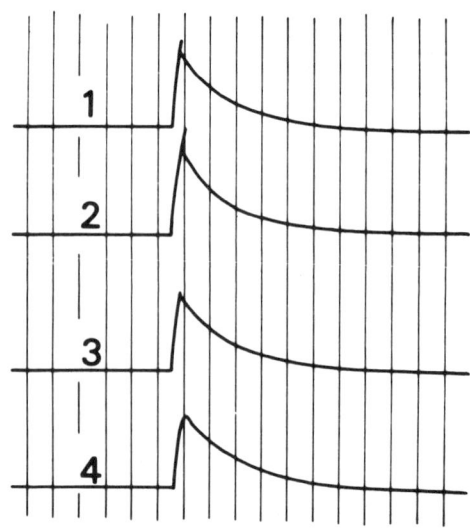

damping (neither overshoot nor undershoot) is desirable. Overdamping is in any event unacceptable. Also apply a train of rapid square-wave pulses of such an amplitude as to produce a trace deflection of about a millimetre. Surprisingly, channels which gave a satisfactory and equal response at higher amplitudes of deflection may show a marked loss of sensitivity to low-amplitude signals, and this will be reflected in a lack of sensitivity to low-amplitude fast activity (Fig. 6.6). If one does not have reason to expect that damping will need to be adjusted, these tests can be combined with checks for sensitivity and linearity (see Sections 6.2.10 and 11 below).

Adjustment: Damping is produced by friction in the galvanometer bearings and between pen tip and paper, and in some cases electrical feed-back within the galvanometer. Only this latter, electrical damping, can be set up accurately. Paper-pen friction can to some extent be adjusted by bending the stylus or by a screw controlling pen pressure. The other components of damping cannot readily be altered. The underdamping of jet galvanometers is not apparent when the signals are limited to the bandwidth normally used for EEG recording and no adjustment is necessary, or indeed possible.

Fig. 6.6. Non-linearity at low amplitudes of deflection. Test signals: (*a*) 200 μV at 100 μV/ cm, (*b*) 100 μV at 100 μV/cm, (*c*) 10 μV at 200 μV/cm. Note that the non-linearity of the second channel was not apparent during calibration at large deflections.

6.2.9. Hysteresis

A failure of the pen to return to its zero position following a deflection may be seen on some machines with moving iron galvanometers and may produce distortion of low-amplitude signals. Gross hysteresis sometimes indicates that the pen is loose on its spindle (Fig. 6.7) or that the amplifier is defective.

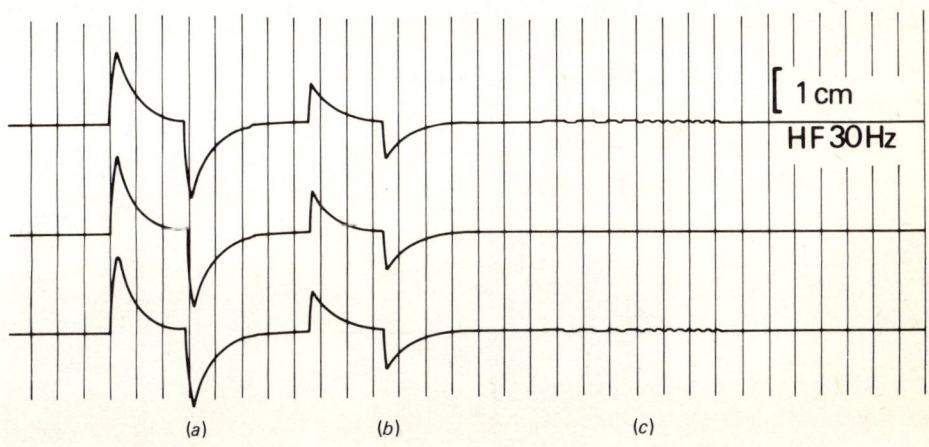

[1 cm

HF 30 Hz

(a)   (b)   (c)

Test: At low or zero chart speed, inject a square-wave test
signal to produce a high-amplitude excursion. The pen should
return to its previous zero position. This test can on many
machines conveniently be combined with those for alignment
and centering.

Adjustment: Unless due to a loose pen, hysteresis cannot be
corrected, but may indicate that the galvanometer needs to be
replaced.

6.2.10. Sensitivity

The trace excursion for a given input amplitude should be
known and equal between channels. There is no agreed convention as to the appropriate sensitivity setting for routine use.
Apart from the fact that one must take into account the amplitude of the EEG being recorded, the choice of setting will
also depend on the dynamic range of the write-out system and
on the spacing between the traces: a sensitivity of 50, 70 or
100 μV/cm is usually appropriate. Unless there is some good
reason for doing otherwise (as in the case of jet galvanometers –
see below), sensitivity should be calibrated at the setting which is
most likely to be used for the recording.

Fig. 6.7. Hysteresis.
Channel 3 clearly fails
to return to zero posi-
tion after a large de-
flection: minimal hy-
steresis is also present
on channel 1 following
the downward deflec-
tion.

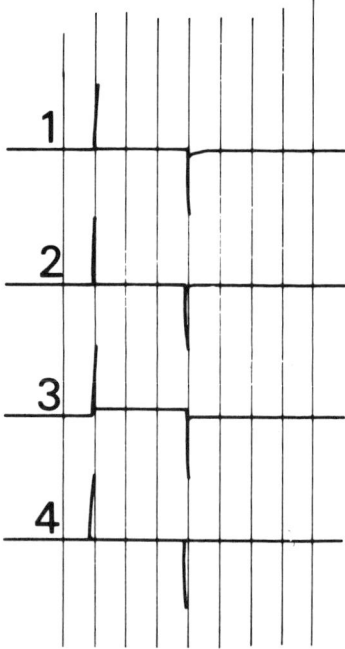

Test: At the sensitivity setting routinely used for recording, in-ject a square-wave test signal of such an amplitude as to pro-duce the largest deflection possible within the linear response range of the write-out system. On many pen recorders this will be 10 or 14 mm (e.g. 100 μV at 70 μV/cm). With jet galvano-meters and the better pen-recorders an excursion of plus or minus 2 cm may be used. Obviously the larger the deflection the more accurately it can be measured. The paper speed should be high enough (30 or 60 mm/s) to allow any over-shoot clearly to be distinguished from the main square-wave excursion. In fact a square-wave is a very unsatisfactory test signal for measuring sensitivity, as it contains high frequency components which are reduced to greater or lesser extent de-pending upon the high frequency response of the recorder. At an HF setting of 70 Hz and a time constant of 0.3 s the ampli-tude of a square-wave is reduced by nearly 10%. If the EEG machine has DC recording facilities, which is rarely the case, when DC is selected the square-wave excursion can reach its true value (Fig. 6.5). Otherwise, until manufacturers of EEG machines routinely provide sine wave calibration signals, the best compromise is to perform a test with HF filters switched out and at a time constant of 0.3 to 1 s. In the case of jet galvanometers, which have an almost linear high-frequency response to 500 Hz or higher, switching out the filters will increase the noise level so markedly that the tracing cannot easily be measured. This problem is overcome by calibrating at a much lower sensitivity setting (e.g. 1 mV calibration signal at 500 μV/cm). Generally the amplitude of the deflec-tion should be checked by means of a pair of dividers set to the expected value. Many machines sometimes produce de-flections which are unequal above and below the baseline. The most satisfactory solution here is to measure the peak-

Fig. 6.8. Use of plastic cursor to measure peak-to-peak amplitude if calibration signals pro-duce deflections which are unequal above and below the base-line.

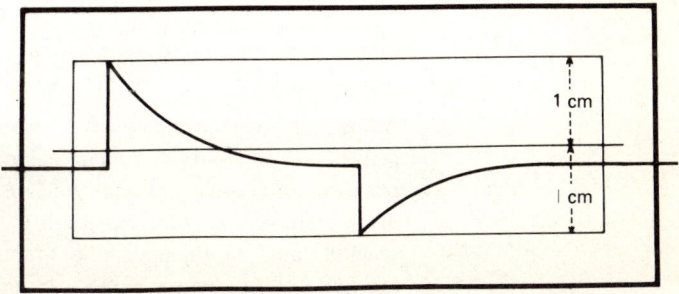

to-peak excursion by means of a cursor specially designed for this purpose (Fig. 6.8).

Adjustment: controls for adjustment and equalization of sensitivities are provided on all channels: sensitivity should be set up to within an accuracy of 5% before every recording.

6.2.11. Linearity

On an ideal EEG machine the output deflection at constant recording sensitivity would be proportional to the amplitude of the input signal. Some recorders achieve this to a very close approximation over virtually the entire range of trace deflection; others show a marked reduction in sensitivity at pen-deflections greater than 10–15 mm.

Test: Linearity may be checked by injecting a series of square-wave pulses of diminishing amplitude whilst the sensitivity is held constant. The largest test signal should give an excursion close to the maximum of which the system is capable, the smallest an excursion of about 1 mm (this last may be used to check damping at low amplitudes of excursion, see Section 6.2.8). The deflections recorded should be proportional to the amplitude of the test signal. Linearity cannot readily be adjusted; a marked deterioration may indicate impending failure of a channel.

6.2.12. Stepped attenuators (gain controls)

After the sensitivity has been set up at a particular value, one should check that correct values are obtained at other settings.

Test: It is worthwhile checking at least those sensitivity-settings which are likely to be used during the forthcoming recording. To be sure that the result of this test is not affected by any non-linearities of the channels (see Section 6.2.11) the testing should be carried out at a constant trace excursion, for instance by injecting a 140 μV signal at 140 μV/cm, 100 μV at 100 μV/cm, 70 μV at 70 μV/cm, etc., thus giving a constant deflection of 1 cm.

Adjustment: The accuracy of the stepped gain controls depends on the stability of a chain of resistors, which may be assumed to be highly reliable, and on the good functioning of the switch. An anomalous result therefore usually reflects a switch fault and the appropriate remedial action is to clean the switch by moving it rapidly to and fro or if necessary (and if recommended by the manufacturer) to apply an aerosol contact cleaner.

6.2.13. Low-pass (HF) filters

The only accurate way to check the high-frequency sensitivity and the functioning of the HF filters is by injecting a test signal with an oscillator and plotting a frequency characteristic. It is worthwhile performing this test on a new machine and possibly as a routine check at monthly intervals, or more often on a machine with electrical frequency compensation which is known to be unstable (not unfortunately a rare situation).

Test: For routine testing it is sufficient to observe the effect of different filter settings on the write-out of a square-wave test signal. With the filter switched out the excursion should show a small overshoot or be critically damped (see Section 6.2.8). Successively lower filter settings should produce a rounding of the waveform which should be similar on all channels (Fig. 6.9).

6.2.14. Time constant (high-pass filters)

Similarly, the only reliable test of the time constant is by plotting the low-frequency end of the frequency characteristic.

Test: For routine testing it is sufficient to observe the decay of a square-wave test signal at different time constant settings, and to confirm that this becomes more rapid at a shorter time constant and is similar on all channels. Attempting to measure

Fig. 6.9. Effects of low-pass filters on response to square-wave calibration signal. Note that the machine in question had galvanometers and final amplifiers of modern design and was critically damped; had there been any under-damping the overshoot would have been much more marked when the filter was off.

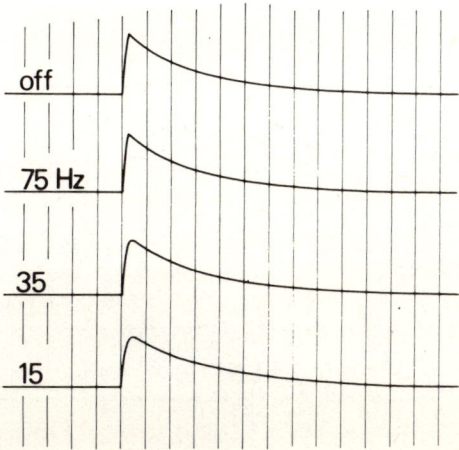

the time constants graphically (Fig. 6.10) may be an instructive exercise but is not accurate. Note, however, that when this is done, the time constants may sometimes appear to be longer than they should be, as the calibration signal is usually applied at the input to the amplifiers but some manufacturers include the capacitance of the headbox and input cable when specifying time constants.

Adjustment: A time constant cannot ordinarily be adjusted. An anomalous, usually very long, value on one channel commonly reflects a switch fault, not necessarily in the time constant control.

6.2.15. Noise

The noise level at an HF setting of about 70 Hz should not exceed 2 μV.

Test: Select the maximum sensitivity and the HF setting closest to 70 Hz and calculate the amplitude of the noise written out. Note that if the HF filters are completely

Fig. 6.10. (*a*) Graphical measurement of time constant. Knowing the paper speed one can calculate from the distance (*d*) the time taken for the calibration signal to decline to 37% of its peak value. (*b*) Effects of different time constant settings on the decay of a square-wave calibration signal. Clearly it would be impossible to check the time constants graphically with any accuracy unless each measurement was performed at such a paper speed as to give a waveform like that on channel 3.

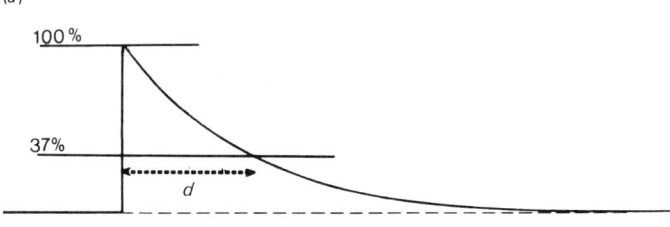

(*a*)

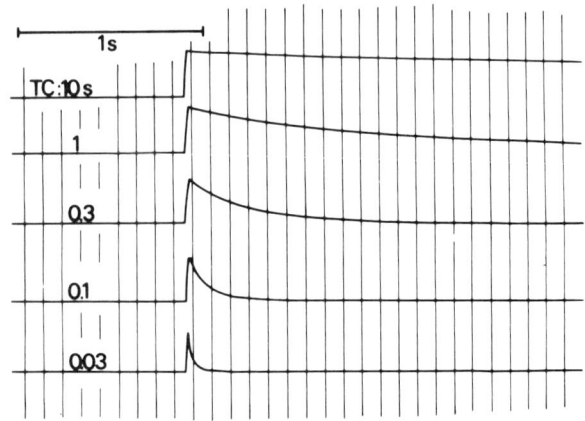

(*b*)

switched out, machines with jet galvanometers, which give a very good high-frequency response, will exhibit a noise level considerably above 2 μV.

Adjustment: Noise levels cannot readily be adjusted but an abnormally high value commonly indicates impending amplifier failure.

6.2.16. Time marker and paper speed

A design fault of some older EEG machines was to derive the time marker from the motor which powered the paper drive. Consequently if the paper speed was incorrect, the marker pulses still appeared at the right spacing on the chart, so the defect easily escaped notice. On modern machines, the time marker is driven by an independent oscillator, so the problem no longer arises. A more common and more important fault than a slight error in the speed of the paper drive is fluctuation in paper speed, generally due to a slipping capstan, but sometimes due to the underside of the paper sticking to inky rollers. This 'judder' has the effect of producing spiky wave forms every time the paper slows up, and, if not recognized, can lead to misinterpretation.

Test: either time marker or paper speed can be checked over a period of 30 s or 1 min with the help of a stop-watch. However, a more convenient test may be deliberately to induce 50 Hz mains interference, for instance by switching a channel to open circuit. The length of chart occupied by 50 cycles of the signal corresponds of course to 1 second. This information can be used to establish the reliability of the time marker which can in turn be used to check the lower paper speed settings at which the 50 Hz signal becomes unreadable. Paper judder is easily demonstrable by the same test, as it produces transverse striations on the chart, due to alternate bunching and spreading of the waves (Fig. 6.11).

Adjustment: paper judder can sometimes be cured by cleaning capstans, rollers or paper guide plates which have become soiled with ink. Correction of the paper speed or time marker requires the help of a service engineer.

6.2.17. Testing unorthodox machines

The above tests are applicable to most conventional machines. However, some recent models have features which may demand different procedures. One important development is the introduction of machines with pre-amplifiers in the headbox for each electrode socket. With apparently one exception, these machines have an internal calibration signal which is injected only into the main amplifiers, and it is therefore impossible without additional test equipment to check the pre-amplifiers. However, if one does apply the calibration signal at the electrode sockets, the write-out on each channel is determined by the combination of the main amplifier on that channel and two pre-amplifiers. When the montage is changed, different electrodes, and hence different pre-amplifiers, will be connected to each channel and different gains may result. The problem may be more theoretical than practical, for headbox pre-amplifiers are generally very reliable and stable. If a machine with headbox amplifiers is used for an application in which accurate calibration is essential (for instance involving data processing), the entire system should be tested with signals injected at the headbox and with the montage to be employed for the subsequent recording. One manufacturer provides a facility for injecting a test signal into each channel before the pre-amplifiers during recording. Alternatively, the pre-amplifiers can be checked by applying a signal of several millivolts between the patient and the EEG machine (on a recorder with a suppressor amplifier this can easily be achieved by a modification of the suppressor circuit). This signal will be rejected by the differential amplifiers (as it is in common mode) and, provided that the gains of the pre-amplifiers on each channel are equal, it will not appear in the tracing.

A newer development is the replacement of conventional switches by solid-state electronics controlled by a micro-computer. This should eliminate the problems of switch faults but may create new requirements, for instance, for testing of the microprocessor itself.

Fig. 6.11. Paper judder. (a) Transverse striations appear on the write-out of a 50 Hz sine wave if the paper speed varies. (b) Judder may be suspected from close inspection of the time marker channel but produces spiky waveforms in the EEG which could readily be misinterpreted.

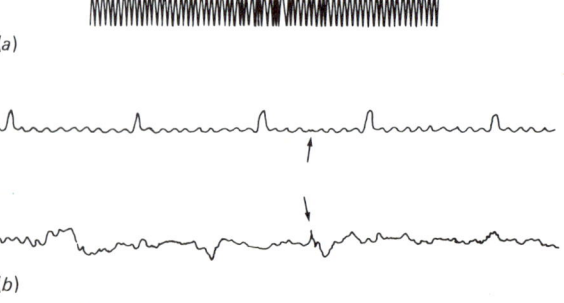

6.2.18. Routine calibration

All the above tests should be carried out daily before the arrival of the first patient. The tests should be repeated before and after every tracing and a permanent paper record of the results kept and stored with the EEG. Sensitivity should be measured and if necessary, set up, to within 5% accuracy, and the other functions at least checked by eye. Depending upon the machine in use, an optimum sequence can be devised so that one test leaves the controls set up for the following item in the sequence, thus minimizing switching operations (see Appendix III). For instance, at the end of the check on stepped attenuators the sensitivity setting is maximum and this is a convenient moment to check the noise level. Though we have often heard a contrary opinion from experienced technicians who have not worked out how to perform the procedure efficiently, the entire battery of tests described above can be performed on most EEG machines within 40–60s, excluding the time taken for measuring the results. Detailed calibration not only helps to optimize the machine performance but, no less importantly, provides a permanent record of the state of the apparatus which guides the assessment of apparent abnormalities in the EEG. It also provides valuable documentation for the service engineer required to investigate an intermittent fault. Failure to devote 1 minute at the beginning and end of a half-hour recording to calibration is merely slovenly practice for which there can be no excuse. In Appendix IV some more complex tests are suggested which may usefully be performed when a new machine is delivered, and repeated at intervals of 1 to 6 months.

6.3. The clinical recording

6.3.1. Reception of the patient

If the preparations as described above have been carried out before the patient arrives in the department, the technician concerned will have established that the apparatus to be used is in working order, will be acquainted with the clinical problem and any previous EEG findings, and will have some idea of the recording procedure which is likely to be appropriate. It is easy to forget that an investigation which is a daily routine for the technician is an important and unnerving event for some patients. Many laymen have little idea of what an EEG involves except that it has something to do with electricity and the brain, and approach it with more apprehension than say a chest X-ray. The co-operation of the subject is necessary to obtain a satisfactory tracing, and the technician must endeavour to gain the patient's confidence and establish a rapport within the short time available. Apart from the normal courtesy and kindness which are mandatory it is also important to display professional competence. The first impression is more likely to be favourable if the technician is evidently aware of the circumstances leading to referral and explains the test and why it is being done.

All stages of the procedure, from application to removal of electrodes, should be carried out by the same technician, preferably working alone. In the case of the physically or mentally handicapped or psychiatrically disturbed patients, the help of a colleague or nurse may be essential. In dealing with small children the presence of a parent is often helpful but can be a considerable hindrance. If a parent seems over-eager to accompany the child to the recording suite, this may generally be taken as a warning that she is worried and likely to make the child anxious too. For recording from unconscious patients the help of a nurse familiar with EEG practice is invaluable, and the permanent staff of any department dealing with large numbers of unconscious patients should include a trained nurse. When recording an EEG outside working hours it is also advisable to have assistance at hand and, for his own protection, a male technician should insist on a chaperon when working with a psychiatrically disturbed female patient.

6.3.2. Preparations for the recording

Electrode application should where possible be carried out with the patient seated in the middle of a well-lit room on an upright chair. This may be done in the recording suite but more effective use can be made of machine time if a separate electrode application area is available. If the patient is unconscious or unable to sit up, the electrodes may be applied after he has been moved to the recording couch. The measurement of the head and application of electrodes provide the opportunity for conversation with the patient, partly to put him at ease, but also to elicit information to supplement that on the request form. Experienced technicians are proficient at eliciting historical data concerning the limited range of problems commonly seen in an EEG department. In the course of the investigation the patient is encouraged to relax and may volunteer important information not mentioned during a hurried out-patient interview.

Children are often frightened of electrode application particularly if compressed air is used to dry the collodion on disc electrodes. To give reassurance one may first demonstrate the procedure on the head of a doll, on the back of one's own hand or on the hand of the patient. Abrasion of the skin and application of electrode jelly are disagreeable if not actually painful. If the child has been co-operative up to this point, he should be warned before the jelly is applied; children are more tolerant of discomfort than of betrayal of their trust.

Any useful information elicited should be added to the request form and in addition the following particulars should be written on the EEG chart prior to the recording.

(1) Name and age: these must be entered without fail. It is all too easy to mix up EEGs in a busy department.

(2) Present drug regimen: often this will differ from the information provided on the request form, either because the patient is not following medical advice or because he is receiving additional medication unknown to the referring physician.

(3) Recent events which may affect the EEG and which may have occurred since the request form was completed: the date of the last seizure if any, recent carotid angiography, electroconvulsive therapy, etc.

(4) Cranial abnormalities, notably gross asymmetries which may effect interpretation of the record, and scalp or skull defects (burr-holes, craniotomy scars etc.) which may help to explain localized EEG abnormalities.

(5) Mental state: level of awareness (e.g. drowsiness, stupor), any evidence of confusion or disorientation, failure to co-operate, and any other abnormality of behaviour.

(6) Other clinical observations, such as obvious neurological deficit, mental subnormality (often omitted from the request form), pallor, sweating, hyperventilation, seizures during electrode placement, etc.

(7) The patient's own statement as to whether he is right- or left-handed or ambidextrous, or, if he is uncertain of this, his hand preference for writing, drawing, etc.

(8) Date of last menstrual period if attacks are said to occur particularly in association with menstruation.

During recording the patient should be relaxed, and this is best achieved in a recumbent position on a bed or couch. Some elderly subjects or those with respiratory or cardiac disorders are more comfortable in a semi-recumbent or sitting position.

For purposes of observing minor seizures or for certain specific tests of psychological function, investigation of pattern sensitivity, etc. (see Chapter 7) it may be more convenient for the patient to be sitting upright. Considerable flexibility may be achieved by the use of an adjustable dental chair, cardiac bed or an airliner seat (obtainable second-hand from aircraft breakers). Extremely restless patients or those liable to frequent seizures should be placed on a low bed with 'cot sides' unless continuous nursing supervision is available. Attention to the comfort of a patient includes specifically enquiring whether he wishes to empty his bladder before the start of the recording, removing shoes and loosening restrictive clothing, and providing a blanket if necessary. If self-retaining electrodes are used the patient's head should rest on a thin pillow. Where pads are employed, it is necessary to support the back of the neck by means of a small firm cylindrical pillow some 10 cm in diameter so that the occipital electrodes are held clear of the bed.

With deaf patients it may be necessary to agree a system of signals (e.g. a tap on the foot to open the eyes and a hand gesture to close them).

Before the beginning of the recording the electrode resistances should be tested (except in the case of needles, see Chapter 3) and should not only be low but also if possible equal. Stick-on electrodes should have a resistance not more than $5k\Omega$ and preferably of the order of 2 or $3k\Omega$; with pads $5 - 10k\Omega$ is acceptable. Most modern machines employ an alternating current of about 10 Hz to test electrode impedance. On some older apparatus a DC source is used and this carries the risk of electrode polarization if a current is passed through any electrode for more than a few seconds in one direction. The problem may be overcome by testing the electrodes in pairs, e.g. A and B, B and C, C and D . . . Again the method of display varies: on older machines there is simply an ohm meter on the console; with more modern apparatus there may be a write-out on the chart indicating electrode impedances, and there may also be a meter or a display of LEDs (light-emitting diodes) on the headbox, which is helpful when adjusting the electrodes. Some departments have constructed devices for testing electrode resistance in the preparation room before the patient is connected to the machine. Attempts to reduce an inexplicably high electrode impedance may be frustrating for the technician and distressing for the patient. However, the effort is worthwhile; proceeding with the record in the hope that the electrode contacts will improve usually proves futile.

If a machine has been properly set up before the arrival of the patient, a calibration check as described in the preceding section can be completed in less than a minute and provides a permanent record of the state of the machine at the time of the investigation. This test should be followed by a 'biological calibration'. At control settings likely to be used during the subsequent recording all channels are connected to the same pair of electrodes. The derivation selected should be one which will give a wide range of different frequency components and both high- and low- amplitude waves. A fronto-occipital or centro-temporal derivation is suitable, and if there is a lack of high-amplitude slow activity the patient may be asked to blink a few times. Small differences in the performance of channels, particularly in high-frequency response, may be more obvious during biological calibration than when a square-wave is used.

6.3.3. The clinical recording

Nothing reflects the different attitudes of various departments more clearly than the approach to the actual EEG recording. Some departments receive many referrals for routine EEG 'screening', often without carefully formulated clinical questions. Such practice is not confined to unsophisticated settings but is found also in many well-known institutions. EEG investigation simply to exclude cerebral disease gives a very small yield of useful information and this in turn is taken to justify the performance of a very limited recording which will show only the grossest EEG abnormalities. Those departments where EEGs are requested to answer clearly formulated and appropriate questions, have more reason to strive after excellence, but they too adopt various approaches. One method of trying to ensure good quality EEGs is to adopt a complex and rigid procedure which is followed in every patient. A lengthy series of preset montages is used each with standardized sequences of eyes open and eyes closed and the procedure is not adapted in the light of the findings. Somatosensory stimulation is for instance employed to block a possible mu-rhythm, even if there is none, and an elaborate photic stimulation routine designed to establish the frequency range of photosensitivity is performed regardless of whether the patient is in fact photosensitive. This approach may produce work of above average quality but the present authors do not view it with enthusiasm. Not only is it stultifying for intelligent people to work in this way, but also the very redundancy of the procedure discourages any initiative in adopting measures which may increase the value of the EEG, for instance, the use of extra electrodes or non-standard montages, investigating possible provocative factors in epilepsy or detecting momentary lapses of awareness (see Sections 7.9 and 7.10).

There is in any department a sequence of montages and control settings which is employed in the first instance unless either the clinical problem or previous EEG findings dictate a different procedure. The filter settings should allow the widest bandwidth compatible with a reasonably artefact-free recording. Thus in patients who do not produce a great deal of EMG activity an HF setting of 70 Hz is acceptable. Some departments favour the use of a time constant of 1 s or longer. This gives a 3 dB cut-off point of about 1/6 Hz, far below the limit of the frequencies normally recorded in the EEG. The use of a very long time constant may be something of a technological *tour de force* as it is possible to obtain a readable recording in this way only if the tracing is virtually free of electrode artefacts. However, it also renders the system very susceptible to blocking, notably from movement artefacts during seizures, with consequent loss of information of diagnostic importance. A shorter time constant of 0.3 s is therefore more generally recommended. This gives a 3 dB point of a little less than 0.5 Hz, which is adequate for conventional EEG tracings.

The high- and low-pass filter settings may be manipulated in order to highlight particular frequency components of the EEG, although their importance for this purpose is sometimes overrated. Reducing the HF setting to a value of the order of 15 Hz will substantially attenuate the beta activity and in theory this may be a worthwhile manoeuvre if profuse beta obscures slower components. This is rarely necessary, however, and the main reason for using HF positions below 70 Hz is to reduce muscle artefact or 50 Hz mains interference. It should be stressed that the use of the HF filter for this purpose is a measure of last resort and attention should first be directed to reducing the artefact itself (see Chapter 8). Filtered EMG potentials can be mistaken for beta activity or spikes and a danger of misinterpretation therefore arises. The time constants may be used to reduce slow components of the EEG and highlight others. Large amounts of slow activity render assessment of alpha and of faster components difficult and in a patient with a large amount of asymmetrical posterior slow activity it is useful to record briefly at a time constant of 0.1 s or less in order to check the symmetry of the alpha rhythm. Note that after filtration by a very short time constant a steeply rising delta wave may have the appearance of a spike. The use of a long time constant is often recommended if one wishes to examine more closely a slow wave focus. In fact, increasing the time constant beyond 0.3 s has little effect on the amplitude of the delta activities commonly encountered in abnormal EEGs although it is essential for recording event-related slow potentials (see Sections 12.3 and 13.4). In some departments it is standard practice to record with various EEG channels at different filter settings. This is not usually recommended but may be acceptable if homologous channels from opposite sides of the head are recorded with the same filter settings and if the technician and the electroencephalographer appreciate the implications for interpretation. Activities which are attenuated by high- or low-pass filters also undergo a phase shift. Fast components at the upper limit of the recording bandwidth are delayed; slow waves close to the lower limit appear earlier with respect to other activities (Fig. 6.12). A machine which is to be used in an environment where there is a high level of interference may require an additional 'notch' filter tuned to the frequency of the mains or of an interfering radio source. These filters often produce a very marked phase shift.

The choice of sensitivity will depend upon the dynamic range of the write-out system, the spacing of the galvanometers and the amplitude of the EEG. It is desirable to use the highest sensitivity (i.e. the lowest value of $\mu V/cm$) which keeps the signal within the dynamic range of the recorder and does not cause the pens to cross. For the average waking subject 70 $\mu V/cm$ is usually appropriate. On those machines with more than usually widely spaced pens 50 $\mu V/cm$ is an acceptable routine setting. If the EEG is of continuously high amplitude, for instance in a child, or during sleep or coma, a lower sensitivity will be required. Intermittent increases in amplitude, for instance due to epileptic discharges, may require that part of the record be recorded at reduced sensitivity, so that waveform and distribution of the paroxysmal events can be studied. On a machine with 16 or more channels it is often advantageous in this situation to duplicate some derivations at both routine and reduced sensitivity settings. An increased sensitivity is necessary when the EEG is of

Fig. 6.12. The effects of various control settings on the waveform of a spike-wave discharge.

(a)

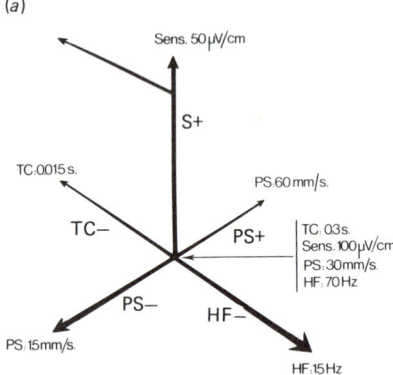

Sens. 50 μV/cm

S+

TC: .0015 s.

PS: 60 mm/s.

TC−

PS+

TC: .03 s.
Sens. 100 μV/cm
PS: 30 mm/s.
HF: 70 Hz

PS−

HF−

PS: 15 mm/s.

HF: 15 Hz

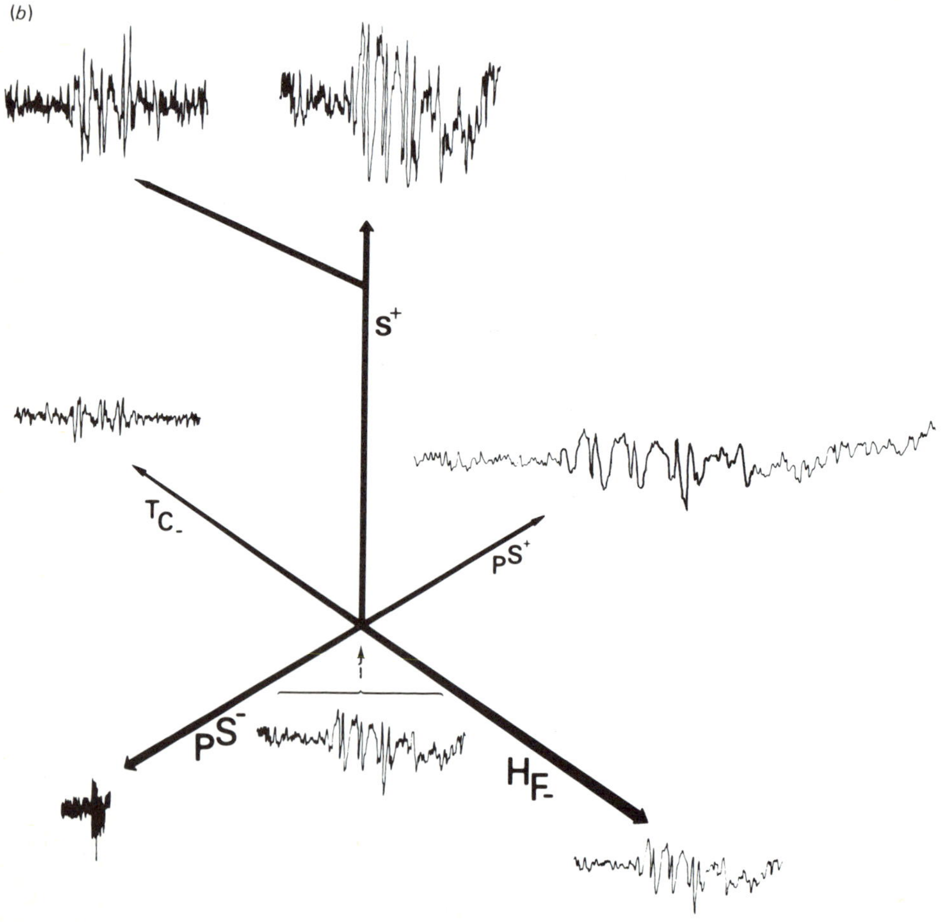

(b)

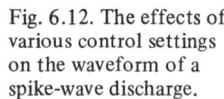

S⁺

TC−

PS⁺

PS⁻

HF−

unusually low amplitude and is mandatory when an apparently isoelectric tracing is obtained during the investigation of possible brain death (see Chapter 9). It should be noted that the frequency composition of the low-voltage EEGs obtained from tense subjects, or from those normal people who simply have little alpha activity, is different from that of a more usual tracing. Consequently, if the sensitivity is increased to give a write-out of normal amplitude, the appearance may be unfamiliar. EEG waveforms are most easily recognized when the ratio of the height to the width of each wave on the chart is about 3 to 2. On some small portable machines with closely spaced channels and a limited pen excursion it may therefore be advisable to combine a low recording sensitivity with a slower than usual paper speed, thus retaining the usual wave shape.

The paper speed generally adopted for EEG recording is 30 mm/s. The routine use of lower speeds may save paper but impairs legibility, except possibly on machines with a very fine line-thickness. A speed of 15 mm/s may nevertheless be used if one wishes to keep the machine running whilst waiting for a particular occurrence, such as the onset of sleep, and is also acceptable for long-term monitoring over a period of several hours, where one is interested in detecting rather obvious events such as the occurrence of epileptic discharges or the changing levels of sleep. Indeed, Osselton (1970) suggests that sleep staging can be carried out from a tracing run at only 3 mm/min. A paper speed of 15 mm/s or less may also be useful for demonstrating periodicities in the EEG, for instance features recurring at intervals of some tens of seconds. Reduction of paper speed to 15 mm/s may render delta waves more easily visible and may assist estimation of the distribution of alpha activity. An increased paper speed, usually of 60 mm/s, may improve the visualization of faster components and in particular helps one to identify suspected mains interference by measuring its frequency. The time relations of rapidly occurring events, such as multiple spike discharges, may be more easily assessed at high paper speeds and errors due to poor pen alignment are reduced.

The consequences of changing several controls simultaneously should be noted. For instance if one wishes to inspect the beta activity, the use of a very short time constant (e.g. 0.015 s) to reduce the amplitude of the slower components not only renders the beta activity more prominent but may also allow a much higher recording sensitivity to be employed. Conversely, if one has elected to use a low paper speed for long-term monitoring and is not interested in the faster components, it is logical also to reduce the HF setting to attenuate muscle potentials which otherwise produce an illegible band of ink. The effects of various combinations of control settings are illustrated in Fig. 6.12.

The recording characteristics of different methods of derivation were discussed in detail in Chapter 4 and will not be considered further here. However, it should be noted that for a routine screening of the EEG for features of possible interest the simplest montages are generally the most satisfactory. A minimum requirement is the use of montages incorporating anteroposterior and transverse bipolar chains and the use of common reference montages which, in combination, involve all of the electrodes. As the number of possibilities for significantly different common reference montages is less than for bipolar combinations, the number of reference montages routinely used will generally be less and each should be run for a longer period than the bipolar. As indicated in Chapter 4 the routine use of a particular electrode for reference purposes is difficult, as the choice of reference must depend upon the EEG findings. Thus for routine purposes common average or source reference may be more suitable. If nonstandard control settings have been used, so far as is compatible with legibility, they should be reset to the standard positions before the start of each new montage. The control settings and montage should be noted on the chart at the beginning of each new pattern and a comment made on the behavioural state of the patient. Unless one is attempting to achieve drowsiness it is useful to instruct the patient to keep his eyes open whilst the chart is being annotated and to close them shortly after the start of each montage. The eyes should be opened and closed at least once in the course of recording each montage in order to observe the effect of visual attention. Immediately following opening or closing of the eyes the EEG is in a somewhat unstable state and may change markedly over the succeeding 5 to 10 s. The eyes should therefore generally be kept open or closed respectively for some 20 s. At a recording speed of 30 mm/s and with pages 30 cm wide, eye opening and closure can conveniently be synchronized with the chart so that the changes in state occur in the middle of the left-hand page when the EEG is unfolded like a book. Such niceties increase ease of interpretation and are among the hallmarks of a skilled technician. Whenever the patient is instructed to open or shut the eyes this fact should be recorded on the chart and the timing indicated by the use of the marker control. If the patient is slow to respond due to drowsiness or possibly an absence attack this should then be apparent in the tracing. Spontaneous opening and closure of the eyes and all other events or changes in the state of the subject should also be entered.

Whenever recording is commenced with a new montage the technician should closely inspect the first few pages to determine whether there is any apparent anomaly of distribution of activity, particularly of eye movement artefacts, which may indicate a technical fault: incorrect switching, unequal filter or gain settings on different channels, a defective electrode, or incorrect plugging of the electrodes in the headbox. For this reason alone it is well worthwhile learning to recognize different types of eye movement artefacts rapidly and reliably so that any anomalous distribution can be quickly identified (Fig. 6.13). An abnormal distribution of EEG activity should be regarded as spurious until proved otherwise. A reasonable procedure to follow in the event, for instance, of detecting an apparent alpha asymmetry is the following:

(1) Check all control settings visually, and move each switch to ensure that good contacts have been made.

(2) Re-test sensitivity calibration.

(3) Re-check electrode resistances and plugging at the headbox, if necessary by touching each electrode in turn and determining whether an artefact is produced on the appropriate channels.

(4) Check the plugging of the input cable into the machine.

(5) On a machine with a 'sindex switch' reverse the right- and left-sided channels.

(6) If a pre-selected montage is in use set up the same pattern on independent selected switches.

(7) If the anomaly appears on a bipolar montage check this with common average reference or vice versa.

The length of the routine resting EEG varies between departments and may be from 2 to 60 minutes. There is however within any particular department usually a reluctance to vary the duration of the routine record according to the clinical problem and the EEG findings. For instance, as epileptiform activity generally occurs intermittently, it is unacceptable to claim that any person with suspected epilepsy has a normal waking record without recording for at least 30 to 40 minutes. Conversely, a tracing of only a few minutes is adequate to establish that someone with altered behaviour is not in status epilepticus, that a patient with porto-systemic encephalopathy has deteriorated, or that a child with the Lennox-Gastaut syndrome still has profuse epileptic activity. To some extent the duration of the 'routine record' may be influenced by the number of channels on the machine. With 20 channels, fewer montages will be required to explore all regions of the scalp than with only 8. However, often the length of the investigation is determined by the time required for the patient to relax, for drowsiness to develop, or for episodic phenomena to appear.

As the tracing proceeds the technician will increasingly depart from the routine procedure and will select montages particularly appropriate to highlight any features of interest which have been found, or to detect features which are expected in the light of the clinical problem or past EEG findings. Additional electrodes

Fig. 6.13. Anomalous distribution of eye movement artefact. Electrode P_4 has become unplugged.

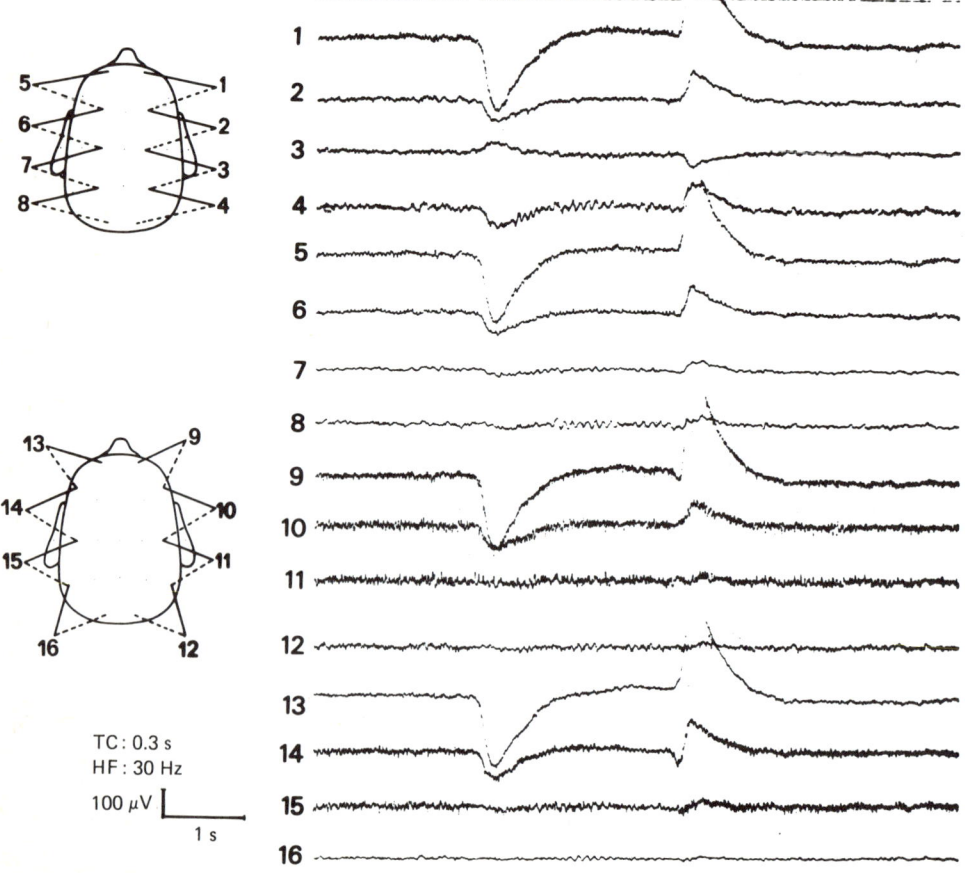

TC: 0.3 s
HF: 30 Hz

100 μV

1 s

may need to be applied and the state of awareness varied, for instance by letting an alert patient become drowsy or trying to arouse a person who is in stupor. Supplementary procedures will be adopted as appropriate (see Chapter 7) but hyperventilation and intermittent photic stimulation are routinely performed after the resting record in most departments unless there is some clear contra-indication. In tense patients hyperventilation often encourages relaxation and may therefore be usefully carried out at an earlier stage. Similarly photic stimulation may be used to soothe some infants or subnormal patients. In order to save paper, sometimes the chart is turned over half way through the recording so that the reverse side can be used. It is a false economy, for paper thick and opaque enough to be used in this way is much more expensive than that which can be employed if one writes on only one side.

6.3.4. Procedures after completion of the recording

The calibration check previously described should be repeated at the end of the recording. If the machine has facilities for registering electrode resistances on the chart it is also worthwhile repeating this test to confirm that the electrodes were still functioning satisfactorily. The electrodes will usually be removed in the application area. In the case of disc electrodes attached with collodion a solvent will be required to assist the removal. Acetone is most suitable and is sometimes mixed with small amounts of olive-oil, which avoids leaving the hair unpleasantly dry. After the electrodes and the larger pieces of collodion have been removed, the hair should be combed whilst at the same time the remaining fragments of collodion are loosened with an acetone-soaked swab. Finally the combing is repeated with a fine-tooth comb of the type used for removing lice. It is not acceptable for the patient to leave the department with visible pieces of collodion on his scalp, but he should be told that tiny particles will fall from his hair for the next few days giving the appearance of dandruff. If a child becomes distressed during electrode removal (and many find the acetone fumes disagreeable) it may be unwise to try to get rid of all the collodion but the parent or escort can be advised how to complete the procedure at home using nail-varnish remover. Some patients are less troubled by the acetone if the scalp is cleaned whilst they are still lying down. To remove electrode jelly or bentonite paste, rubbing with a dry swab should be sufficient. When removing needle electrodes the technician should avoid contact with the needle points.

On completion of the recording the patient may enquire after the results or seek advice about his medical condition. This should be politely refused, but one may reasonably assure him that the tracing will be read shortly by an EEG specialist and may indicate how soon the report is likely to be in the hands of the patient's doctor. It may be added that the significance of a laboratory test depends on the total clinical picture and that the person best qualified to assess this is his own physician. Some departments have the agreement of the referring clinicians that they may at their own discretion make appointments for further diagnostic EEG investigation, for instance sleep recordings. If so, any further appointment should if possible be made before the patient leaves the department. Otherwise, if further investigation seems likely, the technician should mention that this possibility exists but will be decided by the referring doctor. This advice helps to avoid the situation in which a patient recalled for further investigation assumes, either that the first EEG was unsuccessful, or that something serious has been found. The future co-operation of a child patient may be encouraged by the gift of a few pages of *normal* EEG tracing to show to his schoolfriends or the invitation to come again another day and play with the toys in the waiting room etc.

If any procedure has been performed which may affect the fitness of an outpatient to return home (drug-induced sleep recording etc.) the technician is responsible for checking that adequate arrangements have been made for transport, for an escort, and for continued supervision after arrival. If there is any doubt as to whether a patient is fit to leave the hospital he must first be examined by a doctor.

The technician's duties do not end with the departure of the patient. It is good practice to tidy the recording area immediately after the investigation, change soiled linen, replenish supplies of ink and paper, and clean the electrodes. The record should then be annotated more fully, made up into a book or placed in a large envelope. Depending upon the system of documentation used, the EEG should be given a number and entered in the day book or index system and other paper work such as filling in health insurance claim forms should be completed. A factual report (see Chapter 10) should be written whilst the details of the clinical problem and of the findings are fresh in the technician's mind. If either the nature of the referral or the EEG findings suggest that urgent interpretation of the record is necessary, the technician is responsible for informing the electroencephalographer concerned.

6.3.5. Care of acutely ill patients

An EEG technician should have some knowledge of elementary first aid and of basic nursing procedures, such as how to help a disabled person from a wheelchair to the recording couch or to assist the patient to use a bedpan. He should also at least be aware of the dangers and problems presented by such apparatus as i.v. infusions, urinary catheters, tracheotomy tubes, etc. A week spent on a general medical ward forms a useful part of the introductory training of a technician. Discussion of such matters as the first-aid treatment of cardiac arrest is outside the scope of the present text, but mention should be made of two problems which occur especially often in the EEG department: unconsciousness and seizures.

Two main dangers confront the unconscious patient, asphyxia and injury, the one because the reflexes required to maintain the airway may be depressed, the other because he may react inadequately to pain. In the absence of skilled assistance, it is advisable that any patient who is deeply unconscious should be nursed in a semi-prone position. This helps to prevent the jaw and tongue falling backwards and obstructing the airway and helps to ensure that saliva or vomit run out of the mouth and are not inhaled. If difficulty is experienced in keeping the patient in this position, the uppermost leg should be bent at the hip and the knee, and a pillow wedged between the thighs (Fig. 6.14). The prevention of injury in an unconscious patient includes making sure that if his eyes are open his corneae are not abraded by bedclothes, and that if he is wheeled about the department on a trolley a limply dangling hand is not crushed against a doorpost. There is also a danger of bedsores or damage to nerves if the patient remains lying in the same position for a long time. Pressure against hard objects, bed-rails etc. should be avoided and the patient should be turned from one side to the other every half hour.

If the patient suffers an attack, whether epileptic, hysterical or otherwise, although the first concern of the technician must be for his safety, important secondary considerations are to obtain as much clinical and electrophysiological information about the event as possible. If, as is usually the case, the seizure is accompanied by high-voltage EEG activity and/or artefacts, the recording sensitivity should be reduced, the time constant set to not more

than 0.3 s and possibly shorter, HF filters introduced if necessary
to prevent damage to the pens and the paper speed possibly increased. Every EEG department should have an alarm system
which can be activated by the technician sitting at the machine.
One cause of a seizure is cardiac arrest. If the ECG is not being
monitored and the patient is deeply unconscious and pallid, the
carotid pulse should be checked. Assuming that the attack is not
in fact of cardiac origin, one then takes steps to prevent the
patient from suffering injury and to observe as closely as possible
the clinical manifestations. Contrary to the recommendations of
the older nursing textbooks introducing any object into the
mouth to prevent the patient from biting his tongue or cheeks
is not only useless but also dangerous. During the tonic phase of
a major seizure the strength of contraction of the jaws renders it
impossible to prise them apart, and in the clonic phase the violent
movements ensure that any attempt to introduce a spatula or gag
is likely to result in broken teeth, laceration of the tongue or
cheeks or injuries to the fingers of the person trying to do it. In
the tonic phase of a seizure there is also a cessation of respiratory
movements and administering oxygen to overcome the cyanosis
is useless. During a seizure and particularly during automatisms
or post-ictal confusion one is better employed trying to prevent
the patient from suffering injury, for instance due to falling from
the couch or walking into obstacles. The very restless patient is
probably best placed on the floor, with a pillow under his head
and clear of any furniture or apparatus. If after an initial convulsion the patient remains cyanosed or appears to have obstructed
breathing, then it may well be necessary to administer oxygen
and to place him in the stabilized position recommended above
for unconscious people in general. A succession of seizures without intervening recovery of consciousness amounts to *status
epilepticus* and demands urgent medical help. In any event a
physician should be called to examine any patient who has had
a major seizure in the department. The technician should record

Fig. 6.14. A patient in
the semi-prone or
'stabilized' position.

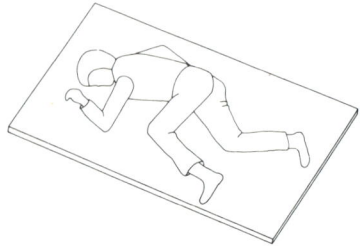

in writing any clinical observations on the seizure pattern and, without becoming an amateur neurologist, may usefully learn to carry out some basic neurological tests such as observing the position of the eyes, eliciting pupilary reflexes, checking the symmetry of muscle tone, and examining the plantar responses. This information may help to differentiate between the epileptic and the hysterical seizure and between generalized and partial epilepsies.

A patient who has been incontinent during a seizure may be too embarrassed to report it. Check therefore, and keep a supply of spare clothing in the department for this eventuality.

7. Procedures to supplement the routine recording

It is often necessary to supplement the resting EEG registration by various additional procedures. Some of these will be carried out in the course of the 'routine' recording at the discretion of the technician, others are performed only at the request of the responsible physician and may require a special appointment, and in some instances medical supervision. These techniques include so-called 'activation procedures' which may unmask abnormalities not seen in the resting record. Other supplementary procedures may be directed to investigation of provocative factors (e.g. exercise or visual stimulation) in patients with seizure disorders, or to seeking possible clinical correlates of paroxysmal discharges. The most used activation techniques are hyperventilation, photic stimulation and diurnal sleep recording.

7.1. Hyperventilation

Hyperventilation (HV) is an increase in respiratory effort and, as it is employed in the EEG laboratory, its purpose is to increase respiratory exchange, breathe out carbon dioxide (CO_2) more rapidly and thus reduce the amount of CO_2 in the blood. In practice this is most effectively achieved if the patient attempts deep, rather than rapid, breathing and in particular concentrates on emptying the lungs as far as possible. The effect of a lowered CO_2 concentration is a fall in blood pressure with simultaneous constriction of cerebral blood vessels; consequently the blood-flow through the brain becomes less and the availability of oxygen and glucose to brain cells is reduced (Meyer *et al.*, 1967; Sugioka and Davis, 1960). Due to reflexes which control respiration, the normal reaction to this state of affairs is to stop breathing until the CO_2 concentration returns to normal; thus effective hyperventilation requires effort on the part of the subject. If HV is performed well some mildly unpleasant side-effects are experienced, including a feeling of light headedness, tingling of the hands and feet and around the mouth, and sometimes painful cramps of the extremities (tetany). These symptoms are normal, but may alarm the patient or indeed the technician; it is amazing how few technicians have themselves hyperventilated in order to experience these sensations at first hand. Some patients become frightened, feel breathless and, paradoxically, continue hyperventilation after being told that they may stop!

A casual request to breathe deeply will rarely produce the necessary effort on the part of the subject. The technician should explain the procedure in detail, laying stress on the importance of concentrating on breathing out and may usefully give a short demonstration of what is required. The patient should be made comfortable; if necessary the bladder should be emptied and tight clothing loosened. HV is usually done with the patient lying down; in a sitting position EEG activation is often much more rapid and marked (Billinger and Frank, 1969). It is also necessary to encourage the patient at frequent intervals, and to record on the chart whether the patient is overbreathing effectively. If HV is carried out vigorously 3 minutes are sufficient to produce marked EEG changes; if the effort appears inadequate the procedure should be extended to 5 minutes. There is little or nothing to be gained by a longer period of HV. Children below the age of six will not generally hyperventilate satisfactorily to command, but can be pursuaded to do so if the task is made into a game, for instance blowing a small paper windmill, or trying to inflate a leaky plastic bag. Gay and Muras (1969) describe a toy animal whose eyes light up when the child blows upon a microphone; this often encourages children as young as three years to overbreathe effectively. There are a number of medical contraindications to HV, notably respiratory or cardiac disease, cerebral vascular insufficiency, or any acute disorder which may be accompanied by oedema, raised intracranial pressure, or vascular changes in the brain. In general HV should not be performed in subjects above 65 years of age without medical approval and is in any case rarely useful. Reactivity of cerebral blood vessels in the elderly is minimal and reduced blood CO_2 is unlikely to produce effective cerebral vasoconstriction. The EEG recorder should be turned on about 1 minute before the start of HV to establish a baseline, as the state of the patient may have changed during explanation and preparations. The recording should continue for at least 2 minutes after HV or until any resultant EEG changes have disappeared. If the findings are equivocal, there is no contraindication to repeating HV after a few minutes. Overbreathing is usually done with closed eyes, but some patients show more marked activation with eyes open.

In normal subjects the EEG changes accompanying HV are most marked in childhood and diminish with increasing age. A normal response comprises an increase in theta activity, sometimes slowing and increasing amplitude of the alpha rhythm due to slight drowsiness and bursts of rhythmic delta activity in subjects up to 35 years of age (Binnie, Coles and Margerison,

1969). Typically the delta activity commences over the front of the head and remains maximum in amplitude in this region, but in children it may begin posteriorly and spread to the frontal regions. Abnormal responses may be localized or generalized, but the most dramatic is the appearance of 3/s spike wave activity in patients with absence seizures. Failure to produce EEG changes during hyperventilation is not abnormal, but in a young subject indicates that the task was performed inadequately. The EEG ordinarily returns to its resting state within 1-2 minutes after HV but frequently the subject falls directly into drowsiness, which may provide the opportunity to obtain a spontaneous sleep recording (see below). In the early days of clinical EEG much importance was attached to the degree and duration of responses to hyperventilation (Heppenstall, 1944) and, as a very marked response in a normal subject may be seen if the blood sugar is low (hypoglycaemia), it was customary to check the blood sugar levels in all subjects showing marked slowing on HV or sometimes to repeat the procedure after administration of 50 g glucose by mouth. This is no longer a usual practice, but if a marked delta response persists for several minutes after HV hypoglycaemia should be considered.

As the change in the EEG is dependent upon the effectiveness of HV in producing a fall of blood CO_2 concentration, it may sometimes be desirable to monitor the procedure. The most reliable method is by measuring CO_2 concentrations in expired air by means of an infra-red gas analyser, but this is not routine practice. The rate of breathing can be monitored by means of a thermocouple or thermistor placed close to the mouth, or by a variable resistance (usually a mercury filled rubber tube) around the patient's waist. In routine clinical practice these measures are unnecessary and there is a close correlation between an experienced technician's rating of performance as 'good', 'average' or 'poor' and the change in blood CO_2 concentration (Binnie *et al.*, 1969).

7.2. Intermittent photic stimulation

Intermittent photic stimulation (IPS) involves presenting to the subject a series of, usually regular, light flashes. At low frequencies each flash produces a visual evoked response (see Section 12.3) and at flash rates from 4 to 20/s or higher one observes photic following, EEG activity at the same frequency as the flashes, or at harmonics of the flash rate. IPS is performed:

(1) To observe photic following and determine whether it is symmetrical and whether it occurs over the normal range of frequencies.

(2) To elicit epileptiform activity in photosensitive subjects.

(3) To observe possible suppression of pre-existing EEG activities during stimulation.

Photic stimulators are available commercially from the manufacturers of EEG equipment and are more satisfactory than industrial stroboscopes which often produce electrical interference. The flashes are ordinarily presented by a lamp placed directly in the front of the patient's eyes at a distance of 30 cm from the nasion. A number of ingenious alternatives have been described, as for instance spectacles containing photo-luminescent panels (Montagu, 1966), but these have not been adopted for routine use. Manufacturers are often curiously vague about the intensity of their stroboscopes but, in order to elicit epileptiform activity reliably in susceptible subjects, a maximum intensity of at least 0.4 joules or 400 nit-s per flash should be available. The appropriate units and methods of measurement are debatable, see Drasdo (1975). The effectiveness of IPS for producing epileptiform activity is also substantially increased (assuming luminance to be unchanged) by the presence of a grid or grating pattern over the front of the lamp (Jeavons, Harding, Panayiotopoulos and Drasdo, 1972; Wilkins *et al.*, 1979). Claims have been made to the contrary but these were based upon studies in which no correction was made for the reduction in brightness due to the grid. Intensity and flash rates are controlled by a unit which should be accessible to the technician seated at the EEG machine. As IPS can elicit seizures in susceptible subjects it is essential that the technician should be prepared to terminate stimulation immediately if epileptiform activity appears. The EEG machine must therefore be running throughout the procedure and a useful safeguard is to have a spring-loaded ON–OFF switch so that flashes are delivered only so long as it is depressed by the technician's finger. An output should be provided from the stimulator to record the flashes by pulses on the marker channel of the EEG machine. If this facility is not available, IPS can be monitored by means of a photo-cell placed close to the patient's face and connected to one channel of the recorder.

The procedure is usually well tolerated but some patients may find it somewhat alarming. It is not acceptable to thrust a lamp in front of the patient's face and commence stimulation without first explaining what is going to happen. Moreover, to obtain reliable results it is necessary to carry out the procedure in a carefully controlled manner. In particular it is essential that the lamp be correctly positioned directly in front of the patient's eyes and that he should fixate on its centre and not turn his head to one side during stimulation. After the lamp has been positioned the room lighting may be dimmed, but it is necessary to be able to see both the patient and the EEG, and not only by the light of the stimulator. Many patients are indeed more sensitive to IPS when the level of background illumination is high, and if a negative result is obtained in a subject expected on clinical grounds to be photosensitive it is worthwhile repeating the procedure with full room lighting (Klass and Fischer-Williams, 1976; van Egmond, Binnie and Veldhuizen, 1980).

Over the years, a variety of different photic stimulation procedures have been advocated, including the use of paired flashes, irregular stimulation, and the use of lights of different colours. There is little evidence that any of these provide information of value in relation to the clinical objectives indicated above. Mention should also be made of a method employed in many departments which has little to commend it, namely the use of continuous IPS over some 20-40 s, whilst the flash rate is slowly increased and then decreased again. Since photic following can not usually be demonstrated satisfactorily when the rate of change of stimulation exceeds one flash/s/s, and as the frequency controls on many photic stimulators are non-linear it is difficult to achieve the slow and steady change of frequency necessary to obtain following over the higher flash rates. This method is also unsatisfactory for eliciting paroxysmal activity, which may require stimulation for several seconds at constant frequency and/ or the combination of stimulation at each frequency with the act of eye closure. Some patients are indeed photosensitive only with closed eyes, others only with the eyes open and in particular there are many in whom epileptiform activity can be elicited only if stimulation is administered at the moment of eye closure (Panayiotopoulos, 1974). Any procedure to screen for photosensitivity is inadequate unless it allows these three conditions to be tested. The most satisfactory method is probably to deliver a train of flashes at constant frequency commencing at the moment of eye closure. After some 8 s the subject is asked to open the

eyes and the stimulation continued for a further 8 s. If epileptiform activity is elicited stimulation at the frequency in question is
terminated. If not, the eyes are kept open and the following train
of flashes, again commencing with eye closure, is delivered after
an interval of 5-10 s. Unless there is reason to suppose that the
patient is highly photosensitive it may be convenient to
commence the stimulation at 18 flashes/s, the frequency most
likely to elicit epileptiform activity in sensitive patients. This
preliminary screening will indicate whether or not epileptiform
activity is to be expected at other frequencies. Little useful
purpose is served by testing a large number of closely spaced flash
rates. For routine screening the following sequence of frequencies
is suggested: 1 (to demonstrate individual evoked responses), 55,
6, 50, 8, 40, 10, 22, 12, 16, 20. Taken in pairs, these values
correspond to the 10th, 20th, 40th, 60th and 80th percentile
points of the frequency distribution curve of photosensitivity
found by Jeavons and Harding (1975) in a large population of
IPS-sensitive subjects and will conveniently discriminate between
high, moderate and mild sensitivity. The range of frequencies to
which a patient is sensitive is fairly stable and appears to correlate
with seizure incidence and with the effect of anti-epileptic drugs
(Rowan *et al.*, 1979). In order to measure the sensitivity range it
is desirable to administer the various rates alternating between the
higher and lower frequencies gradually converging on 18 flashes/s.
When the upper and lower limits have been defined the procedure
may be terminated. The choice of intensity setting
depends on the stimulator, but in non-photosensitive subjects
should be the highest which is tolerated without distress. Patients
who wear spectacles are sometimes more sensitive with, and
sometimes without, their glasses – so both conditions should be
tested.

In normal subjects IPS typically produces symmetrical
depression of on-going rhythmic activity. In addition, photic
following may be seen which is maximal over the occipital
regions. The amplitude of the following response is very variable
and probably of no clinical significance, except in uraemia and
in some children with rare degenerative diseases in whom
extremely high-amplitude responses of $100-300\,\mu V$ may be
seen (Pampiglione and Harden, 1977). Slight asymmetries of
photic following are common and usually parallel those of
the alpha rhythm. An amplitude difference of more than 50%
is seen in about 5% of normal subjects (Kooi, Eckman and

Thomas, 1957) and asymmetries which change with flash
frequency or between the eyes open and closed states may
also occur in normal subjects (Lansing and Thomas, 1964; Klass
and Fischer-Williams, 1976). The amplitude of photic following is
generally maximal at about the alpha frequency and diminishes
above 10-12 Hz. It has been claimed that marked following at
frequencies above 18/s is typical of patients with migraine (Golla
and Winter, 1958), but subsequent work has not confirmed this
(Liske, 1965). The presence of harmonic components at twice or
half the flash frequency is of no established clinical significance
but is often particularly striking in those subjects who also
exhibit epileptiform activity during stimulation. IPS sometimes
induces rhythmic contractions of the muscles of the face, scalp
and neck and shoulders synchronous with the flashes. This
phenomenon of 'photomyoclonus' is demonstrable in some 50%
of normal adults with a stimulus more powerful than that used
in routine practice (Bickford, Sem-Jacobsen, White and Daley,
1952) but may be misinterpreted as an epileptic discharge. The
most dramatic epileptiform response to IPS, the 'photoconvulsive
reaction', (Bickford et al., 1952) consists of generalized,
bilaterally synchronous irregular spike or polyspike wave activity,
of maximum amplitude over the fronto-central regions and often
outlasting the stimulus. However, a variety of less marked and less
generalized responses may be seen, including occipital spikes or
sharp waves synchronous with the flashes, and irregular spike
wave activity confined to the back of the head. The literature
concerning the clinical significance of photosensitivity is
extremely confused, chiefly because some authors describe
photomyoclonus, high-frequency following, marked harmonics,
and other normal phenomena as photosensitivity. This has
resulted in misleading claims that a large proportion of normal
subjects are photosensitive. Clear generalized spike-wave discharges
during IPS are virtually confined to people with epilepsy and
their relatives. Some 60% of people showing such responses give
a history of visually-induced epileptic seizures (Jeavons and
Harding, 1975; Stefansson et al., 1977).

7.3. Sleep

Recording during drowsiness and sleep is widely used in diagnostic
EEG, particularly in the investigation of epilepsy, although the
usefulness of sleep tracings has been questioned (Gloor, Tsai and
Hadded, 1958; Maulsby and Markand, 1972). Sleep may occur

spontaneously during routine EEG recording, and natural sleep can also be studied at night. Sleep may be induced during the daytime either by the use of drugs or by keeping the patient awake during the previous night (sleep deprivation).

Success in obtaining sleep during the daytime depends in part on the recording environment and on the technician. The illumination of the recording room should be dimmed, the surroundings quiet, and the patient reclining and relaxed. Attention to his comfort should include checking that he is sufficiently warm. Many people even when fully dressed, require a blanket to keep them warm lying inactive at a normal room temperature. Stick-on electrodes are necessary for sleep recordings; pad electrodes become increasingly uncomfortable and dry out too rapidly, needles and discs attached with bentonite may come loose if the patient sleeps restlessly. ECG and possibly EMG or additional scalp electrodes should be applied at the start of the investigation. The attitude of the technician is most important; it should be suggested that the patient may doze off, but over-emphasizing the need to sleep may prevent relaxation.

During sleep the EEG follows a very constant pattern and the depth of sleep may be classified on the basis of the EEG and other findings. The system most widely used is that of Dement and Kleitman (1957) and was described in Chapter 2.

Sleep recording is useful for a number of purposes (Silverman, 1956):

(1) To induce paroxysmal activity in patients with epilepsy. Focal discharges commonly increase in amount or appear during drowsiness or light sleep. Generalized discharges increase in amount during the deeper sleep stages. During REM sleep generalized discharges are rarely seen; focal epileptiform activity may be reduced but often persists in substantial amounts, particularly when of temporal lobe origin.

(2) Non-epileptic types of abnormal activity are only occasionally activated by sleep recording and indeed often disappear (Schoppenhorst and Kubicki, 1973). It was formerly claimed that the depth of a tumour could be assessed by the persistence or disappearance of focal delta activity during sleep (Silverman and Groff, 1957) but this has since been disputed (Daly, 1968).

(3) Abnormalities of the activities normally associated with sleep may reflect disease. For instance unilateral cerebral pathology may produce asymmetries of sigma activity and

K-complexes. Patients with diencephalic damage or diffuse degenerative disorders such as Alzheimer's disease (Letemendia and Pampiglione, 1958) may show poorly formed low-amplitude K-complexes and anomalies of sleep spindles. The actual pattern of sleep is rarely of clinical interest, except in some patients with narcolepsy (attacks of an irresistable desire to sleep), who may pass into REM or stage III within a few seconds of falling asleep (Roth, 1976). Quantitative analysis of sleep patterns is however carried out extensively in connection with research on centrally acting drugs, many of which change the sleep pattern, particularly by suppressing REM.

Where sleep does not occur spontaneously it may be induced by drugs, which must be given under medical supervision. Some people become nauseated and may vomit after taking sleeping tablets in the daytime and patients must therefore be asked to fast for 3 hours before the investigation. If a waking record has already been obtained it may be convenient to give the medication at the start of the tracing. This will allow some 15-20 min to check the previous findings and to carry out hyperventilation which is itself conducive to sleep. The drugs most widely used for sleep EEGs are medium-acting barbiturates such as quinalbarbitone (Seconal). The typical adult dose is 200 mg by mouth and an additional 100 mg may be given after 25-30 min, if the patient shows no sign of sleeping. For children a liquid preparation is preferable to capsules; the dosage depends on age, weight and other factors and must be determined by a physician. A repeat dose given three quarters of an hour or more after the first is rarely effective. Barbiturates induce beta activity in the EEG, and although this may change the record, it may also provide information of diagnostic value, as asymmetries of barbiturate-induced fast activity often reflect asymmetrical cerebral pathology (Pampiglione, 1952). Various other drugs are sometimes used for sleep recordings, including chloral hydrate and diazepam. Chloral hydrate acquired an early and undeserved reputation for producing relatively little beta activity. It is, however, a gentle hypnotic drug and is particularly useful in young children. Diazepam may suppress generalized epileptiform activity, which can be an advantage, for instance if the purpose is to demonstrate a focus. Diazepam and other benzodiazepines tend to produce large amounts of beta activity which may obscure other elements in the EEG. It has been claimed that short-acting intravenous barbiturates such as methohexitone (Brietal) are particularly effective in activating the EEGs of some patients with epilepsy, but whether they are any more provocative than natural sleep is questionable (Sherwin and Hooge, 1973). Their routine use as a time-saving way of inducing sleep is to be deprecated, as it is just the gradual passage through light drowsiness and stage I that most often provides information of diagnostic value.

A sleep tracing should be no less interactive than a waking record. At different stages of sleep, changes of montage may be necessary to display both sleep phenomena and EEG abnormalities optimally. Unless the patient is having difficulty going to sleep, auditory stimuli should be given from time to time (tapping with a pencil on the EEG machine or using a phono-stimulator) to elicit arousal phenomena. As features of clinical interest may appear on awakening, it is important to continue recording whilst one awakes the patient.

7.4. Sleep deprivation

Night sleep deprivation (NSD) is not only a means of causing a patient to sleep during the daytime; it is also an activation procedure in its own right. An adult should stay awake all night (preferably without the help of caffeine-containing beverages) and the EEG should be recorded as early as convenient in the morning. In the case of a child below the age of ten the patient should be kept awake for 4–5 hours after his normal bedtime and then awakened early. For an outpatient the same precautions must be taken as for drug-induced sleep recording; for the journey both to and from the hospital an escort and transport must be provided. If no responsible person is available to ensure the patient is kept awake, it may be convenient for him to be admitted to a hospital ward the previous evening.

After NSD, epileptiform activity, particularly focal discharges, may appear when not previously present or may be greatly increased in amount. Photosensitivity may also appear or be enhanced and the response to HV may become abnormal. There is little evidence that sleep deprivation for 24 hours produces EEG abnormalities in normal subjects, apart from those changes which may be attributed to drowsiness (Bennett, Ziter and Liske, 1969; Spadetta, 1971; Welch and Stevens, 1971). Most clinical studies of NSD have been based upon selected patients in whom waking and drug-induced sleep records had previously failed to establish a diagnosis of epilepsy (Scollo-Lavizzari, Pralle and de la Cruz, 1975; Bechinger and Kornhuber, 1976). The yield of diagnostic findings in epileptic patients with previously normal waking and drug-induced sleep tracings may be as high as 40% (Pratt, Mattson, Welkers and Williams, 1968). NSD increases seizure liability and close medical supervision is essential if NSD is used in patients with large amounts of epileptiform activity in previous tracings or in those with a high seizure incidence. It follows that NSD should not be used as a routine screening procedure in patients suspected of epilepsy until at least a resting recording has been examined.

7.5. Special forms of visual stimulation

Some 50% of patients who are sensitive to IPS give a history of epileptic seizures induced by viewing television (Jeavons and Harding, 1975; Stefansson *et al.*, 1977). In a patient with a history of possible television epilepsy the finding of sensitivity to IPS may be regarded as evidence which supports the diagnosis, but further confirmation may be obtained by EEG recording during television viewing. For this purpose a black and white set with a large screen is most suitable. A moving TV picture is not necessary but the set must be in good working order and must have a 'synch' signal, either from a television transmission or from a closed-circuit TV system. Whilst the EEG is monitored, the patient should first view the television from a distance of 2 to 3 m and if no paroxysmal activity is induced should gradually be brought nearer to the set until viewing from the nearpoint of vision (300 mm). If the patient requires spectacles to see the television clearly these should be worn. TV can induce seizures in susceptible subjects as readily as IPS; stimulation must therefore be carried out with caution and there must be some means of turning off the set or covering the screen immediately if a discharge is induced.

The incidence of seizures induced by visual pattern is uncertain, partly because an association with environmental pattern stimulation is less easily recognized than for instance one with television. However, some 70% of IPS sensitive patients are sensitive also to visual pattern. Where a history of pattern-induced epilepsy is in question, pattern stimulation in the EEG laboratory may be considered appropriate. However, to induce epileptiform activity in the EEG the stimulus must conform to strict criteria. The optimum pattern for EEG activation in sensitive subjects comprises a grid of equal black and white stripes of high contrast. Each stripe should subtend a visual angle of about 15 minutes of arc and the whole display should subtend at least 15° but preferably more. A high level of illumination is required. These conditions may be met by means of a card 300 mm wide, with 2.5 mm black and white stripes, viewed at a distance of half a metre and brightly illuminated by means of a spotlight or slide projector. For further details see Darby, Wilkins, Binnie and de Korte (1980a).

Patients giving a history of seizures associated with sudden changes in environmental illumination (e.g. on going out of doors) should also be tested simply by turning the room light on and off. Sometimes this is more provocative than IPS (Klass and Fischer-Williams, 1976).

About a quarter of photosensitive patients induce EEG discharges or even seizures in themselves by blinking. To demonstrate this phenomenon it is necessary to record for some tens of minutes with the eyes open and in a well-lit room (Darby, de Korte, Binnie and Wilkins, 1980b).

7.6. Combined hyperventilation and photic stimulation
In some departments if neither hyperventilation nor IPS have produced a marked reaction the two activation methods may be applied simultaneously. There is little evidence that this technique has any advantage over HV and IPS carried out separately.

7.7. Tests of vasomotor lability
In the older EEG literature it was suggested that EEG changes or ECG slowing on reflex stimulation of the vagus nerve, either by massaging of the carotid sinus or by pressing on the eyeballs were of value for identifying patients with a liability to fainting or vaso-vagal attacks. Indeed a cerebral form of carotid sinus syncope was described, characterized by EEG changes on carotid massage without any associated change in heart rate, but is no longer accepted (Gurdjian, Webster, Hardy and Lindner, 1958). The manoeuvre of Valsalva (straining to breathe out against the closed glottis) was also proposed as a test of vasomotor instability, as was recording the EEG whilst the patient was abruptly raised from supine to a vertical position on a tilting table. These techniques have been generally abandoned in Anglo-American practice, as they give positive results in many normal subjects

who do not suffer from fainting and negative results in many who clearly do. However, they continue to be widely used on the continent of Europe. As carotid massage can cause a cerebrovascular catastrophe and eyeball pressure, a detached retina, the present authors can see no justification for their use except possibly in the most carefully selected cases and in collaboration with a cardiologist. Significantly, both are omitted from the relevant section of the comprehensive *Handbook of Electroencephalography and Clinical Neurophysiology* (Naquet, 1976).

7.8. Tests of insufficiency of the great vessels
In patients with a history of transient neurological symptoms apparently brought on by sudden change of posture or by head movements it may sometimes be useful to induce an attack under EEG and ECG control. Note however, that this problem most often arises in elderly people with so-called 'drop-attacks' due to degenerative disease of the basilar or vertebral arteries usually combined with osteoarthritis of the cervical spine. In these patients such manipulations carry a risk of neurological damage, are unlikely to be of diagnostic value and are not justified.

If carotid ligation is being considered in a patient with an arterial aneurysm, some neurosurgeons prefer to evaluate the adequacy of blood flow from the great vessels by compressing the ipsilateral carotid artery for a period of some five minutes. Development of localized slowing or neurological signs may indicate that the patient will not be able to tolerate the surgical procedure. The test carries some risk to the patient and unfortunately produces both false positive and false negative results. If it is performed, strict medical supervision is essential.

7.9. Trigger factors in epilepsy
Other provocative factors in epilepsy may need to be investigated. For instance, some patients give a history of seizures principally in association with exercise. To investigate these one may record the EEG during 10 minutes vigorous exertion on a bicycle ergometer. Recording should continue for at least 20 minutes thereafter, as activation of epileptiform activity is seen much more commonly during recovery than during the period of exercise itself (Kuyer, 1978).

Trigger factors in reflex epilepsies such as eating, reading or listening to particular music are easily investigated in the EEG laboratory. In the case of reading epilepsy it is worth noting that the seizures often commence with the jerking of the lower jaw and the submental EMG should therefore be monitored. An acurate history is important, for the type of reading material which elicits seizures may be highly specific. The duration of reading is also a factor, and it may be necessary for the patient to read for an hour or longer before a seizure or EEG activation is seen.

7.10. Investigation of clinical correlates

A recurring problem in EEG practice is presented by the patient with repeated generalized epileptiform discharges in whom few or no clinical seizures are observed. Close observation or psychological testing shows that in some subjects impairment of awareness occurs during brief discharges, that is, the patients are actually having seizures which in many instances require treatment. A number of simple tests of psychological function or attention may be applied. Firstly it is useful to record with the patient sitting upright and possibly with the arms outstretched. During the discharges one may then observe a loss of tone, a falling away of the arms or nodding of the head which were not recognizable in the recumbent position. Simple tests of attention include asking the patient to count aloud, press regularly on a switch connected to the marker channel of the EEG machine or to recite poems or nursery rhymes. Auditory attention may be checked by the technician counting out loud or himself reciting and asking the patient to repeat what was said after the discharge is ended. There are, however, some subjects in whom impairment of awareness can be demonstrated only by more sophisticated tests requiring the advice of a clinical psychologist.

7.11. Drug activation

Apart from being employed to produce EEG changes by induction of sleep, drugs are sometimes used to provoke EEG abnormalities of possible diagnostic significance. Various agents have enjoyed popularity, including drugs which cause lowered blood sugar levels (e.g. tolbutamide) and particularly drugs having a direct convulsant action on the brain, notably pentylenetetrazol (Metrazol or Cardiazol) or bemegride (Megimide). With an anaesthetist in attendance, the drug is injected slowly over a period of some 10 minutes with continuous monitoring of EEG, blood pressure, and heart rate (Merlis, Hendriksen and Grossman,

1950). The subject becomes anxious, alpha activity is diminished and theta increases and finally various types of paroxysmal activity appear. The results reported in the literature are confusing and inconsistent, due in part to the lack of standardized methods of administration. In general the dose required to produce paroxysmal activity is less in patients with epilepsy than in others but the incidence of activation in normal subjects is considerable (Baker and Klass, 1957). A variation of the technique was to combine the pentylenetetrazol injection with photic stimulation ('photo-Metrazol test') and to determine the threshold dose required to induce photosensitivity. In view of the high incidence of activation in normal subjects and of irrelevant findings in patients, these forms of activation have rightly fallen into disuse (Driver, 1962; Schwamb, Clausen and Summer, 1956). They may still be indicated in highly selected patients, usually in the course of a detailed diagnostic work-up, often with depth electrodes prior to neurosurgical treatment of partial epilepsies. Even here the findings must be regarded with considerable scepticism unless any paroxysmal discharge is accompanied by a clinical attack typical of the patient's own habitual seizure pattern (Bancaud *et al.*, 1968). The concordance between the EEG patterns of spontaneous and drug-induced seizures is poor (Weiser *et al.*, 1979).

7.12. Drug suppression tests

In patients with partial epilepsies, secondary generalized discharges may obscure any focal epileptiform activity. Where it is thought that this may be the case, the generalized discharges can be suppressed by a slow intravenous injection of diazepam, 1–2 mg/min up to a dose of 10 mg. Suppression of the generalized discharges may then unmask a focus. The effect on the EEG must be closely monitored during the injection, as too large a dose will simply abolish all epileptiform activity. This drug can suppress respiration, even in small amounts, and the means of supporting respiration must be at hand. Intravenous diazepam produces drowsiness and the opportunity therefore arises to combine this investigation with a sleep recording.

8. Artefacts and interference

Because of the high sensitivities required for EEG recording, problems frequently arise from the registration of unwanted signals. These may be divided into electrical interference from the surroundings, instrumental artefacts arising anywhere within the recording system (from electrodes to the final ink tracing), and phenomena of biological origin. This classification is not rigorous as, for instance, defects in instrumentation increase susceptibility, to environmental interference and movement of the subject may lead to artefacts arising at the electrodes.

8.1. Environmental electrical interference

8.1.1. Electromagnetic interference

Except in the rare circumstances where EEGs are recorded in the open air, mains frequency electromagnetic fields are almost always present in the environment. The strength of these fields will be greatly increased in the vicinity of mains apparatus, particularly if this contains unscreened electric motors, solenoids, transformers, etc. The strength of the field is determined by the current, thus a powerful lift motor will present a far greater problem than the coil of an electric light bulb. The fields due to equal currents flowing in opposite directions tend to cancel each other out, so mains cables will not usually cause severe electromagnetic interference. The fluctuating magnetic flux will induce an e.m.f. in the circuit formed by the pair of leads on each channel of the EEG machine and the patient's head. The size of this e.m.f. will be determined by the rate of change of magnetic lines of force passing through the circuit. The principle may be illustrated (and in practice an electromagnetic field may also be conveniently investigated) by means of a coil of wire connected to the input of one channel of the EEG machine. When the loop is positioned in a plane at right angles to the magnetic field the interference recorded is maximum, and if the loop is positioned parallel to the field so that no lines of force pass through it the pick-up will be minimal. Applying the same principle to electromagnetic interference during EEG recording, it follows that interference will occur most readily when the electrode leads are widely spread over the pillow, forming a loop with a large area, and can be reduced by bunching them closely together and if necessary tying them into a bundle with adhesive tape. There will also be an optimum orientation of the leads which minimizes electromagnetic pick up (Fig. 8.1). It should be noted that interference arising in this way produces an out-of-phase signal at the input to the EEG machine and thus the use of differential amplifiers provides no protection against it.

Electromagnetic interference can also occur in the much larger inductive loops formed by earth connections between the patient, the EEG machine, and other apparatus. These arise particularly in the intensive care unit or operating theatre, but may also be a consequence of attempts to eliminate electro-static interference (see below) by means of additional earth connections, for instance to a patient's bed. Note that in this case the electrodes and their leads are in parallel with respect to the induced e.m.f. and therefore, provided the electrode resistances are equal, the interference (E) will appear in-phase at the input and will be largely eliminated by the differential amplifiers (Fig. 8.2).

Fig. 8.1. Effect of positioning of leads on electro-magnetic pick-up. (a) The amount of electro-magnetic interference is determined by the number of lines of force passing through the loop formed by the leads, the electrodes and the head. (b) Reducing the cross-sectional area of this loop by bunching the leads together will reduce the electro-magnetic pick-up. (c) Re-orientating the leads so that they lie parallel to the electro-magnetic field will also reduce interference.

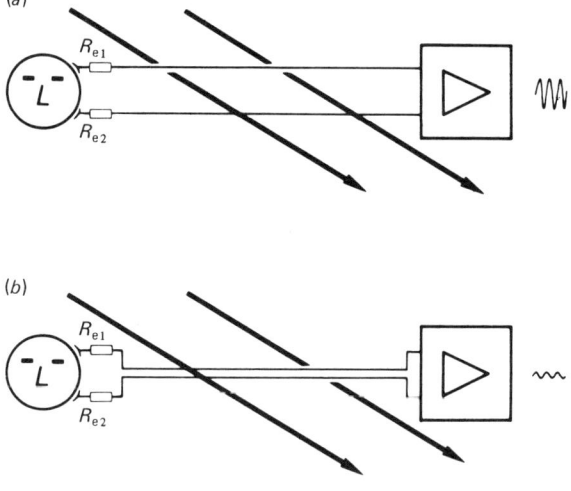

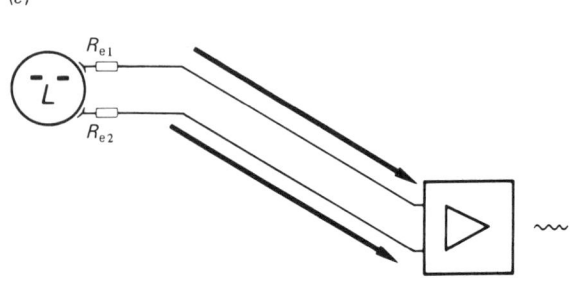

Some hospital paging systems make use of an inductive loop running around the buildings; they produce interference which can generally be recognized by its intermittent character. Electromagnetic fields from mains-operated apparatus frequently contain harmonic components at twice the mains frequency. At suitable control settings and on a machine with an adequate high-frequency response this component can be detected in the interfering signal and may help to give a clue to its nature.

8.1.2. Electro-static interference

If a conductor has a fluctuating potential with respect to earth, then a similar potential will be induced by capacitance in other nearby conductors separated from it by an insulating medium such as air. The body and the electrodes are such conductors and will pick up capacitative potentials from sources in their vicinity. By contrast with electromagnetic induction capacitative interference is dependent on the voltage of the interfering source and not upon the current. The potential induced on the patient will depend upon the impedance between his body and the source of interference and on the impedance between the body and earth, these two forming a potential divider circuit (Fig. 8.3). Thus the higher the resistance of the subject to earth and the closer his proximity to the potential source, the greater will be the induced potential. Mains-frequency electro-static induction arises from a variety of electric apparatus but slower, irregular potentials are also picked up from charged objects moving in the vicinity of the patient. The commonest cause of this second type of interference is personnel wearing rubber or plastic shoes and dressed in synthetic fabrics, and is aggravated by the use of insulating floor coverings or wax polish.

Fig. 8.2. Electromagnetic pick-up by earth loop. Electromagnetic induction may occur within the loop formed by the electrode leads and earth connections.

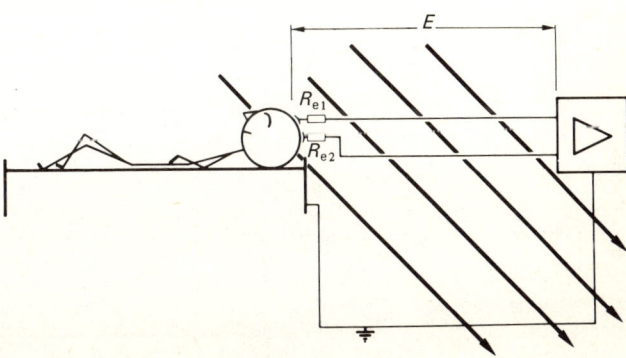

Sources of electro-static interference may be investigated by means of a simple dipole aerial attached to the input of the EEG machine (Fig. 8.4). Again the magnitude of the induced potential is affected by the distance from the source and the orientation of the aerial. In practice this means that such interference can be reduced by moving the patient away from interfering sources and

Fig. 8.3. Electrostatic interference. (a) E.m.f. (E) induced between a conductor and earth by capacitive coupling to an adjacent conductor attached to an AC source. (b) The size of the induced e.m.f. (E_1, E_2) is influenced by the distance (D_1, D_2) between the conductor, in this case the subject, and the source of interference. (c) The situation during EEG-recording: the subject is so far as possible grounded through the resistance of the earth-electrode (R_{eg}) and, provided the resistances of the recording electrodes (R_{e_1}, R_{e_2}) are equal, the interference will appear as a common mode signal at the inputs to the recorder.

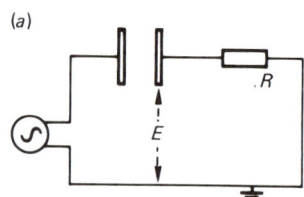

(a)

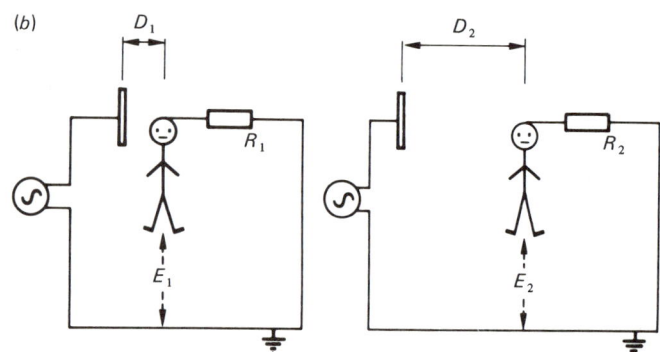

(b)

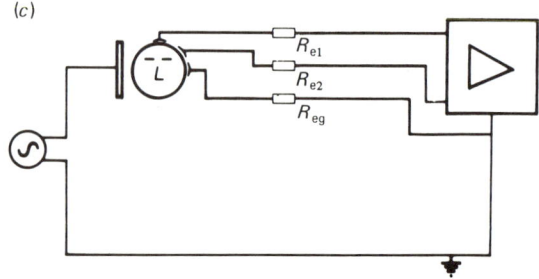

(c)

by determining an optimal orientation so that the induced potentials at all the electrodes are so far as possible equal and therefore in-phase at the input to the differential amplifiers. Lowering the resistance of the patient's earth connection will also reduce the size of the induced potential. Note however the possibility of picking up electromagnetic interference if additional earth leads are carelessly trailed around the recording area. The best method of earthing the patient is through an electrode plugged directly into the earth-socket of the headbox. In those countries where three-pin mains plugs are not used this type of interference can sometimes be reduced by re-inserting the plugs of mains operated apparatus, so that the live and neutral connections are interchanged.

Conductors near the patient may themselves act as aerials picking up electro-static interference from other objects and inducing a potential in turn in the subject. The commonest cause is a metal bedstead and the solution is to earth it (preferably to the headbox and certainly not to the patient). Sometimes the offending conductor is a person standing close to the patient, possibly to give an injection or perform some other nursing procedure. The solution is to equip him too with an earth lead or, if the bed is already earthed, to ask him to grip the bedstead firmly with one hand.

A form of capacitive interference can be produced by movements of the wires in the input cable, this should therefore be arranged tidily in a position where it will not be knocked or trodden on.

8.1.3. Radio-frequency interference

Radio-frequency (RF) signals are far outside the bandwidth of EEG recorders. They are however often modulated at lower frequencies which can appear in the tracing. For example diathermy equipment, both surgical and that used in physiotherapy, often produces

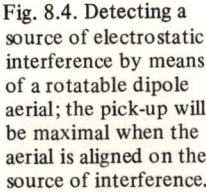

Fig. 8.4. Detecting a source of electrostatic interference by means of a rotatable dipole aerial; the pick-up will be maximal when the aerial is aligned on the source of interference.

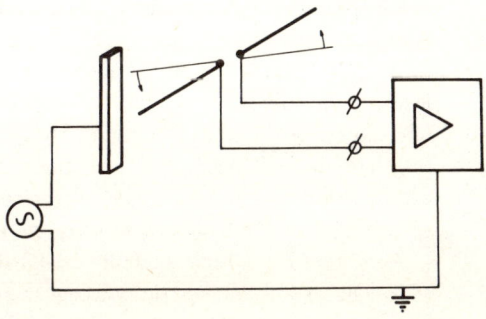

radio-frequency interference modulated at 50 or 100 Hz. Other sources include hospital paging systems and mobile transmitters used by police and ambulance services. The modulation frequency is not necessarily a harmonic of the mains, and RF interference should be suspected if signals of a constant high frequency, say 120–400 Hz, appear abruptly and intermittently in the tracing. RF signals can also cause trouble by interference effects with the carrier frequency of some amplifiers. The possibility of RF interference should be considered when selecting a location for an EEG department, and areas adjacent to a department of physical medicine, an operating theatre suite, or a transmitter used for a paging system or ambulance services should be avoided. In the event of intractable RF interference or indeed the need to record in environments where it is unavoidable, such as operating theatres, RF filters may be fitted to the EEG machine.

8.1.4. Mains-borne interference

EEG machines are generally tolerant of small, slow fluctuations in mains voltage, as may occur in rural areas, or in a building with an inadequate mains supply when apparatus drawing a large current is suddenly switched on. If the mains voltage changes by more than 10% the gain of the machine may well fluctuate and common mode rejection deteriorate.

Greater problems are presented by high-voltage spikes on the mains, usually produced by defective apparatus on the same circuit.

These difficulties can be overcome by the use of a mains filter for spikes and even a stabilized power supply if the voltage fluctuates. However they are best avoided in the first place by ensuring that a proposed EEG department has a separate mains riser.

8.1.5. Reduction of external electrical interference

As a rule modern EEG machines with a common mode rejection ratio of 10 000 to 1 or higher are not seriously affected by the levels of interference that can be expected in a normal ward, laboratory, or office environment. Excessive interference should in general be dealt with at source; arcing switch contacts on a lift can be fitted with a suppressor, small electrical appliances should be properly earthed, electric motors and the like screened.

Persistent offenders which are easily overlooked include fluorescent lights and automatic switchgear of all kinds, notably in thermostats (air conditioners, coffee-makers, refrigerators, etc.).

Attempts to screen the recording area, for example by the use of a Faraday cage, are not only expensive but also often unsuccessful. When a site for an EEG department is being chosen or if interference occurs repeatedly during recording of portable EEGs in a particular area, a simple inductive loop and dipole aerial may be used (as described in Sections 8.1.1 and 8.1.2 above) to detect and identify possible sources of interference.

8.2. Instrumental artefacts

8.2.1. Electrode defects

The ways in which electrodes can produce artefacts were discussed in Chapter 4. It should be noted that in practice there is an interaction between various factors. For instance the e.m.f. in the input circuit produced by two electrodes with slightly differing potentials will not ordinarily cause trouble during recording with AC coupled amplifiers. However, if the contact resistances also vary, for example as the subject moves, then the combination of an e.m.f. and a varying resistance will produce a fluctuating current in the circuit and therefore a varying potential across the input impedance of the amplifier. This will appear as interference. Large standing potentials in electrodes will also tend to produce marked switching artefacts or even temporary blocking of the machine when montages are changed. This effect can be reduced by machine design, either by connecting each input lead to earth through a resistance of 1 to 2 MΩ or by the provision of automatic deblocking facilities.

Unequal electrode resistances will also increase the susceptibility of the EEG machine to electro-static interference. Capacitative coupling of the subject to a source of changing potential will ordinarily produce potentials at the electrodes which are equal and in-phase, and should be rejected by a differential amplifier. However, if the electrode resistances are unequal then the currents flowing to earth through the electrode leads and the input impedance of each side of the differential amplifier will also be unequal; consequently the interfering signal becomes unbalanced and will appear in the tracing.

Apart from the contact potentials and resistances of the electrodes themselves, another source of standing potentials and of sometimes variable resistances is found in the junction between the electrode and its lead. For instance, often a copper lead is connected to a silver electrode by means of a solder containing tin and lead; when this junction becomes contaminated with electrode jelly a voltaic cell is created by the different metals immersed in electrolyte. A similar effect occurs when a clip, possibly of nickel-plated steel or brass is attached to the stem of a pad electrode. Moreover, in this case the contact resistance of the oxidized surfaces of the metals is quite high and movements of the patient will cause the clip to scrape against the electrode changing the resistance. 'Clip artefacts' have a fairly characteristic waveform but can be mistaken by the unwary for spikes. Examples of various commonly occurring types of electrode artefacts are shown in Fig. 8.5.

Faults in electrode leads and plugs may also produce spiky artefacts. If the resistance is very high or electrical continuity completely broken, mains interference often appears. The effects on the recording of a broken electrode lead or plug which has not been properly inserted into the headbox are varied and depend

Fig. 8.5. Electrode artefacts. (From Binnie and McClelland, 1977.)

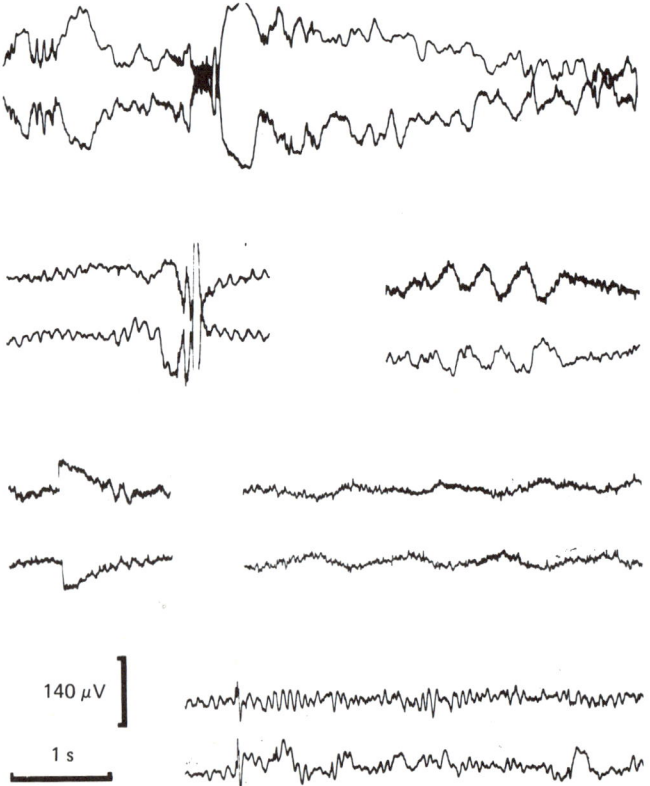

140 µV

1 s

upon the detailed design of the EEG machine. For instance, on some apparatus all the headbox input sockets are automatically connected to earth when no plug is inserted. This may result in the input lead associated with an unplugged electrode effectively being connected to the earth electrode; if this is located on the forehead, eye movement artefacts will be picked up on the affected lead. On some machines the input leads are grounded through a high resistance to reduce the effects of standing potentials when changing montages (see above). In this case the lead associated with a disconnected electrode assumes a potential approximating to that of a common average reference and will therefore pick up the higher amplitude activities recorded at other electrodes, notably eye movements and alpha rhythm.

In general, artefacts associated with electrodes and their leads are confined to a single input. They can then be readily identified, as they occur on just two adjacent channels of a bipolar chain or, in the case of reference recording, on either one channel or on all if they arise at the reference. Locating the fault is nevertheless difficult if the artefact is at an electrode not attached to a black lead but nevertheless included in a common average reference. The classical 'mirror-image' appearance of the electrode artefact occurring in the middle of a bipolar chain is not always immediately apparent if the on-going EEG activity is of high amplitude. Where the cause is movement of the subject it is possible for several electrodes to be affected simultaneously. EEG phenomena localized to only one standard electrode are very uncommon but can occur. In case of doubt it is advisable to apply additional electrodes adjacent to that picking up the suspicious activity.

Electrode lead sway produces relatively slow potentials probably due to the movement of the leads through the earth's magnetic field. These may appear on many channels during recording from a moving subject, particularly under conditions of telemetry. The problem may be solved by using leads as short and light as possible for this type of recording and securing them with adhesive tape. The effects of lead sway will be minimized if the electrode impedances are low (Gatzke, 1974). The Teflon-coated wire used on needle electrodes readily becomes electrostatically charged and may give rise to spiky artefacts if the leads move.

8.2.2. Machine faults
Total failure of a machine to run is often due to loss of mains

supply. If there is an illuminated indicator associated with the mains switch, such a fault will be quickly identified. Otherwise one should check the mains socket, plug and lead. Alternatively a fuse may have blown. Often there is a single mains fuse together with secondary fuses to protect individual circuits. If one unplugs the mains lead from the socket outlet and measures the resistance between the live and neutral pins, with the machine switched on, a value above 1000 Ω will indicate either that the lead or plug is defective, that the mains fuse has blown, or, less probably, that there is a fault in the winding of the mains transformer. Failure of secondary fuses may be suspected if some parts of the machine work and others not. For instance the pens may move when switched on but the paper drive may not respond. Machines with jet galvanometers have a mains cut-out which prevents the apparatus being run with an empty ink bottle. If such a machine is left running, for example on a ward, attended by nursing personnel not familiar with this feature, they may assume that some serious fault has developed. The technician should know the locations of the fuses on the apparatus which he routinely uses and be able to change them. If the fuse blows again shortly after being changed, a fault, and possibly a safety hazard, is present and the apparatus should on no account be used again until it has been checked by a qualified engineer.

Apart from total failure of the machine to run, and the various faults which have already been discussed in connection with calibration (Section 6.2) the other types of machine failure which commonly occur during recording may produce any of the following effects:

interference at mains or sometimes other frequencies
high noise level
abnormal (usually long) time constants
unstable baseline or sustained deflection of a channel
transient artefacts (mostly spiky in character)
inappropriate distribution of bio-electrical activity (e.g. two channels identical or eye movement apparently at the back of the head).

All of these faults can arise either from defective switches or from amplifier failure. The first step is to check all the switches in the affected channel or channels. They may be rotated rapidly to clean possibly dirty contacts or re-set to different values. When performing this test do not forget master controls such as the switch used to choose between calibration, preselectors and independent selectors, or switches associated with deblocking, electrode resistance measurements, etc. If these measures do not locate the fault, the next step is to replicate the derivation and control settings of the defective channel on another channel. If this fails to reproduce the fault, indicating that it probably arises in the electrodes, headbox or input cable, one may exchange amplifiers between affected and unaffected channels. This will generally indicate which, if any, amplifier module is faulty. Interchanging amplifiers generally takes some minutes and many EEG machines are equipped with a reserve channel which can be switched in to replace one which is defective. In this case one may complete the investigation and attempt to trace the fault afterwards.

8.3. Biological artefacts

A variety of bio-electrical phenomena of non-cerebral origin may be recorded together with the EEG. From the standpoint of obtaining a legible EEG tracing these may be regarded as artefacts but, under other circumstances, they are useful biological signals which one may indeed wish to record (see Chapter 9). Even where purely incidental findings, they may assist the interpretation of the EEG. For instance slow lateral eye movements are a valuable sign of drowsiness; eye opening and eye closing artefacts record on the trace precisely the point in time where the patient opened or shut his eyes; frequent blinking and a large amount of myogenic activity may indicate the subject is tense; short bursts of EMG activity may mark the occurrence of myoclonic jerks; above all, eye movements provide a valuable test signal for checking the functioning of the entire recording system.

8.3.1. Eye movement artefacts

The cornea is some tens of millivolts positive with respect to the retina, the exact value depending upon, amongst other factors, the brightness of the ambient lighting. With an AC coupled recording system this potential is not apparent as long as the eyes and lids remain stationary. If the eye is rotated, the electrodes towards which the cornea is moving undergo a positive change with respect to the others; conversely the electrodes from which the cornea recedes will change in a negative direction. Thus, for instance, when one looks to the right, F8 undergoes a positive change with respect to its neighbours and F7 a negative change. Similarly an upward eye movement will cause both prefrontal

Fig. 8.6. Oculographic artefacts recorded with (*a*) bipolar and (*b*) common average reference derivation. The movements are in order upwards, downwards, right, left, eyes shut and eyes open. Note that in order to enhance the legibility of this illustration a lower than usual sensitivity has been used; at a more normal setting the larger movements will produce artefacts outside the dynamic range of the recorder. (*c*) Myogenic artefacts thought to arise from the lateral rectus muscle and associated with involuntary lateral eye movements.

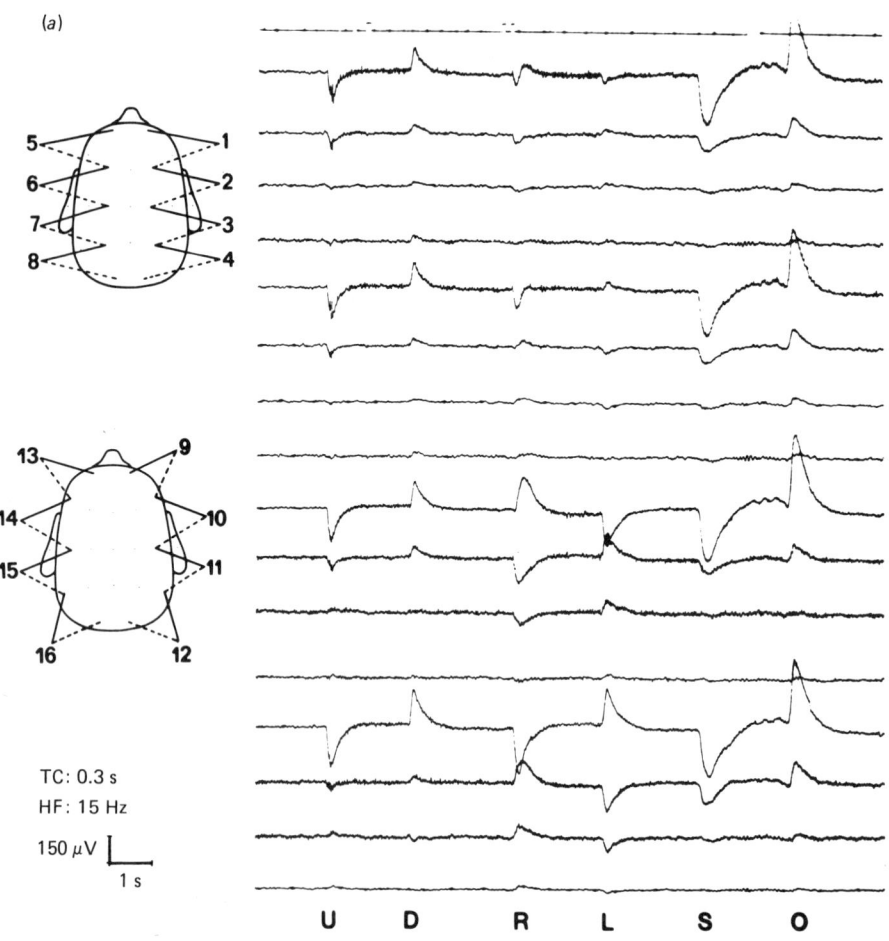

(*a*)

TC: 0.3 s
HF: 15 Hz

150 μV

1 s

U   D   R   L   S   O

(b)

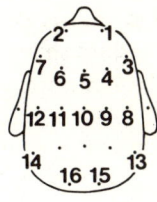

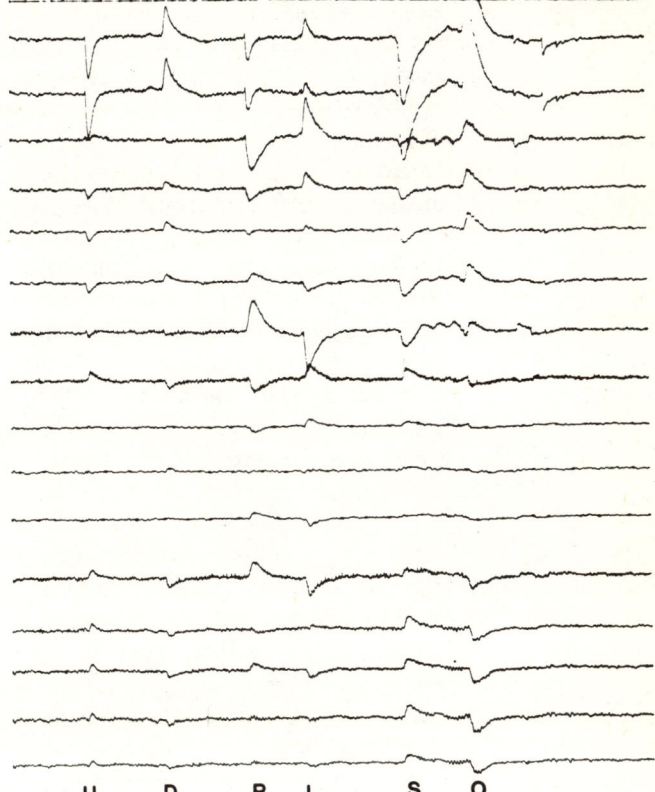

TC: 0.3 s

HF: 15 Hz

150 μV ⌐

1 s

U   D   R   L   S   O

(c)

TC: 0.3 s

HF: 70 Hz

70 μV ⌐

1 s

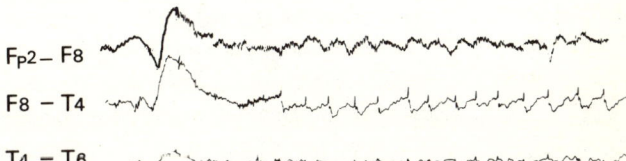

$F_{P2} - F_8$

$F_8 - T_4$

$T_4 - T_6$

$T_6 - O_1$

electrodes to undergo a positive change which will also be detected but less markedly at the superior frontal electrodes. A useful exercise of both theoretical and practical value which a student technician should be asked to carry out within the first few weeks of training, is to record voluntary eye movements in vertical and horizontal directions with standard bipolar and common reference montages (Fig. 8.6) (Nelligan, 1964).

Closure of the eyes produces a positive-going change at the frontal electrodes for two reasons: firstly the eyes reflexly roll upwards (Bell's phenomenon) and secondly, because the resistance of the eyelids is lower than that of air, there is an increased spread of the corneal potential over the forehead (Zao, Gelbin and Rémond, 1952). During blinking only the second of these factors applies (Stones, Whitehead and MacGillivray, 1967) and the distribution of the potential change produced by blinking is slightly different from that of eye closure. Every technician of more than a few weeks experience should be able, on sight, to recognize the different types of eye movement artefacts. Unless one eye is diseased (or absent) or there is paralysis of the external ocular muscles, eye movements and the artefacts they produce are symmetrical. Any asymmetry should be regarded with suspicion (as evidence of possibly asymmetrical electrode placement) and grossly anomalous distribution (Fig. 6.13) almost always indicates a technical fault.

If one is familiar with the appearance and distribution of eye movement potentials it is usually not difficult to distinguish these from frontal slow activity. On a machine with a reserve channel or when the montage does not require the use of all available channels, it is convenient to monitor eye movement, for instance between an electrode placed 10 mm above the outer canthus of one eye and another 10 mm below the outer canthus of the other. It must not be forgotten that such a derivation will also pick up electrical activity of cerebral origin. If in doubt one may ask a colleague to place the fingers upon the patient's closed lids with a light downwards pressure, both to reduce, and to monitor, eye movements. If one is working alone, the patient can sometimes himself prevent eye movement by placing his fingers on the lids, or small coins balanced upon the closed lids of a recumbent subject may render the eye movement easily visible to a technician seated at the machine. Various mechanical eye movement transducers have been devised for use during routine EEG recording (Papakostopoulos, Winter and Newton, 1973). However, most require one eye to be covered and are uncomfortable or likely to worry an anxious subject.

All of these measures are likely to change state of awareness and may therefore influence the EEG and particularly the occurrence of frontal slow activity. In the few circumstances where doubt remains, one should apply additional electrodes below the eyes if the suspected movements are vertical, or adjacent to the external canthi, if they are lateral. Derivations can then be taken from electrodes on opposite sides of the orbit to a remote, occipital reference. When the eye moves, the cornea approaches one electrode of the pair and recedes from the other producing opposite potential changes and consequently opposite deflections. By contrast, slow activity at the front of the head will probably affect these electrodes approximately equally and the deflections will be of like polarity (Fig. 8.7). The suspected frontal slow activity can also be compared with known eye movements by asking the patient to look up and down, from side to side, or open and shut the eyes.

Lateral saccadic eye movements are sometimes accompanied by tiny EMG spikes from the lateral rectus muscle (Fig. 8.6). Once

Fig. 8.7. A montage suitable for distinguishing vertical eye movements from frontal slow activity. Note the phase reversal between the infra-orbital (channels 11, 12) and prefrontal (channels 9 and 10) electrodes. Frontal slow activity will be in-phase between such derivations.

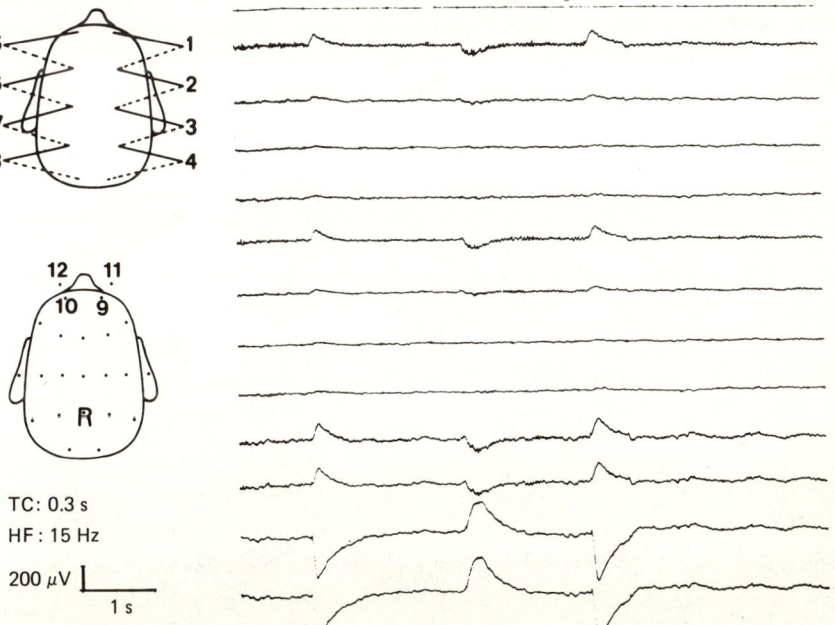

TC: 0.3 s
HF: 15 Hz

200 μV

1 s

the relationship with eye movement is recognized the likelihood of misinterpretation is small.

8.3.2. Myogenic potentials

Electromyographic activity is recorded in the scalp EEG chiefly from the temporalis, masseter and occipito-frontalis muscles and it is therefore most prominent at prefrontal, temporal and occipital electrodes. It is also very troublesome at some electrode sites off the scalp, on the chin and neck in particular. Continuous myogenic activity generally indicates a tense patient. Short bursts of diffuse high-voltage EMG artefacts are seen in association with swallowing, and rhythmic bursting at about 2/s during chewing (a problem which seldom arises except during long-term EEG telemetry). EMG artefacts can generally be identified by the very short duration of the spikes in relation to their amplitude and the irregularity of waveform and frequency (Fig. 8.8). However on occasions the distinction between EMG and EEG spikes may be impossible, particularly during myoclonic jerks or an epileptic seizure where movement, muscular activity and cortical discharges may occur simultaneously.

Myogenic activity due to tension may be reduced by helping the patient to relax, both mentally and physically, adjusting his pillow if necessary and asking him to let the mouth fall slightly open. If all else fails, it may be advisable to stop the recording, offer him a glass of water, and spend some more time talking

Fig. 8.8. EMG artefact. (a) Two examples, showing regular, and irregular, waveforms. (b) Characteristic brief wide-spread EMG artefact together with an eye-blink associated with swallowing. (c) Repeated brief bilaterally synchronous EMG artefacts characteristic of chewing movements.

(a)

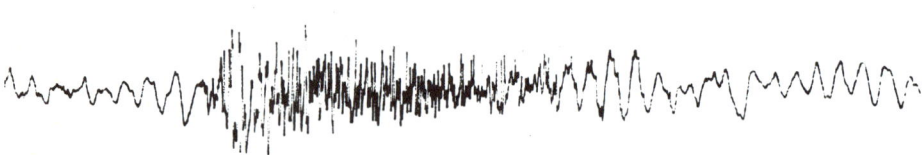

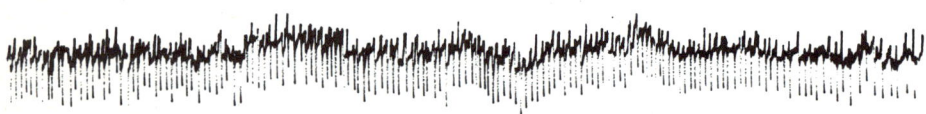

with him. One must also check that the patient is not in discomfort due, for instance, to an arthritic hip or a full bladder. The use of HF filters to reduce myogenic activity is a measure of last resort; it may protect the pens from damage and prevent ink being spattered about but it does not greatly enhance the legibility of the EEG. After filtration, myogenic potentials may be even more difficult to distinguish from beta activity or cerebral spikes than they were before. If the machine has jet galvanometers, which both have a good high-frequency response and do not present the risk of damage to the pens by high-amplitude signals,

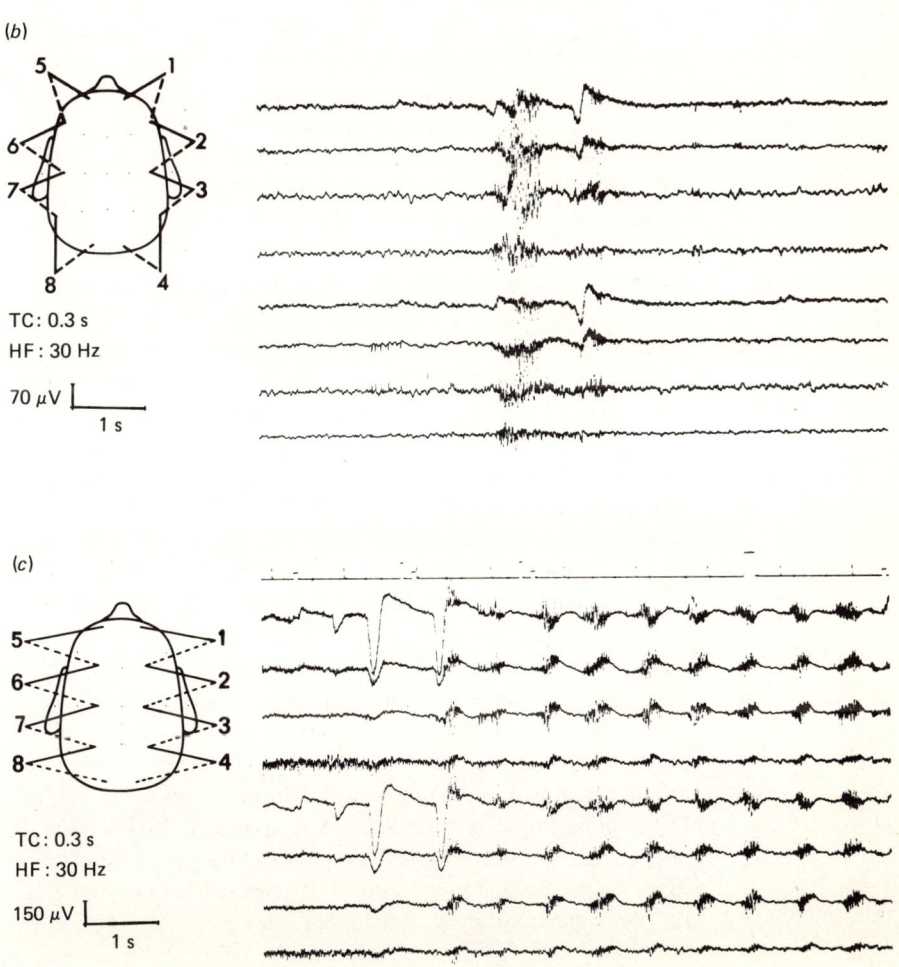

(b)

TC: 0.3 s
HF: 30 Hz

70 μV

1 s

(c)

TC: 0.3 s
HF: 30 Hz

150 μV

1 s

it is preferable to tolerate a certain amount of EMG artefact than to attempt to filter it out.

8.3.3. Electrocardiographic artefact

The orientation of the electrical field of the heart in normal subjects is usually such that the potential gradients which it produces over the scalp are quite small. Consequently ECG pick-up does not often present major problems in bipolar EEG recordings with closely-spaced scalp electrodes. However, when derivations are made between widely-spaced electrodes, as happens with common reference recording, and particularly if the reference electrode is not on the scalp but over the mastoid process, neck or chin, the ECG is readily picked up. Prominent electrocardiographic artefacts also occur in the EEG when the electrical field of the heart is abnormal. This may arise as a result of cardiac disease (for instance left ventricular hypertrophy in a patient with high blood pressure) or may be a consequence of physical rotation of the heart due to obesity, pregnancy, lung disease, fluid in the abdomen, or just an unusually broad or narrow build.

Electrocardiographic activity can generally be recognized by its wave form, frequency and regularity (Fig. 8.9), but should always be checked by simultaneous recording of an ECG with electrodes on the wrists, chest or shoulders.

Little can be done to reduce ECG artefact apart from changing the posture of the patient if it is due to physical rotation of the heart. The ease generally of recognizing an ECG artefact in the electroencephalogram is no excuse for failure to monitor the ECG itself. In particular, extrasystoles have an abnormal ECG field and may therefore appear in the EEG as isolated spikes or sharp waves which are not regular and will not be correctly identified without simultaneous ECG monitoring. In some departments the ECG is therefore recorded throughout the EEG investigation and indeed an ECG channel may conveniently split up a 16 or 20 channel montage and assist the electroencephalographer to interpret the trace without having to count individual channels. If the ECG is not recorded throughout, ECG electrodes should be applied at the beginning of the investigation so that an ECG can be immediately registered if necessary. If one waits until the patient becomes drowsy and exhibits some suspicious sharp waves, belatedly applying electrodes will arouse him and the phenomenon of interest may disappear.

8.3.4. Mechanical artefacts of cardiac origin

The pulsations of an artery in the scalp underlying an EEG electrode may produce a regular artefact, generally consisting of rounded or saw-tooth slow waves at the same frequency as the pulse. The chief offenders are the superficial temporal and posterior auricular arteries and therefore the mid- and posterior-temporal electrodes are most often affected. The identity of the artefact can be confirmed by simultaneous ECG recording (Fig. 8.10). Pulse artefact can sometimes be reduced by re-applying the electrode, but usually it must be displaced. If this is done one must of course take the abnormal electrode location into account when interpreting the EEG.

A more widespread rhythmic artefact is also sometimes produced by a ballisto-cardiographic mechanism, that is to say, by the vibrations of the entire body produced by cardiac action. The artefact is generally of very low amplitude, and therefore most often seen in iso-electric recordings taken in the intensive care

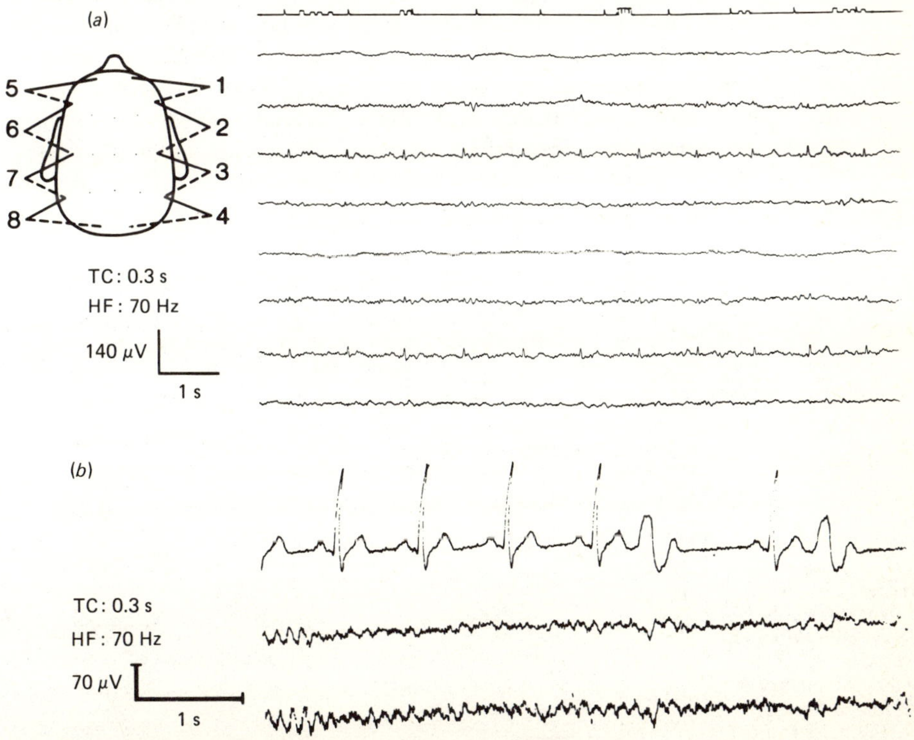

Fig. 8.9. ECG artefact. (a) A fairly typical distribution with maximal amplitude over the temporal regions. (b) An abnormal ECG complex may produce transient artefacts in the EEG even when no continuous ECG artefact is present; in this patient ventricular extrasystoles were associated with apparent theta waves on the EEG.

(a)

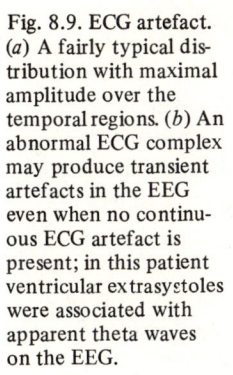

5 — 1
6 — 2
7 — 3
8 — 4

TC: 0.3 s
HF: 70 Hz

140 μV

1 s

(b)

TC: 0.3 s
HF: 70 Hz

70 μV

1 s

unit. It generally appears over those electrodes which are in contact with the pillow. The synchrony with the ECG should enable the artefact to be identified but is not always obvious, partly because many of these patients have an irregular cardiac action, but chiefly because the waveform is often bi- or triphasic and therefore not obviously at the cardiac frequency (Fig. 8.11).

This artefact can readily be mistaken for cerebral activity in a situation where it is vitally important to establish whether cerebral activity is, or is not, in fact present. It can be eliminated or its distribution altered by repositioning the patient so that the affected electrodes are no longer in contact with the pillow.

8.3.5. Movement artefacts

Movement of the subject may result in a varying electrode contact resistance, particularly when pad electrodes are used, and also in swaying of electrode leads. Movement artefacts thus result from a combination of instrumental and biological factors. They can to some extent be reduced by good electrode application, the use of self-retaining electrodes rather than pads, and, during telemetry, by the use of leads which are light and as short as possible. Movement artefacts are recognizable by the relationship to the observed activity of the subject, but if reliable observation presents dif-

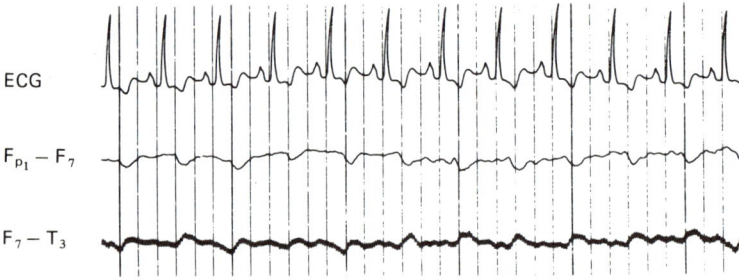

ECG

$F_{p_1} - F_7$

$F_7 - T_3$

Fig. 8.10. Pulse artefact. This cannot be identified by its regularity and waveform alone, but must always be established by simultaneous recording of the ECG (note similarity to fifth example of Fig. 8.5).

TC: 0.3 s

HF: 35 Hz

140 μV

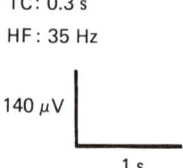

1 s

ficulty this may be improved by the use of a tremor transducer. These artefacts occur particularly at electrodes in contact with the pillow or headrest, and this helps to indicate their origin. A further clue is given by the fact that they are often accompanied by myogenic potentials. Nevertheless, under circumstances where paroxysmal EEG activity may be expected in association with movement (for instance during a tonic-clonic seizure or accompanying myoclonus) reliable identification of movement artefacts can be extremely difficult. The use of a tremor transducer at least allows the timing of the recorded waveform to be closely compared with that of the movement.

Two particular instances of movement artefact may be noted, the rhythmic activity sometimes seen in association with tremor and the slower undulating changes occurring with respiration, particularly during hyperventilation (Fig. 8.12). Changes in the skin potential may also contribute to the artefacts during

Fig. 8.11. Ballistocardio-graphic artefact. The triphasic waveform does not immediately suggest an artefact of cardiac origin, but increasing the gain (at arrow) reveals that it is phase-locked to an EEG artefact. Without this clue ECG recording (below) would have been essential to identify the phenomenon. The EEG was in fact iso-electric.

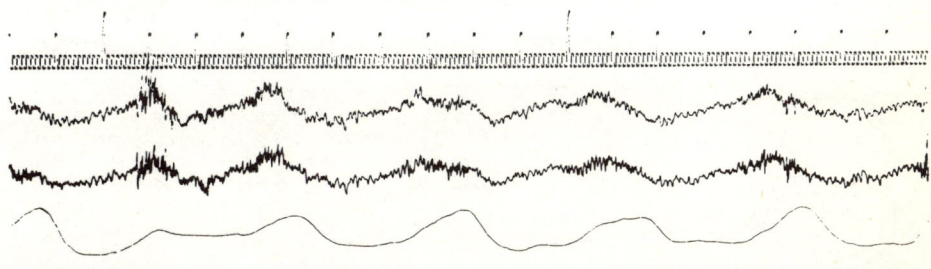

70 μV

1 s

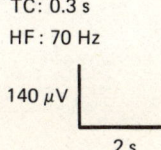

Fig. 8.12. Respiration artefact. Bipolar derivations $F_{p_2}-F_8$, F_8-T_4 compared with output of respiration monitor (thermocouple in nostril). Respiration rate was about 20/minute (note reduced paper speed).

TC: 0.3 s
HF: 70 Hz

140 μV

2 s

hyperventilation. If there is any doubt about the origin of a poss-ible tremor or respiratory artefact, tremor or respiration respec-tively should be monitored (see Chapter 9).

8.3.6. Cutaneous artefacts

Changes in sweat glands or in the capillaries of the skin produce alterations both in the resistance and potential of the skin. These may indeed be intentionally recorded as the 'psycho-galvanic skin reflex' (see Chapter 9). During EEG recording with time constants of the order of 0.3 s the phenomena become prominent only when the patient is obviously sweating (Fig. 8.13). The solution is to attempt to cool the subject by the provision of a fan or moistening his brow with ether.

Fig. 8.13. Sweat artefact on channels 9 to 12 and 16. Note that this was recorded at the time constant of 0.3 s, with a longer setting the artefact would have probably been even more marked.

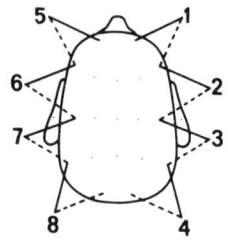

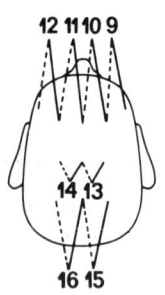

HF: 70 Hz
TC: 0.3 s

140 μV

1 s

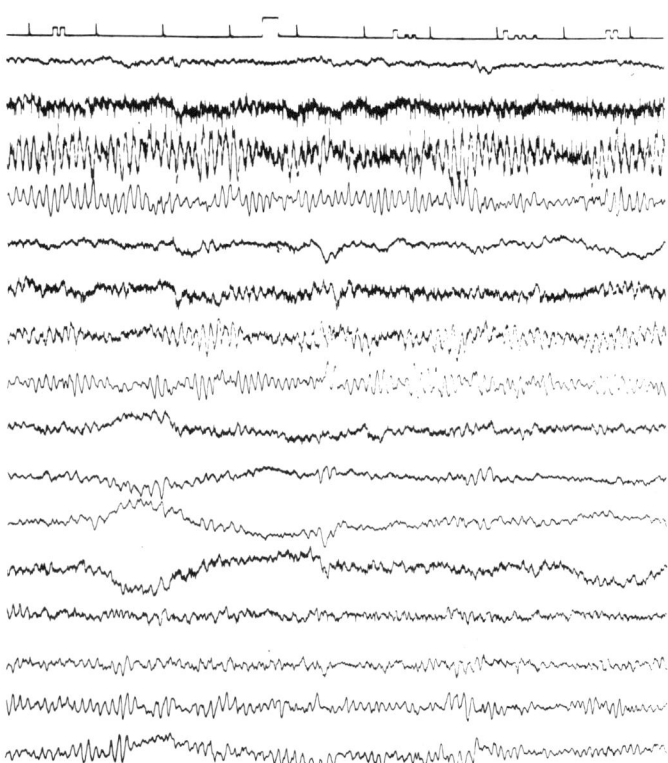

8.3.7. Rarer types of artefacts

Unusual artefacts are a happy hunting ground for the collector
of EEG exotica. They include photochemical effects arising at
the surfaces of electrodes during photic stimulation, spikes due to
electro-statically charged drips falling in an infusion apparatus,
bursts of irregular spikes or slow waves seen when bubbles form
in the tubing of an artificial ventilator, spikes due to bi-metallic
effects produced by dissimilar filling materials in the subject's
teeth and a low-amplitude activity in the theta range produced
by vibration of the bed. Fig. 8.14 illustrates some examples.

The best rule is to assume that all unusual EEG phenomena are
artefactual until proved otherwise, but at the same time not to
accept that the phenomenon is artefactual without trying to
obtain supportive evidence. An account by Radcliffe, Darby and
Tierney (1969) of a patient with an unusual fast activity at almost
50 Hz, which was not due to mains interference, provides an
interesting cautionary tale.

Fig. 8.14. Some unusual
artefacts: (a) Bilaterally
synchronous slow waves,
produced by move-
ments of the tongue.

(a)

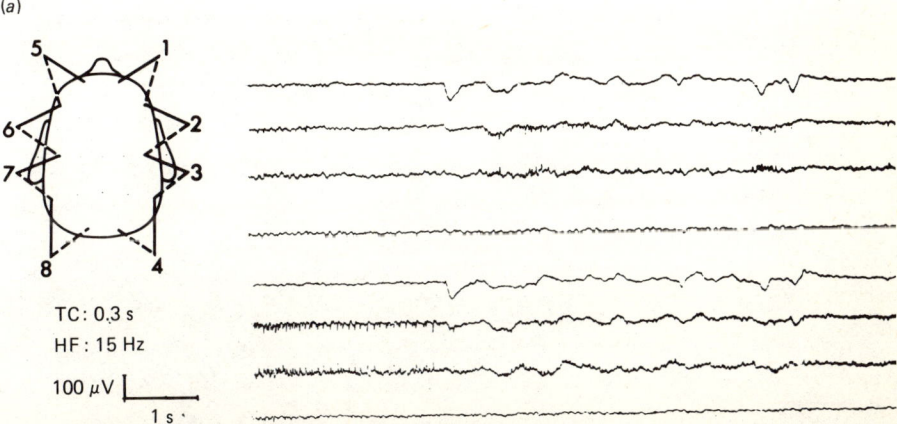

TC: 0.3 s
HF: 15 Hz

100 μV

1 s

Fig. 8.14. (cont.) (b) A rhythmic activity at about 6 Hz on channel 4 of the otherwise very low-amplitude EEG of a moribund patient in an intensive-care unit. This activity was due to vibration of the bed in contact with electrode O_2; the last 3 seconds of the extract show the disappearance of the artefact after a pillow had been placed under the patient's neck to prevent contact of the electrode with the bed (from Binnie, 1975b).

(b)

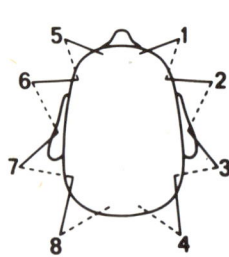

HF: 70 Hz

TC: 0.3 s

140 μV

1 s

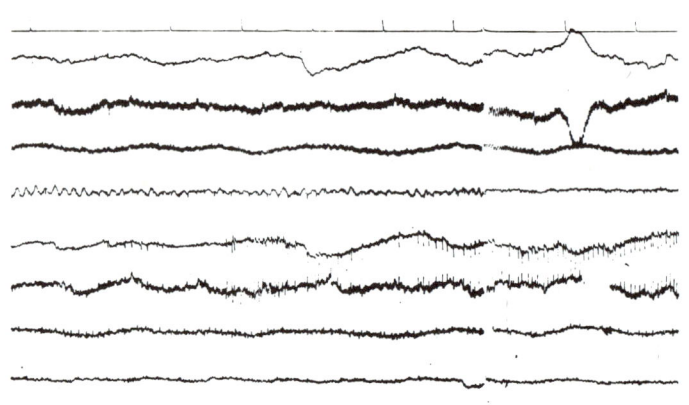

Fig. 8.14. (cont.) (c) Movement artefact superficially resembling epileptiform activity during a simulated tonic convulsion in a healthy subject. The unusual waveform and distribution would arouse the suspicion of any experienced observer. Note, however, that this illustration was deliberately recorded at a low sensitivity; at a more usual setting the waveform and distribution might have been difficult to determine (from Binnie, 1980).

(c)

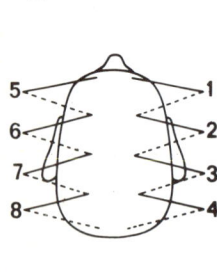

TC: 0.3 s

HF: 30 Hz

150 μV

1 s

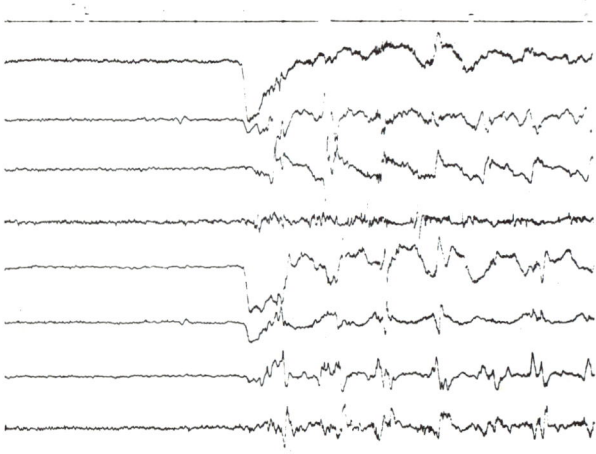

Fig. 8.14. (cont.) (d) Intermittent high-frequency interference from hospital paging system (middle and lower channels) with 50 Hz main interference for comparison (upper channel).

(d)

140 μV

1 s

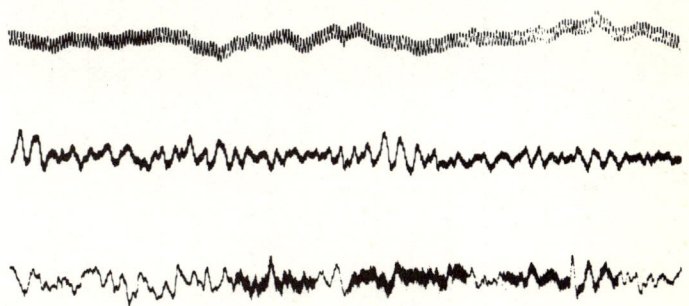

Fig. 8.14. (cont.) (e) Periodic bursts of spiky activity due to air bubbling through condensed fluid in the plastic tube connecting an unconscious patient to a respirator. This phenomenon closely resembles EEG wave-forms which may occur under similar clinical circumstances (from Binnie, 1975b).

(e)

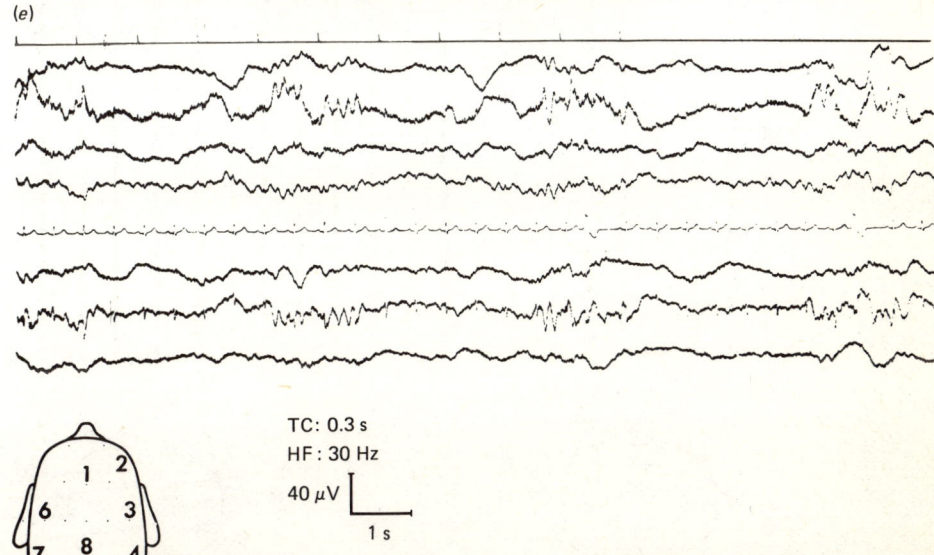

TC: 0.3 s
HF: 30 Hz
40 μV

1 s

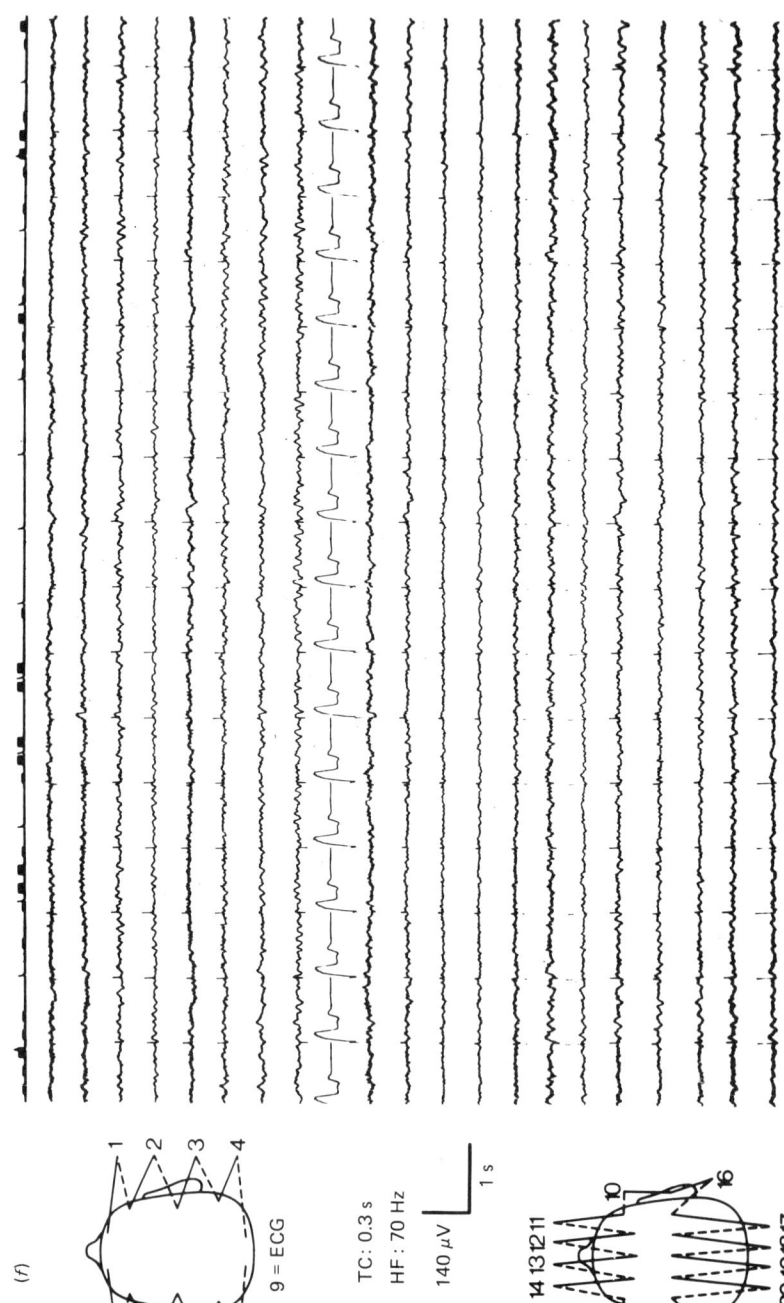

Fig. 8.14. (cont.)
(f) Artefact from
cardiac pace-maker.
Note wide-spread
prominent artefact
synchronous with ECG
but of very short
duration; ECG is itself
abnormal.

(f)

9 = ECG

TC: 0.3 s

HF: 70 Hz

140 μV

1 s

9. Special recording procedures

9.1. Intensive care

EEG recording in an Intensive Care Unit (ICU) is one of the most interesting, worthwhile, and difficult tasks with which the EEG technician is confronted. The findings may be literally life-saving, not least when the EEG justifies continued support of a patient who, on clinical grounds, would have been abandoned as beyond help. The technical difficulties are threefold. Firstly, the EEG signals themselves may be of extremely low amplitude demanding high recording sensitivities, and indeed one of the most exacting tasks is to establish in a case of suspected brain death that EEG activity is absent. Secondly, there are a multiplicity of mains-operated electrical devices in the environment of, or attached to, the patient, any of which may be sources of severe electrical interference especially when a high recording sensitivity has to be used. Finally, the situation is made yet more difficult for the technician by the need to disrupt as little as possible the intensive nursing procedures and often also cope with doctors, nurses or relatives requesting an immediate interpretation of the findings.

Generally a portable or at least transportable EEG machine will be used for ICU recordings, and this may be equipped with some special facilities either to reduce interference (mains frequency notch filters) or for enhanced patient safety (isolated input). A comprehensive kit of all materials and accessories required for emergency mobile EEGs should be kept permanently with the machine in a box or on the trolley. Some suggestions are given in Appendix V but note in particular the need for respiration and tremor transducers and an earth lead. The technician should be assisted either by a colleague, or, ideally, by a nurse with experience both of intensive care and of EEG procedures. The value of this type of expert help in coordinating the EEG investigation with the nursing procedures is considerable. The normal documentation provided by the request form and the technician's notes (see Chapter 6) should be supplemented by detailed information concerning vital functions, therapeutic procedures, medication, etc. and it is generally useful to use a proforma for this purpose (see Appendix V).

Both the urgency of the investigation and the need to minimize the disturbance to other activities in the ICU demands that the EEG team work fast. One technician may therefore calibrate the machine whilst the other measures the head and they may apply electrodes together. If the second member of the EEG team is a nurse she too should learn the necessary technical skills.

The choice of electrodes will depend upon the clinical situation. If the patient is unconscious and immobile, needles can be most quickly applied. The theoretical objection that these shorten the time constant of the recording system is immaterial as it does not in practice result in loss of information within the bandwidth of EEG recording. Nevertheless, for this reason needles are not considered acceptable for EEGs recorded as an aid to establish brain death. Before needles are used it is necessary to check that the patient is not likely to have an abnormal bleeding tendency (due for instance to anti-coagulants, liver failure, septicaemia, etc.). Where needles are not suitable disc electrodes should be used. They can be applied marginally faster with bentonite than with collodion and this may have some advantages if the patient is moving little. Pad electrodes are in general unacceptable for intensive care recording. It will generally be necessary to turn an unconscious patient, to apply the electrodes first to one side and then to the other, and the technician must be prepared to modify his usual procedure and sequence of electrode application.

In the majority of intensive care units, when the EEG machine is switched on, profuse mains-frequency interference may be anticipated. With experience the technician learns to accept this as a matter of routine rather than as a cause for dismay. It is then necessary systematically to check, and so far as possible, eliminate, sources of interference. If some electrode resistances, though within the acceptable range are higher than the others, they should be reduced (assuming that needles are not in use), electrode leads scattered over the pillow should be bunched close together; various positions of the mains cable and of the EEG machine may be tried in order to reduce interference. So far as possible all the equipment attached to the patient should be connected to a single mains distribution panel and in particular trailing leads and portable distribution boards should be avoided. With the consent and help of the nursing staff the mains cables in the vicinity of the patient can thus be tidied up. The less vital items of equipment can be switched off and unplugged to determine whether or not they contribute to the interference (electric blankets, rectal thermocouple, ripple bed, electric fans, etc.). Then, again with the co-operation of the nursing staff, certain life-support or monitoring equipment may be briefly disconnected. The ECG can be recorded on one channel of the EEG machine and the ECG monitor turned off, and the ventilator pump replaced by a manually operated Ambu bag. The possibility of multiple earth connections should be checked, not only to reduce interference, but also in the interests of safety. The patient is probably earthed at least through the ECG machine, and possibly through a rectal temperature monitor, a blood pressure transducer, or antistatic bedding. Sometimes the solution is to disconnect the earth electrode of the EEG machine; often it is better to provide an improved earth, or to earth conductors in the vicinity of the patient, such as the bedstead. After mains interference has been minimized, one may then set about identifying and reducing other artefacts. The commonest are those due to ECG or respiration. Others may arise from tremor, shivering when the patient is cooled, other unvoluntary movements, the ballistocardiogram, vibration of the bed, electrostatically charged drips in an infusion, and bubbles of condensed fluid in the plastic tubing of a ventilator (see Chapter 8). It is not acceptable, particularly where brain death is in question, to accept any phenomenon as artefactual simply because of its appearance. In all cases the appropriate function (ECG, respiration, tremor, etc.) must be simultaneously monitored on the chart.

Minimal technical criteria for EEG recording in connection with the establishment of brain death have been proposed (Silverman, Masland, Saunders and Schwab, 1969). These include low electrode resistances, the use of maximum bandwidth compatible with a legible EEG recording, a sensitivity of at least 20 μV/cm, and the use of both bipolar chains and also montages with large inter-electrode distances. The recording should last at least half an hour and various stimuli including pain should be applied to see whether or not there is any behavioural or EEG response. If one suddenly approaches the patient to apply a painful stimulus a capacitative artefact will generally be seen and the best method is to earth oneself to the bedstead with one hand, grip one anterior axillary fold (the fleshy part in front of the armpit) with the other, and when artefacts have subsided apply strong pressure. All stimulation should be noted on the chart and the single-handed technician will need to use a remote event marker.

Careful clinical observation and annotation of the chart are even more important than in more routine EEG practice. Changes in state of awareness, small twitches which may represent epileptic seizures, and irregularities of respiratory rate should all be noted, and where possible monitored with the appropriate transducers.

For most purposes requiring EEG recording in the intensive

care unit, it is desirable that the person required to interpret the EEG should be present during part of the tracing. Therefore, after technical problems have been solved and some 15 minutes of tracing obtained, it is appropriate to call the electroencephalographer concerned. If the EEG findings suggest a condition requiring immediate treatment for which EEG monitoring might be required, for instance status epilepticus, on the spot interpretation should be requested before the electrodes are removed.

On completion of the recording it may be useful to establish whether a further tracing is likely to be required within the next 24 hours and if so, again with the agreement of the nursing staff, it may be reasonable for stick-on electrodes to be left in place. Though one must be guided by common sense and the interests of the patient rather than by a strictly legalistic approach, in general the technician should refuse to offer any interpretation of the EEG findings no matter who asks. He does however have the responsibility to ensure the record is interpreted by a qualified person with such urgency as the situation may demand.

Any account of the EEG in the intensive care would not be complete without mentioning the possible use of simple devices such as the Cerebral Function Monitor (Maynard, Prior and Scott, 1969) to measure the amount of EEG activity over a long period of time and provide an indication of any trends. This provides a valuable supplement to more comprehensive EEG recordings. Evoked response studies (see Section 12.3) are sometimes also performed in a deeply unconscious patient as an aid to establishing whether or not cerebral electrical activity can be demonstrated. For this application a mobile special-purpose evoked response system is used incorporating both stimulators and an averager.

9.2. Recording in the operating theatre

The problems of recording in the operating theatre are not dissimilar from those encountered in the ICU. Again, one may anticipate many sources of electrical interference and EEG recording will have to be coordinated with the work of others. The anaesthetist and the theatre sister are usually responsible for organizing the activities of the paramedical personnel during an operation and the technician should consult them in advance about the location of the EEG machine and the most convenient time to apply electrodes etc.

Certain apparatus used in the theatre may present an unusually powerful source of electrical interference, sufficient indeed to

cause damage to the EEG machine. This includes surgical diathermy, defibrillators, pacemakers, and fibrillators (used to stop
cardiac action during some heart operations). It is possible to record whilst any of these are in use, but only by the addition of
RF-filters or other modifications of the EEG equipment. When a
machine without these features is used it may be prudent to
suspend the recording and disconnect the input lead during the
use of diathermy or the defibrillator. The patient will in any event
have one earth connection provided for surgical diathermy and in
order to reduce interference it may be better to use this as the
earth for EEG recording rather than a separate electrode on the
scalp. Subject to the agreement of the anaesthetist, the most
satisfactory time to apply EEG electrodes may be after anaesthesia
has been induced and whilst the patient is being positioned on the
table and prepared for operation. Considerable skill and speed
on the part of the technician may be required. Application of EEG
electrodes to the conscious patient often causes alarm and it is
probably not helpful to draw the attention of someone about to
undergo open heart surgery to the fact that the operation may
affect his cerebral function. Even if for the purposes of EEG
monitoring a small number of electrodes appears to be sufficient,
additional electrodes should generally be applied, because access
to the head during the operation may be restricted and the only
solution to malfunction of electrodes may be to change the
montage.

Sterilization of the EEG apparatus is impractical but the theatre
staff may well wish to wipe the machine, and particularly the
wheels, with disinfectant. If EEG recording is performed routinely
during operations, a separate EEG room may be provided, separated
from the theatre by a window and with communication by
intercom.

Simple monitoring devices as described in the preceding section
may be more suitable than the conventional EEG for registering
the level of anaesthesia and detecting cerebral catastrophies.

9.2.1. Electrocorticography

Electrocorticography, recording from the exposed surface of the
brain, is the most exacting form of EEG recording in theatre. The
course of the operation may depend upon the findings; immediate
interpretation of the record and close collaboration and communication between the surgeon and the EEG personnel are
therefore vital. From this point of view, it is most satisfactory for

the recording apparatus to be in the operating theatre. However, if this is not acceptable, good two-way communication must be provided so that the electroencephalographer can see the operative field, and the surgeon the EEG chart. This may be achieved either by a large window or by closed circuit television. Detailed annotation of the whole procedure is desirable, conversations between the surgeon and the electroencephalographer may be recorded or taken down by a stenographer. Sketches and possibly photographs should be made of the electrode sites, usually by the surgeon himself, or by the electroencephalographer.

The characteristics of the electro-corticogram (ECoG) differ from those of the EEG in some important particulars and these have consequences for technique and instrumentation. The ECoG is in general 5–10 times greater in amplitude than the EEG but in particular the fast background activities and the fast components of spike discharges are much more prominent. Conversely, slow activities are relatively less important and the quantity of low-frequency artefacts greater. ECoG phenomena may be very sharply localized and thus, though the operative field is relatively small, a large number of electrodes and a greater number of channels may be required than in routine EEG practice. Though it is possible to obtain adequate ECoGs with a conventional EEG machine, the ideal apparatus would have some 30 or more channels, a rather better high-frequency response than many EEG machines, a short deblocking time, preferably automatic deblocking, and possibly a greater choice of time constants in the range 0.3–0.05 s. ECoG electrodes (Fig. 9.1) are of two main types. Some consist of chlorided silver balls on wire arms which in turn are swivel-mounted on one or more straight or semi-circular bars, bolted to the skull at the margin of the operation site. Though the springy wires are generally sufficient to ensure good contact with the surface of the brain, this may sometimes be improved by the addition of small wicks soaked in saline. The other type of electrodes are mounted on one or more pieces of thin plastic membrane. Sometimes these are produced by printed circuit technology using sputtered gold. They are considerably quicker and easier to apply and there is less room for confusion concerning their location. However, they have the considerable disadvantages that the inter-electrode distances are fixed and it is not possible to explore an area of interest with a single electrode, visibility of the operative field may be impaired, and in particular part of the cortical surface becomes inaccessible to electrical stimulation.

Application of the electrodes is the responsibility of the surgeon. There is no rigid placement system for ECoG electrodes. Generally each individual electrode is identified by a number and the electro-encephalographer will devise on an ad hoc basis whatever montages may be appropriate; these must be carefully documented.

Stimulation of the cortex is carried out by electrical pulses of 0.1–10 ms duration at a constant current generally between 0.5 and 10 mA. The stimulating electrode is operated by the surgeon who is of course responsible for the entire procedure. Suitable cortical stimulators are commercially available. The problems of identifying and reducing artefacts have been considered above and in Chapter 8. Bates (1963) gives a helpful account of the types of artefacts which may arise in electro-corticographic recordings.

The scope of conventional electro-corticography may be further extended by the introduction of depth electrodes, either for chronic or acute registrations. This is beyond the scope of the present text and the reader is referred to Bancaud (1975).

9.3. Long-term recording from a mobile subject
It is sometimes necessary to record from a subject who is, to greater or lesser extent, free to move about and indulge in every-day activities. Apart from research applications, such records are

Fig. 9.1. Electro-corticography electrodes. Above: conventional electrode holder showing clamp for attachment to skull and one of the two arms bearing movable sockets for the electrodes, one of which is in place. Below: electrodes mounted on thin plastic film.

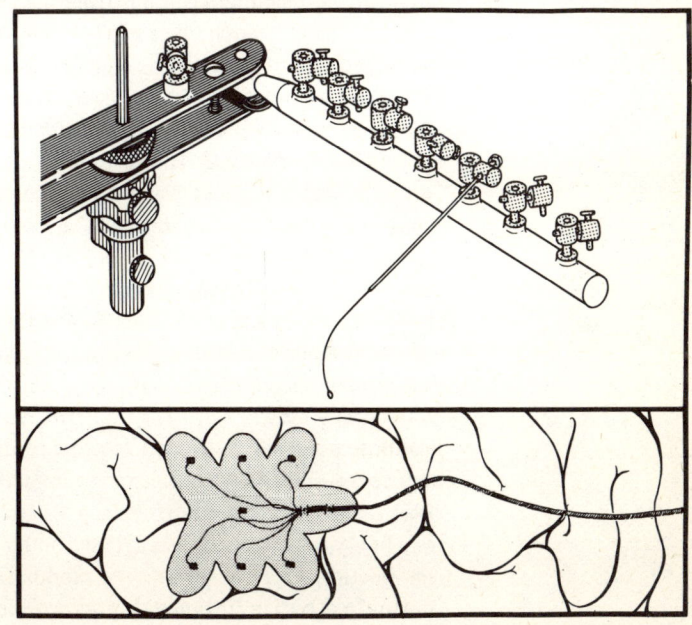

generally required in order to monitor known or possible seizures and may be of many hours or even of several days duration. Depending upon the degree of mobility required, recording may be carried out in various ways:

(1) *No additional equipment*. The patient or the technician moves the headbox as necessary. This is a good deal less inconvenient than might be supposed and indeed even during 'routine' recordings one should always be ready to adopt this approach when appropriate. For instance when a child becomes difficult he may be removed from the couch to the mother's knee or if minor seizures are suspected these may be observed most conveniently with the patient sitting upright on a chair.

(2) *Use of a modified headbox*. The headboxes provided as standard by the manufacturers of EEG machines are generally some 20 cm wide and weigh about a kilogram. Though it may be less convenient for plugging in electrodes, a miniaturized headbox can easily be attached to the patient's clothing and will greatly increase mobility. Such a device is surprisingly useful for recording from the sitting, fairly active subject, for instance during the administration of a psychological test or investigation of trigger factors in epilepsy (see Section 7.9).

(3) *Impedance matching amplifiers*. The usefulness of a miniaturized headbox can be further increased if it is equipped with impedance matching amplifiers. These provide no gain, but the impedance of the input is high (preferably over $10 \, M\Omega$) and that of the output low ($100 \, \Omega$ or less). There is a separate amplifier associated with each electrode, and the montage is still set up at the EEG machine itself. The construction of such a headbox with 16 to 20 electrode sockets and a weight of not more than 300 g should be within the capability of any department of medical electronics, but they do not yet appear to be commercially available. The high-input impedance helps to reduce artefacts arising at the electrodes and their leads, whilst the low-output impedance reduces the pick-up of interference in the input cable which can therefore be increased in length to some 10 m or more.

(4) *Cable telemetry*. If the miniaturized impedance matching headbox is further developed to provide amplification, the signals may be transmitted over some tens of metres and one has in effect a cable telemetry system. If the signals are multiplexed the need for a heavy multicore cable is avoided and if they are also digitized (see Section 13.1) or pulse code modulated they can easily be transmitted over a distance of a kilometre. Cable telemetry is

comparatively inexpensive and for many purposes it is more satisfactory than radio telemetry, although the latter has been much more widely used. Applications requiring EEG telemetry often demand continuous clinical observation or video monitoring and these necessarily impose some restrictions on the mobility of the subject. If a patient in hospital is being closely observed for the occurrence of possible seizures it is not unreasonable to require that he should remain over a period of some hours within a radius of 50 m and if it is acceptable to interrupt the registration for a few minutes he can move from one building to another before again being connected to the central recording system (Ives, Thompson and Gloor, 1976).

(5) *Radio telemetry*. There are now several EEG radio telemetry systems commercially available. This method provides greater mobility than is allowed by the use of cable but at the price of costly apparatus, rather less reliability, and some technical problems which may not necessarily be anticipated when the equipment is purchased. Radio telemetry apparatus is often bulkier and heavier than that required for cable telemetry and this factor may restrict the patient's activity. Before embarking upon radio telemetry it is important first to establish that the task cannot be performed equally satisfactorily by a more reliable and more inexpensive means such as cable or miniature tape recordings (see 6 below). It is of questionable value to invest in a costly telemetry system and then require the patient to remain in one room for purposes of video monitoring. It is important to check that the system chosen conforms to legal requirements in the country where it is to be used and that the restrictions on permitted frequencies do not for instance limit the number of channels. Radio transmission from different rooms within a hospital may present considerable difficulties, although these can be overcome by the use of multiple aerial locations and a system which automatically switches the receiver to that aerial receiving the strongest signal.

(6) *Miniature tape recorders*. Tape cassette recorders which can conveniently be carried by the subject are now available for EEG recording. They range from 2 to 16 channels; some record for only 1 hour on a standard cassette, others for as long as 24 hours. These are discussed further in Section 13.3. At the time of writing, rapid technological developments are taking place in this area and it is difficult to predict what type of system will appear most satisfactory even a year from now. Currently the choice is

between a recording of many hours on a small number of channels at the price of poor signal quality and low reliability or a rather short recording with more channels and of higher quality. Miniaturized cassette recorders offer great flexibility and are suitable for a number of specific applications. The EEG electrodes can be concealed under the hair and recording may be carried out over several days in the patient's home, at school or at work (Ives and Woods, 1975).

(7) *Long-range telemetry.* It is possible to transmit EEGs over great distances, between continents if necessary, by telephone lines or cable TV systems. Such techniques may find a further clinical application for long-term monitoring of patients in their own homes.

Artefacts can readily arise during recordings from a freely moving subject. Little can be done to avoid those of biological origin, for instance the regular bursts of EMG activity seen during chewing, but attention to technical details can at least reduce those arising from the electrodes and their leads. The headbox or the amplifiers should be located as close to the electrodes as possible; they may be strapped to the patient's head, built into a helmet, or fixed to his clothing at the collar or shoulders. The leads themselves should be as short as the location of the headbox permits and should be made of wire thinner and slightly springier than that ordinarily used. The electrodes themselves should be of stick-on type (possibly recessed) and additionally secured by means of gauze squares attached with collodion; these may if desired be painted with felt pen to match the hair colour. The combination of securely fixed electrodes, short light leads and amplifiers of high input impedance on or near the head, will markedly reduce movement and electrode artefacts even during most sporting activities. Special electrodes have been described offering a particularly low susceptibility to artefacts (Kado and Adey, 1968) and electrodes with built-in amplifiers have also been developed (Hanley, Adey, Zweizig and Kado, 1971). Our own experience does not suggest that these are necessary for clinical applications.

Before embarking upon any form of long-term monitoring it is important to consider how the resulting data will be handled. The visual analysis of 24 hour recordings on paper chart is certainly possible but extremely time consuming and tedious. It is possible to use a tape loop (Sherwood, 1970) or buffer memory to store only the EEG immediately preceding and during an event of interest (see Section 12.5). Alternatively systems are now available to allow tape recorded EEG to be scanned rapidly on an oscilloscope so that the features of interest can be detected. In the future data processing may well provide the solution to the problem of data overload.

9.4. Simultaneous EEG and video monitoring

Video recording of the patient is of special value for obtaining a record of clinical manifestations during epileptic seizures but may also be more generally useful as an aid to interpreting long and complex investigations, involving for instance psychological testing. It is of course important to be able to relate the timing of events on the video recording to those in the EEG. This may be achieved by the use of a digital time marker on the video picture linked to a character generator which indicates elapsed time on the EEG chart (Ives and Gloor, 1978). Alternatively a picture of the subject may be combined with a video display of the EEG itself. This may be obtained by directing a second camera at the EEG chart and, by means of a split effect generator, recording a composite picture of the patient and of his EEG. A more convenient method is to convert the EEG signals to video form and they may then be superimposed as a white or black tracing upon the picture of the patient. At the time of writing, several analogue-to-video converters suitable for this application are commercially available but they are costly, not yet entirely reliable and present various technical problems. An alternative method is the use of a microprocessor with an analogue-to-digital converter and video display interface. This allows the user software control of display format and is the most satisfactory solution for any department having access to microprocessor technology, especially if the signals are already available in digital form from a telemetry system. Multiplexed EEG signals can also be stored on the audio channel of a video recorder (see Section 13.3) and replayed simultaneously with the picture.

The video recorder used should at least have single-frame and slow-motion playback facilities to assist analysis of epileptic seizures. A time-lapse recording capability may also be desirable. This allows the number of frames per second to be reduced from the standard 25 or 30 to 5 or less. By this means a recording of many hours duration may be made on a single tape which otherwise has to be changed at intervals of 60–90 min. Playback is possible in real time, though with a low frame speed the picture will appear jerky. Accelerated playback is also possible, thus one may rapidly search through the tape until the event of interest is identified. A time-lapse recorder used for seizure monitoring may be equipped with a remote control for switching to a normal frame speed when an event of interest is observed. The quality of reproduction of time-lapse of video recordings may be greatly improved by the use of a digital video memory which produces a stable picture between one frame and the next. Video tape recorders are now available for domestic use and a simple basic cassette recorder and camera are fairly inexpensive. However, a system with all the facilities described above, together with monitors, automatic diaphragm, camera tripod and possibly remote controlled zoom, pan and tilt, can easily cost as much as an EEG machine.

Combined telemetric EEG and video systems for prolonged monitoring of patients with epilepsy are now used for routine clinical purposes in a number of centres (Ives *et al.*, 1976; Ives and Gloor, 1978; Penry and Porter, 1977; O'Kane and Sauter, 1977). Such facilities and their use are exceedingly costly and they are justified only for the investigation of carefully selected patients, with appropriate problems. Most typically this method of investigation is required: (i) as an aid to the differentiation of epileptic from psychogenic seizures, (ii) as a means of obtaining an ictal record for the localization of a possible focus in a patient considered for neurosurgical treatment of epilepsy, (iii) for the measurement of seizure frequency in patients with absence attacks, not readily identified by other means, and (iv) for the investigation of provocative factors in people with reflex epilepsies. There have been few clinical evaluation studies of this new and challenging field of electroencephalography, but preliminary results are encouraging (Stålberg, 1976; Binnie *et al.*, 1981).

9.5. Polygraphy

Many bio-electrical phenomena which, in EEG practice, are generally regarded as irritating artefacts are nevertheless sometimes to be considered as important signals. As indicated in Chapter 8, it is often necessary to monitor these phenomena in order to identify reliably the artefacts occurring on the EEG tracing. Moreover throughout this manual it has been emphasized that electroencephalography is of the greatest value when the EEG signals are interpreted in close combination with data from other sources, including other biological signals. Methods of recording some bio-electrical activities other than the EEG have already been discussed in Chapter 8 in the context of artefact identification. These will be reviewed and some further techniques discussed in the following pages. For a comprehensive manual on polygraphic techniques see Venables and Martin (1967b).

9.5.1. Oculography

Eye movement artefacts are typically much larger than EEG signals, having an amplitude of some 10–40 μV per degree rotation of the eye. Ideally oculography should be carried out with DC recording, so that sustained deviation of the eyes is registered as a continuous deflection on the tracing. If DC recording is attempted, electrodes will need to be prepared carefully to ensure great stability and this may be improved by self-chloriding (see Section 3.3.1). Although special electro-oculographic electrodes are available, in the EEG laboratory ordinary silver stick-on electrodes will generally be used to record the EOG. Horizontal eye movements may be recorded monocularly with electrodes placed on either side of one eye or binocularly with electrodes placed adjacent to the external canthus of each eye in the horizontal plane passing through the corneae. Vertical movements can be monitored by electrodes directly above and below each eye in the vertical plane of the cornea.

The amplitude of the EOG is dependent on light adaptation, the location of the electrodes, and individual variation. For quantitative studies it is necessary first to calibrate the system by asking the subject to carry out standardized movements, fixating for instance centrally and then on targets 30° to the left and right.

Mechanical methods of recording eye movements include the use of a drum with a thin rubber diaphragm placed in contact with the closed eyelid and attached to a pressure recording system, and the use of a light-weight tremor transducer directly above the eyelid. More sophisticated methods used for research purposes employ a strain gauge or mirror attached to a contact lens, or involve reflecting ultra-violet light off the corneo-scleral junction.

9.5.2. The electrocardiogram

Electrocardiography is beyond the scope of the present text. It may however be noted that ECG recording is often required during electroencephalography, to help to identify possible ECG, ball-

istocardiographic, or pulse artefacts, as a guide to state of awareness, and to monitor cardiac function during such manoeuvres as
carotid artery compression. A lead I ECG may be recorded with
conventional ECG electrodes strapped at the usual sites. For many
purposes it may be more convenient to attach the electrodes
elsewhere, for instance at either side of the neck or on the
shoulders. Although this does not strictly give a classical lead I
ECG, it is quite adequate for monitoring cardiac rhythm and
detecting gross abnormalities. The paper speed and filter settings
typically used for routine ECG practice are not available on all
EEG machines but to obtain a tracing not unlike a routine ECG
one should use a time constant of the order of a second and a
sensitivity of $100 \mu V/mm$.

Routine ECGs are ordinary only of some tens of seconds
duration. In the course of an EEG recording of half an hour or
longer ventricular extrasystoles will quite often occur in healthy
subjects. Though unsuspected ECG abnormalities during the EEG
recording should generally lead to cardiological referral, an isolated extrasystole as often as once a minute should not give rise
to concern. Note also that sinus arrhythmia (the variation of
heart rate with the respiration which is seen particularly in the
young and in athletic adults) may become very marked during
hyperventilation, and if unfamiliar may be mistaken for an abnormality of cardiac rhythm.

9.5.3. Respiration
Respiration may be monitored in various ways, by detecting the
variations in air temperature close to the mouth or nose with
inspiration and expiration, by monitoring the girth of the chest
by means of a belt incorporating a strain gauge, by measuring
variations in the electrical impedance of the chest, or by asking
the subject to breath through a mouth-piece and measuring the
volume and velocity of airflow.

The simplest method probably is with a thermistor or thermocouple taped in front of the nostrils or mouth as appropriate.
This method registers the rate of respiration but does not indicate
its depth.

A webbing belt may be placed around the chest attached to a
crystal strain gauge transducer, or the belt itself may consist of a
rubber tube filled with mercury, the resistance of which will vary
with the respiratory movements. Some subjects make more use of
thoracic and some of abdominal movements in breathing, but

within any individual a general indication is obtained of any changes in depth of breathing.

Measurement of the electrical impedance of the chest (impedance plethysmography) involves applying a small alternating current between two electrodes on either side of the chest and recording the potential difference across two electrodes placed between these.

Finally, for precise measurements of respiration, use may be made of a pneumotachograph. The patient must breath through a mouth-piece down a tube which contains a pneumatic resistance. The drop in air pressure across the resistance is registered by means of a sensitive strain gauge transducer. With appropriate ancillary equipment this device can give direct registrations of the velocity of airflow or the total volume of air displaced in a certain period.

Respiratory movements are slow compared with EEG signals and should be recorded with long time constants or a DC channel. Those simple transducers which generate an electrical potential (crystal strain gauge, thermocouple, etc.) may be plugged directly into the headbox of the EEG machine. Those which comprise a varying resistance (thermistor or mercury strain gauge) may be used as one limb of a Wheatstone's bridge circuit, and the imbalance signal written out on the EEG chart. Pneumotachographs and impedance plethysmographs are sold with associated amplifiers etc. and sometimes special circuits for differentiating and integrating the signals.

9.5.4. Tremor and body movement

Movements are generally registered by means of a piezo-electric acceleration transducer. These may be rather crudely fashioned from a crystal gramophone pick-up and are also commercially available from the manufacturers of EEG machines. They are usually sensitive to movements in only one direction and must therefore be appropriately orientated to record the movement of interest. Special amplifiers are also available to convert the signals from acceleration to velocity or to displacement, which for some research purposes may be of more interest. For tremor recording a time constant of 0.3 s is generally adequate and the upper frequency of interest is commonly 15 Hz or lower.

Where the movement is due to muscular activity it may also be registered by EMG recording and when detailed qualitative information is required, simultaneous EEG and video recording may be appropriate (see Section 9.4).

9.5.5. Electromyography

For recording a superficial EMG during an EEG recording, silver stick-on disc electrodes may conveniently be used. In the present context the purpose of EMG recording will generally be to monitor the occurrence of muscular contraction, for instance a myoclonic jerk or the voluntary response in a reaction time task. The location of the electrodes will depend upon the muscle of interest. For recording from the larger muscles one should generally find a point over the belly of the muscle midway between its origin and its insertion, and apply two electrodes respectively 25 mm above and below this point. The potential difference between these two electrodes may conveniently be recorded at normal EEG sensitivities with a short time constant and the maximum high-frequency setting available. For purposes of recording changes in muscle tone during sleep, or in association with atonic epileptic seizures, one may choose locations over the chin (in the midline 20 mm above and below the point of the chin) or over the neck (one electrode 30 mm lateral to the second cervical spine and a second 10 mm medial to and 50 mm below this location).

9.5.6. Skin resistance and skin potential

Both the electrical resistance of the skin and the potential between one region and another change in association with variations in activity of the autonomic nervous system. Measurements may be made either of the basal values of resistance and potential or of transient changes in these. Skin resistance is largely determined by the activity of the sweat glands and its measurement is highly complex, the results obtained being dependent upon current density, the use of AC or DC measurements and whether the resistance testing is performed under conditions of constant current or constant applied potential. Discussion of these issues is beyond the scope of the present text and the reader is referred to Venables and Martin (1967a).

Quantitative measurements of skin potential are also complex but for purposes simply of registering change it is sufficient to apply a pair of chlorided silver disc electrodes, one on the palm, generally at the base of the thumb, and the other on the back of the forearm. The forearm electrode may be regarded as a reference point and the skin should be carefully abraded to give it a very low resistance. Electrodes should be as stable as possible and after careful preparation and slow chloriding (see Section 3.3.1) they should be allowed to assume stable potentials by self-chloriding. The resting skin potential between the sites described is of the order of $70\,\mu$V and transient changes of 5 or $10\,\mu$V occur when the subject is startled, emotionally stressed or during various manoeuvres such as sniffing or sneezing. For a more detailed account the reader is again referred to Venables and Martin (1967a).

Manufacturers of EEG equipment often offer a range of transducers and polygraphic modules. Often this is little more than a reflection of the inadequacy of the number of inputs or range of sensitivities available from the headbox. Facilities may be provided for integrating the signals and for displaying or writing out instantaneous frequency of a periodic phenomenon such as the ECG etc. Before investing in any of these the user should seriously consider whether they are needed. A home-made thermocouple, a few EEG electrodes with extra long leads (for ECG and EMG recording) and a simple piezo-electric accelerometer will meet most people's requirements.

10. The EEG report

10.1. Introduction

The end result of the considerable effort and thought which go into an EEG investigation is an EEG report. One might conclude from the foregoing technical discussion that EEG interpretation is a complex task best left to scientists. In fact the skills required to produce a useful EEG report are not so much scientific as literary, in the sense that details of the record must be described in such a way that they can be fully appreciated by the reader who is likely to be non-expert in EEG matters. Accomplishing this is not difficult, so long as the electroencephalographer retains objectivity and remembers that his chief aim is communication with others.

The report usually has two parts: a description of the phenomena which are contained in the EEG, and a conclusion or an interpretation of its significance in the clinical context. In some departments the description, or *factual report*, is written by the EEG technician; in others, probably the majority, by the electroencephalographer. It may seem inappropriate that a technician should be charged with the responsibility of writing any part of a clinical report but the ability of an expert technician to recognize a wide variety of phenomena is put to good use in describing what he has seen. Indeed the technologist, who has seen the EEG recorded and at the same time observed the patient, is in a better position than the electroencephalographer to distinguish abnormalities from artefacts or the effects of changing vigilance. Moreover, an important component of the factual report, which also influences the subsequent interpretation, is an eye-witness account of the state of the patient and of any clinical manifestations such as seizures. Reporting also serves an educational function; it helps to develop visual skills and makes the technologist very aware of the consequences of his techniques for the legibility of the record.

The *interpretation*, by contrast, is unquestionably the responsibility of a doctor trained in electroencephalography and neurology. Unhelpful or misleading reports are more often due to poor clinical judgement than to an inability to recognize EEG phenomena.

10.2. The factual report

How should the factual report be organized? There are a number of methods in use, each with certain advantages and disadvantages. Some departments prefer to describe the recorded phenomena in a stereotyped manner, even to the extent of employing a form for this purpose. Such a form includes headings for various frequency bands, response to hyperventilation and the like, and either short phrases are used or boxes ticked to indicate the presence or absence, amount, amplitude, etc. of the item in question. Summary methods have the advantages of brevity and consistency, are time saving, and allow easy information retrieval. On the other hand, such restrictive formats tend to suppress original thinking about individual clinical problems, producing dull and sometimes misleading reports.

Another method of reporting, and that which the authors favour, is more discursive in style with a more or less individually tailored description for each patient. This method allows freedom to emphasize important features of the record and, in a certain sense, gives a verbal picture of the EEG to the reader. The hallmark of a well-designed EEG report is that the recipient is able to imagine what the record actually looks like.

The first consideration is the state of the patient, for accurate appraisal of the significance of the recorded activity is dependent on this factor. At the beginning of the report, therefore, a statement of the patient's ability to co-operate, and an estimate of his level of consciousness and general condition is essential. Is he alert or drowsy, disoriented or confused, or perhaps lethargic? Can he be easily aroused? He may be in a delirium or in deep coma. Each of these states influences the EEG, sometimes dramatically, and thereby the reader's interpretation of the findings.

Secondly, drugs which the patient is taking also influence to a great extent the EEG picture and should be carefully noted, as the medication may have been changed since the request form was written. Perhaps one of the drugs will account for excessive beta activity, another for slowing. It should also be noted that drugs also influence the patient's state of awareness, perhaps providing an explanation for both clinical and EEG findings.

If the general appearance of the EEG or the course of the investigation is in any way unusual it is better to say so in the first sentence rather than to leave the reader gradually to deduce this for himself as the report proceeds. For instance:

'The record is grossly asymmetrical, faster components being more prominent on the right and those of lower frequency on the left.'

'Thirteen seconds after commencement of the recording the patient suffered a seizure (see description below) and remained in a post-ictal confusional state for the remainder of the investigation.'

'The patient was dyspnoeic, had a severe cough and remained seated in a wheelchair throughout the investigation; consequently there is a considerable amount of movement and muscle artefact and it was not possible to obtain a sleep recording as requested.' If there has been a previous recording, the opening remarks should include some general comments about the similarity or the differences of the two tracings:

'The background activity closely resembles that in the previous tracing, but paroxysmal activity is much reduced in amount.'

'In comparison with the previous record the EEG is considerably slower and higher in amplitude.'

One should then proceed to a general description of the initial or basal state of the EEG before onset of drowsiness or any activation procedures. To describe an EEG phenomenon one may need to give some or all of the following details:

(a) The frequency of an activity or the duration of an isolated wave.

(b) The mean peak-to-peak amplitude of an activity or wave.

(c) The distribution of the phenomenon, with particular reference to its symmetry if it occurs bilaterally; the location of a focal event should be described in the factual report (but not in the interpretation) in terms of electrode sites.

(d) Waveform; established terminology is very limited in this respect and one should be prepared to use whatever vocabulary may be appropriate to describe what is seen.

(e) Incidence: is the activity almost continuous or the paroxysmal event seen on every page, or is the phenomenon rarely present?

(f) Reactivity to stimuli and to eye opening or closure, or to changes in the state of awareness.

(g) Behavioural correlates: does the patient for instance jerk when the transient event occurs or appear unresponsive during the discharge?

As a general rule, the EEG can be imagined to consist of:

(a) A basic background of ongoing activity which consists of components in various frequency bands, mainly posterior dominant rhythmic activity (alpha activity in normal subjects), beta waves, and some intermittent theta activity.

(b) Features which interrupt or disturb the basic ongoing

activity. One might see, for example, a background consisting mainly of alpha activity and, in the left anterior temporal region, intermittent focal theta waves. In such a case one might conclude that the brain as a whole is not diffusely involved by a pathological process but is able to generate normal activity. Thus, as a first statement, mention of a well-organized alpha rhythm gives the reader a base-line from which to judge the significance of the focal theta waves.

As the presence of occipital dominant rhythmic activity is so important to the overall interpretation, it is reasonable to describe it first and in some detail. It sets the stage for all that follows. Whether or not in the alpha frequency range, the essential features of the posterior dominant rhythmic activity, if present, should be mentioned – e.g. its location, frequency, amplitude, symmetry, abundance, and reactivity to eye opening and closure or other stimuli. This rhythm may be very regular and constantly present with no other intermingled frequencies. It would be in this case well organized. It may also be present but irregular due to many intermingled slower components. In an extreme case, few if any posterior rhythmic waves will be seen, and irregular slowing predominates posteriorly. The degree of disorganization of the posterior dominant rhythm correlates roughly with the extent of diffuse cerebral dysfunction, and with the state of awareness of the patient. Thus, accurate appraisal of the posterior rhythmic activity can provide a key to accurate analysis of the record as a whole.

Beta activity, the other major background component, may be described next, usually in a sentence describing its symmetry, distribution, frequency and amplitude. Although beta activity is generally less useful than the posterior dominant rhythm as a guide to the character of the EEG, it sometimes provides essential information and should not be neglected.

The stage is now set for the description of major pathological features of the EEG which may be considered in two main groups: paroxysmal activity and slowing. Some EEGs will contain both, others mainly one or the other. It is not only impossible to describe in detail all possible findings in an EEG, but such an attempt would result in a long, dull, and in the end useless report which would go unread by all but the most tenacious. It is therefore advisable to determine the most important abnormalities and describe them in both qualitative and, in so far as possible, quantitative terms, reporting other features more concisely.

If slowing is the major feature, the first decision must be: is it diffuse or focal. As may be expected, the clinical consequences of this decision can be considerable. In the case of diffuse slow waves, one should study the frequency band of the slowing and determine whether it is mainly in the theta or delta range. Because of the overlap of the observed frequencies, it is wise to refer to the major frequencies present, rather than simply delta or theta activity. Note that diffuse slowing may not be symmetrical or equally distributed over the anterior and posterior regions; these characteristics should be mentioned. Also, the rhythmic or non-rhythmic character of the slowing may have important diagnostic implications and should be stated. Thus: 'There is continuous, diffuse, moderate voltage irregular slowing of 3–5 Hz, most prominent over the temporal regions, left more than right.'; or 'The record contains intermittent diffuse slow activity, mainly in the delta band at 2–3 Hz, with small amounts of intermingled slow theta components at 4–5 Hz. This slowing is most prominent over the frontal regions.'

Focal slowing is treated in much the same way and should be described with reference to the involved electrode(s). For example: 'Over the right fronto-temporal region with a maximum at F_8 but spreading to F_{p2} and F_4, there is continuous polymorphic delta activity at mainly 1–2 Hz.'

The general term *paroxysmal activity* indicates electrical events that suddenly appear and disappear from the record. It may or may not be epileptic in character. This important decision will be indicated in the interpretative report. Considering epileptiform discharges, important features include the wave shape (e.g. spike-wave complexes, spikes, or even bursts of rhythmic slow waves), frequency, and amplitude. If the events occur in series or runs, the length of the discharges should be indicated. In addition, a quantitative or semi-quantitative statement is useful, not only for evaluation of the record in question, but for comparison with other EEGs the patient may have had or will have. The same considerations regarding diffuse versus focal phenomena apply. For example: 'On three occasions there are bursts of high-voltage (amplitude 300 μV) rhythmic 3/s spike-wave complexes lasting from 8–10 s. These are of maximum amplitude over the frontal regions and have a slight right hemispheric preponderance.' In the case of focal discharges one might say: 'Over the left temporal region there is an active moderate voltage spike focus which is focal at T_3 with variable representation at F_7 and

T_5. The spikes reach an amplitude of 100 μV and occur 6–10 times in any 10 seconds.'

If clinical events are observed during the discharges, these must be carefully described as this information is of great diagnostic value. In the case of spike-wave discharges as described above: 'During the discharges the patient was unresponsive and blinked his eyes rhythmically. There were also slight movements of the left cheek. At the end of the discharge he was responsive to questions and did not appear to be confused.'

Following the description of the basic resting record, it is usual to describe the results of activation procedures such as hyperventilation and photic stimulation. The duration and estimate of the quality of effort of hyperventilation should be included, along with a statement of major changes which occur if any. Note that pre-existing abnormalities may be emphasized or new abnormalities may appear. In the latter case a more detailed description is necessary. With photic stimulation the frequency range at which the photic stimulus is delivered is mentioned, along with the presence or absence of the following response. Paroxysmal discharges during photic stimulation are described with reference to the range of frequencies at which they occur. Also note whether paroxysmal discharges are observed with eyes open or closed, the latency of response after the onset of the flash-train and whether they outlast the stimulation.

The foregoing is intended as a general guide and not as a protocol to be slavishly followed. Whenever a non-standard format will assist communication it should be adopted. Most importantly, the significant data must not be lost in a sea of verbiage.

10.3. The conclusion

The conclusion, or interpretation, is the most important component of the EEG report, for it is in this section that the electroencephalographer must come to grips with the problem and state clearly what he thinks about the findings. Often, indeed, it is the only part of the report that the referring physician will read. Sometimes it is easier to describe an EEG event than it is to determine or explain its significance. Although electroencephalographers like to think that they are quite expert at this exercise, the truth is that we can make effective use of only a small part of the data generated during even a very routine EEG examination. Nevertheless, there are often clear-cut conclusions that can be drawn from the EEG, and with care and attention to detail the yield of clinically useful information can be markedly increased.

If the factual report was reasonably concise no detailed summary should be necessary; the conclusion should simply draw together those findings which are relevant to the clinical problem and explain their significance. At this stage a qualitative evaluation is more helpful than the description of EEG phenomenology. 'The EEG shows a mild diffuse abnormality of background activity more severe on the left than the right' is of much more value than repeating what was said already in the factual report, concerning perhaps a slowed alpha rhythm and a left-sided excess of theta activity.

Following the statement of the main findings, the electroencephalographer should if possible attempt a reasonable clinical interpretation, based on his knowledge of the patient, his experience, and the experience of others as reported in the literature. Finally, he should recommend further EEG investigations if appropriate, for example a sleep recording or activation procedure. It is important to recall that the clinician ordering the EEG is seeking help in solving a particular problem. The electroencephalographer may feel his task is complete if he, for example, writes: 'The record is markedly abnormal and contains a left temporal delta focus against a bilaterally disorganized and slow background.' To him, this conveys the idea of a focal structural process which may be in turn affecting the brain as a whole; in other words, such a patient could have an advanced tumour which is beginning to cause increased intracranial pressure. However the report would be of much greater value to most users if one added: 'The findings indicate a structural lesion in the left temporal lobe and suggest diffuse cerebral dysfunction. One should consider the possibility that the patient has increased intracranial pressure.' Another example might be: 'The record is moderately abnormal and shows diffuse moderate voltage irregular theta activity with absence of the alpha rhythm. There is no focal slowing.' This suggests a diffuse cerebral process and not, for instance, a tumour or cerebro-vascular accident. One might then say: 'The findings are consistent with bilateral disease, or perhaps a metabolic disturbance.' If the history included renal disease with an increased blood urea nitrogen, then one might be more definite, and emphasize that: 'The EEG is consistent with a diagnosis of uraemia.' In these cases, serial EEGs may be very helpful in following the clinical course of the patient and should therefore be recommended.

Negative findings may be important. Take the example of a patient entering the hospital with the acute onset of a left hemiplegia. One might expect to find a slow-wave focus in the right hemisphere. Instead, the impression is: 'This is a normal EEG.' Applying this knowledge of pathological processes and their physiological consequences, the electroencephalographer may then say: 'A normal EEG in a patient with this history suggests that the lesion involves either the base of the pons or the internal capsule.' These areas, when damaged, often give rise to no EEG abnormalities although the neurological deficit may be striking. Conversely, it is sometimes necessary to warn the user what conclusions may not be drawn from a normal EEG, for instance: 'The EEG is within normal limits and in particular there is no asymmetry of background activity. It should be noted that these negative findings do not exclude the diagnosis of chronic subdural haematoma as suggested on the request form.'

At this point it should be emphasized that not all clinico-EEG correlations are obvious. The electroencephalographer is sometimes at a loss to explain the findings and how they relate to the clinical problem. A particularly troublesome example is the discovery of an ipsi-lateral slow-wave focus in a patient with a hemiplegia. This is difficult to explain anatomically and, although explanations can be rather artificially constructed, it is perhaps wiser to say: 'The EEG-findings in this patient are at variance with the clinical picture, and the reason is not apparent.' Such a statement also avoids any future uncertainty as to whether there was actually a discrepancy, or merely an error in the EEG report. Incidentally it is always a good idea just to check with the nursing staff or the technician (who should have noted it) to determine if it really was a left and not a right hemiplegia. When the clinical significance of a particular finding is unknown or there are other interpretative or technical difficulties, a good deal of confusion may be avoided by saying so:

'The resting EEG is within normal limits and in particular is symmetrical; nevertheless responses to photic stimulation appear to be confined to the right hemisphere. The significance of this finding in the present clinical context is doubtful but it would probably be worthwhile to check the visual fields.'

'During the seizure no paroxysmal activity is seen; however the record is partly obscured by myogenic potentials and the possibility of low-amplitude spikes can certainly not be excluded.'

There are no general rules concerning how far one should go in trying to offer a diagnosis; some EEG abnormalities are entirely non-specific, others virtually diagnostic for a particular disease, and others may acquire very precise predictive value in a clearly defined clinical context. For instance:

'There is a mild diffuse abnormality of background activity and some sharp waves appear over the temporal regions. These findings are non-specific but as the patient complains of episodic headache it is worthwhile noting that similar EEG appearances may be expected in some 30% of people with migraine.'

'There is a severe and well-localized right parietal abnormality. In the present context of recent subarachnoid bleeding, it should be noted that ruptured intracranial arterial aneurysms do not commonly produce an abnormality at this site and a primary intracerebral haemorrhage or possibly bleeding due to an angioma are more likely diagnoses.'

The conclusion ends with suggestions for any possible further EEG investigations, stating the reasons:

'In view of the discrepancy between the present findings of generalized paroxysmal activity and the history suggesting complex partial seizures, a seconal-induced sleep recording with naso-pharyngeal electrodes is advised to detect a possible focus.'

'The record is diffusely slow and disorganized. Although there is no clear focus the slowing is somewhat more evident in the right frontal region. The findings support the clinical diagnosis of encephalitis. In view of the more localized abnormality a follow-up tracing within 24 hours is strongly recommended because of the possibility of a developing cerebral abcess.'

Finally, one should be cautioned to avoid apparently impressive but actually vague 'neurophysiological' terminology to 'explain' certain findings. For instance, to describe an irregular posterior dominant activity as a 'regulatory disorder', or small sharp transients as indicative of 'cortical irritability' is inaccurate, speculative and explains nothing. This sort of statement leads colleagues, sometimes rightly, to think that the electroencephalographer spends too much time in the laboratory away from the real world.

11. Planning an EEG department

11.1. Location

Major considerations in choosing a location for an EEG department are accessibility to patients and freedom from noise and electrical interference. The site may need to be accessible to bedridden, unconscious or handicapped patients and conversely it may be necessary without difficulty to wheel a transportable machine from the department to the wards. On the other hand, if most of the users are outpatients, easy access from the hospital entrance or clinics may be important. To some extent problems of accessibility can be solved by the provision of a satellite unit to serve the intensive care unit or the neurosurgical ward. The chosen location should not be adjacent to obvious sources of noise (the childrens' ward, the ambulance park), or of electrical interference (physiotherapy, operating theatres, the aerial of the paging system). It is worthwhile to have the site inspected by an expert on electrical interference who will test for electrostatic and electro-magnetic fields.

11.2. Electrical supplies, earthing and interference

Rather than attempting to solve problems of mains-borne interference and inadequate earthing after they have arisen, it is better in the first instance to ensure that the department has an independent mains riser and its own earth busbar with an earth electrode buried in the ground. The resistance to earth should not exceed 0.5 Ω. If use is made of existing mains wiring this should be carefully inspected. Metallic conduit, which should be earthed and continuous with the socket outlet boxes, provides a screen against mains interference and is preferable to the plastic tubing now widely used. However, the practice of using the conduit itself as the earth connection is not acceptable and an independent earth lead should be provided for every socket outlet. When several pieces of apparatus are to be used simultaneously, problems of earth loops (see Chapter 8) are less likely to arise if all devices are plugged into socket outlets mounted in a single distribution box. The number of socket outlets required is readily underestimated and it is not unreasonable to require that each EEG recording area be equipped with a single distribution box containing at least eight sockets.

If the site is well chosen and an independent mains supply and earth connection are provided, special measures to combat interference should not be necessary. However, the possible use of radio-frequency filters, stabilized power supplies, and mains filters has been noted elsewhere (Chapter 8). A sometimes intractable problem even in a well-sited department is capacitative interference from water pipes. A solution lies in the use of plastic pipes.

11.3. Lay-out
Within the department corridors and entrances to clinical areas must be large enough for stretchers and/or hospital beds.

11.3.1. Recording suites
There is no single design for an EEG recording area which ideally meets all requirements and if the department has several suites, these should be so far as possible individually designed for specific applications. There are some advantages in a three-room suite comprising separate areas for electrode application (15 m^2), accommodation of the apparatus (10 m^2), and for the patient whilst the record is performed (15 m^2). As the total time taken by a technician of moderate experience to apply and remove electrodes is not much less than that taken to record a routine EEG, it is possible for two patients and technicians to use the suite simultaneously; whilst electrodes are applied or removed in the preparation room, a tracing is in progress in the recording and machine areas. The preparation room should be equipped with a compressed air supply, air-conditioning or an extractor to remove acetone fumes, and a laboratory sink for cleaning electrodes. There should be an upright chair for electrode application and good overhead lighting. The room should be large enough to accommodate a patient on a stretcher. Other facilities include trolleys and cupboards for electrode application material, racks for storing leads and electrodes, possibly self-chloriding apparatus, clothes hooks for the patient's coat, a mirror so that he can comb his hair after completion of the investigation, a couple of chairs for people accompanying the patient, and some toys which can be used by a child sitting on a chair.

The patient's room should have a restful décor and good acoustic isolation. There should be black-out blinds or heavy curtains, and variable intensity lighting which can be controlled by the technician seated in the machine room. Types of recording couches were discussed in Chapter 6. There should also be a couple of easy chairs for persons accompanying the patient and a table or trolley with materials for adjusting electrodes and for transducers which may need to be used. Otherwise the room should as far as possible be free of equipment apart from the photic stimulator lamp. There should be space enough for a patient on a stretcher or in a wheel-chair to be brought into the recording area without the need to remove the bed. A patient lying on his back has a view of the ceiling and a focal point of interest such as a picture may promote fixation and reduce eye movements.

The machine room should be sufficiently large to accommodate the EEG machine and ancillary equipment, together with supplies of paper, ink, etc. A workbench or table on which the previous EEGs of the patient can be spread out and examined is desirable. The machine area should communicate with the recording room through a large hatch at least a metre high and 1.2 m wide. This should allow the technician a free view of the patient and particularly of his face. The opening should be fitted with a window, preferably double-glazed to provide sound attenuation during sleep recordings, but it should be possible for the window to be widely opened to permit free communication. The use of an intercom to avoid the need of a window which can be opened is unacceptable and tends to create an impersonal atmosphere which can only add to the anxieties of the patient. Below the hatch there must be a hole to accommodate the EEG input cable. It must also be possible to black out the machine room while providing some means of illuminating the chart without producing too much scattered light. Only one manufacturer of EEG machines seems to provide illumination of the chart as a standard feature. It should be remembered that a consequence of blacking out the recording and machine areas may be a reduction of ventilation and a separate extractor fan (electrically screened of course) may be required.

Though a three-room recording suite has certain advantages for controlling the environment, especially for sleep recording, there are also merits in being able to carry out the whole investigation in one large room. Observation of behavioural changes is facilitated when the patient and technician are in the same room, and it is also easier to attend to the needs of an ill patient or reassure an anxious one if there are no barriers. A single-room suite is also convenient for the more interactive procedures, for instance administration of intravenous injections under EEC control, performance of psychological testing during EEG record-ing, or detailed investigation of visual sensitivity. The flexibility of a single recording room will be more fully realized if the allocation of space is generous (e.g. 35 m^2) and if the equipment and furniture are entirely mobile.

The furnishings of the recording area should be conducive to relaxation and not too obviously institutional in appearance. They should also be resistant to the solvents used in EEG practice (acetone, alcohol and ether) and should be made of anti-static materials. In general this implies that natural fabrics and stuffings should be used in the chairs and particularly in the recording couch and that certain floor coverings, notably nylon carpeting and vinyl tiles should be avoided. It may be desirable to have one recording room especially furnished for children and decorated with nursery-rhyme characters, etc.

11.3.2. Other accommodation

The following additional accommodation may be regarded as essential in any but the smallest satellite department:

(1) Waiting room or area, both for ambulant patients and for those on stretchers or in wheel-chairs, and with the means of segregating those who are acutely ill or psychiatrically disturbed.

(2) Administrative area, suitably located for reception of patients and for observation of those waiting.

(3) Accommodation for filing of EEGs and reports.

(4) Work-room for technicians to annotate EEGs, write reports, prepare electrodes , etc.

(5) Staff sitting room, this may be combined with (4) above.

(6) EEG reporting area which may be located in (4) above, in a doctor's office or in a separate room.

(7) Staff and patient toilets.

(8) Storage space for recording materials, electrodes, linen, drugs, etc.

Any substantial department will in addition require some or all of the following:

(9) Offices for medical staff.

(10) Electronics workshop.

(11) Storage for mobile EEG equipment.

(12) Accommodation for micro-film equipment.

(13) Accommodation for data processing facilities.

(14) Room for patients who are acutely ill, recovering from the effects of drugs or undergoing neurological examination.

(15) Area suitable for technician training, possibly combined with (4) or (6) above.

(16) EMG room.

(17) Recording suite with complete blackout and extra sound isolation for evoked potential work.

(18) Area suitable for ambulant patients undergoing long-term EEG monitoring.

11.4. Size and staffing of an EEG department

The smallest independent unit which is viable comprises two machines and three technicians. The failure rate even of modern EEG equipment is such that a department with a single machine cannot reliably provide a continuous service. Moreover with a technician team of less than three, isolation, both physical and intellectual, is bad for staff morale and it is in any event difficult to cover holidays and sick-leave. A one-machine unit functioning as a satellite of a larger department is an entirely different matter, and there may be considerable advantages in providing a machine on the spot to meet the special needs of, for instance, an intensive care unit or hospital for mental subnormality. Regardless of the size of the department, to make effective use of the apparatus the number of trained technicians should exceed the number of EEG machines, in a ratio of 1.5 : 1 or even 2 : 1.

The workload of any EEG department must necessarily depend upon the nature of the referrals and the type of records carried out. As a general guide an annual output of 700 recordings per technician or 1000 per machine is reasonable and corresponds roughly to the recommendations of the appropriate professional bodies in the USA, Great Britain and the Netherlands. The medical staffing required for the minimum EEG department with two machines, three technicians and an annual output of about 2000 records should be equivalent to one full-time electro-encephalographer. These norms are not adequate if the department undertakes research, performs evoked response studies or long-term monitoring, provides a 24-hour emergency service, carries out portable EEGs, or receives large numbers of children or disturbed patients.

11.5. Data storage

EEGs are extremely bulky and routine records of an acceptable length can easily occupy 2 m of shelf length per 100 tracings. They are also heavy and expert advice must be obtained before it is assumed that a floor can support ceiling-high racks of EEG records. As serial EEG changes are important for many clinical applications, it is necessary to store the records for a considerable period, life-long arguably in the case of people with epilepsy. Data storage and retrieval consequently present difficulties for many departments. The simplest method probably is to number and store the records sequentially. After a period determined by the availability of storage space within the department, the older records can be moved in bulk to a passive archive elsewhere. EEG reports typed on cards can be handled similarly. An alternative is to give every new patient an accession number and to attempt to store all his records together. This has the advantage that the entire previous series of records can easily be found when a patient returns for a further EEG, but the practical drawback that a great deal of shelf space must be left free to allow for an unpredictable number of repeat tracings. When the time eventually comes to destroy records or transfer them to a passive archive, it will be necessary in each case to check how recently each patient was last seen. So far as report cards are concerned, it is much less difficult to store all those of each patient together, in a plastic folder or otherwise, but in this case one probably needs a further card-index system or daybook from which individual EEGs can be identified by the date and record number.

EEGs are often microfilmed. The capital investment is modest compared with the cost of space, and if the tedious task of feeding EEGs into a machine designed to film continuous charts is unacceptable to departmental staff, the service is provided commercially by the suppliers of microfilm apparatus. The choice of equipment is easy, for there are few machines on the market capable of reading charts of the width of a 16-channel EEG. A more difficult decision is between the use of microfilm and 'jackets'. The latter are small plastic folders of the size of a postcard into which several strips of microfilm can be inserted. Standard format jackets will typically hold 75 cm of film which is equivalent to approximately 25 m or 75 pages of EEG. Jackets are very convenient to use, they can be individually indexed and stored and any chosen point of the tracing can be reached quickly without the need to scan the preceding film. However, unless the EEGs are very short, several jackets will be required for each tracing. A much more compressed microfiche format is used for computer output and if this becomes available for filming continuous charts it will probably be the method of choice. However, at the present time microfilm, despite the inconvenience of locating the wanted record in a film which is usually 30 m in length, is the most satisfactory compromise. It should be noted that microfilm readers can also produce prints and transparencies for overhead projectors and this may facilitate preparation of material for lectures or publications, though the quality of reproduction is sometimes poor.

However EEG data, both reports and records, are stored, it is important that the documentation should include details of the referral. In interpreting past records it is often necessary to know the circumstances under which they were taken, for instance the time since the last seizure, the medication, etc.

Somewhere in a corner of many EEG departments is to be found a dusty pile of punch cards which represents past and unsuccessful attempts at establishing a data base for scientific purposes. More recently such systems have commonly been computerized but have not necessarily been any more useful in consequence. There are several reasons for failure. Often too much work is required to prepare the data (a 200-item question-aire including the amplitude and frequency of every activity in every region of the head is not likely to be filled in conscientiously, if at all). Alternatively, the data may be unreliable or simply not available (for instance, detailed clinical information). In any event the information so carefully preserved for posterity may be of little interest or value. On the other hand, a well-designed data-storage system can be a valuable asset to any EEG department. Firstly, it can be used for research purposes to identify patients with particular combinations of EEG phenomena, diagnoses, etc. Secondly, it may be used administratively to determine the sources and patterns of referral. A third application, the value of which is not generally appreciated, is for quality control: for instance such a system enables one to determine how often a particular activation procedure provides new information, or to identify sources of referral which give an unusually low yield of clinically useful findings.

12. Data processing in electroencephalography

12.1. Background to EEG data processing

Human observers can become very proficient at reading EEGs; they can scan hundreds of metres of paper tracings, ignoring artefacts, and detect clinically important anomalies representing only a tiny part of the total data presented. On the other hand, they have difficulty in quantifying their observations; for instance, without preliminary training it is difficult to get independent raters even to agree consistently about the gross features of EEGs. Few however have had the courage to publish any detailed study of inter-rater reliability (Volavka *et al.* 1973). Electroencephalographers may be inconsistent in their individual performance but above all have difficulty in communicating their observations objectively so that they may be used by others. It might therefore be hoped that through the quantitative characterization of the signals by data processing techniques the usefulness of electroencephalography could be increased. Moreover, there are many features of the EEG, clearly detectable with electronic aids, which are beyond the resolution of the human visual system. Examples are the subtle relations of phase and frequency between different regions of the head (measurable by use of the 'coherence function') and transient EEG phenomena of low voltage causally related to external events, so-called 'evoked responses'.

Mathematical analysis of the EEG is almost as old as electroencephalography itself. In 1932 Diesch proposed analysing the EEG in terms of its frequency components by means of power-spectral analysis. The 1940s and 1950s saw the development of various devices for EEG analysis, of which the most successful and best known was the Burden Neurological Institute low-frequency wave analyser (Baldock and Walter, 1946). This comprised a parallel array of filters (Fig. 12.1) which separated the various frequency components of the EEG. The amount of activity passing through each filter over a predetermined 'epoch' or period of time, usually 10 s, was written out on the chart. The device was somewhat unstable and required frequent tuning. Although it usually analysed only one or two channels, it nevertheless presented an overwhelming volume of data. If 20 different frequency bands were measured on two channels every 10 s, the number of values produced in the course of a routine clinical EEG recording ran into thousands. Nevertheless, some workers showed that simple but meaningful indices could be derived from this information, such as the mean frequency or the ratio of alpha to theta activity. These measures could usefully be applied to specific scientific problems such as detecting serial changes in the EEG related to metabolic disorders (Laidlaw and Read, 1963), or to physiological processes such as the human menstrual cycle (Margerison, Anderson, Dawson and Lettich, 1964) or even distinguishing normal from abnormal EEGs (Matoušek, 1967). More recently, with the development of small digital computers which may cost less than an EEG machine, it has become possible to carry out EEG signal analysis accurately and reliably, and to present the results in ways which can be easily grasped and interpreted by the electroencephalographer or the referring physician.

Small computers are also used for studies of *evoked responses*. Any sudden sensory stimulus, such as a tone pulse or flash of light, may elicit two types of response in the EEG. There is a non-specific reaction, independent of the sensory modality of the stimulus, consisting of a widespread potential change, usually maximal at the vertex, and sometimes accompanied by attenuation of on-going activities, especially if the subject's attention is attracted. A more specific evoked response occurs with a characteristic amplitude and waveform and constant time course following the stimulus, generally maximal over the cortical area appropriate to

Fig. 12.1. Principle of the Burden Neurological Institute low-frequency wave analyser: block diagram and example of write-out which represents the integrated output of each filter as a succession of pen deflections on the EEG chart.

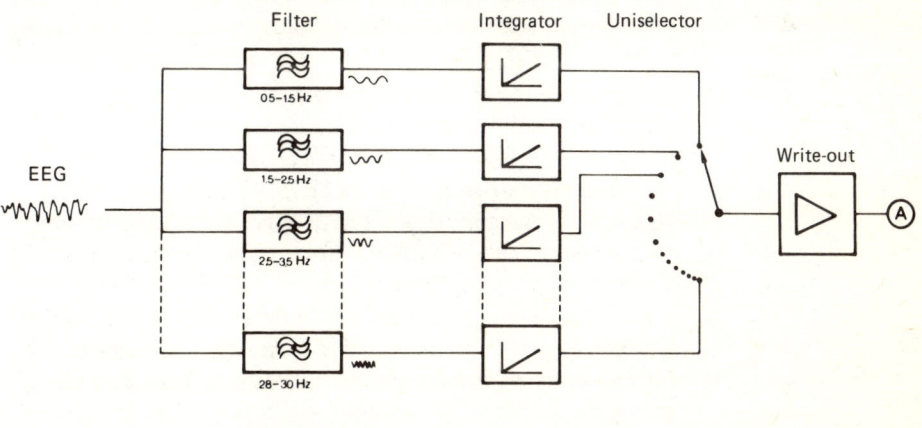

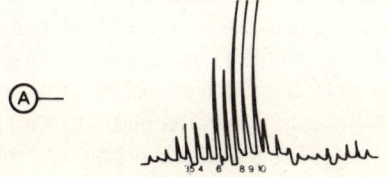

the modality and laterality of stimulation. The largest evoked responses are those elicited by visual stimuli and these can generally be detected in the conventional EEG record, particularly when the stimulus is presented repetitively at a suitable frequency to produce photic following. However, much smaller responses, for instance to auditory or tactile stimuli, can also be detected by 'signal averaging' (Section 12.3.) which is carried out with a computer. This may be a very simple machine intended for this one application, or a general purpose computer capable also of analysing on-going activity.

It will therefore be seen that EEG data processing, from the standpoint both of technique and applications, falls mainly into two categories: (i) the quantification of on-going activity, so-called *time series analysis*, and (ii) the detection of transients, discontinuous events such as evoked potentials and spontaneous epileptiform discharges. The value of both types of analysis may be increased by application of mathematical *pattern recognition* techniques to permit computer-assisted interpretation of the EEG and this is a rapidly expanding field which deserves consideration in its own right.

12.2. Time series analysis

12.2.1. Amplitude analysis

The objective of analysing on-going EEG activity may be just to obtain some simple measure, for instance to detect change in the course of biochemical disease, or the aims may be more ambitious, for example to arrive at a diagnostic interpretation of the record, via a pattern-recognition process. In either case the first step is to describe the tracing in numerical form. It can be argued that so little is known about the physiological mechanisms determining the characteristics of the EEG that there are no *a priori* grounds for selecting a particular method of quantifying the signals, and that one must empirically determine which technique seems to be most appropriate to any specific application. If a very simple index, such as the total electrical power regardless of frequency, is sufficient to answer the question under investigation, there is no reason to adopt more complex measures. In fact, just such measurements of the size of the EEG signals have been used very successfully, for instance to detect the effects and duration of action of various drugs (Drohochi, 1969; Doenicke, Kügler, Shellenberger and Gürtner, 1966). The magnitude of the EEG may itself be measured in various ways: the peak-to-peak excursion of the signals, the average amplitude (after rectification, without which the mean would be zero) or the power, which is the mean of the squared amplitude. This last measure has the theoretical advantage that it is widely used in engineering and its mathematical properties are understood. However, a feature which may sometimes be a disadvantage, is that particularly large waves have a disproportionately great influence on the values obtained.

A so-called 'Cerebral Function Monitor' is commercially available which provides a continuous tracing on a slowly-moving chart of the amplitude of the EEG (Fig. 12.2). The device also incorporates a single-channel EEG amplifier with special features to reduce susceptibility to interference and to check electrode resistance. It has been applied very successfully for following the progress of patients unconscious after acute cerebral anoxia and for monitoring cerebral function during open heart surgery (Prior *et al.*, 1971; Branthwaite, 1973; Prior, 1979).

12.2.2. Fourier analysis

Visual EEG analysis describes the record in terms of amplitude and frequency; established mathematical techniques are available to quantify a signal in much the same way, and have been extensively used in fields as varied as vibration engineering, radio astronomy, X-ray crystallography and seismology. These methods are mostly based on *Fourier analysis*, which in turn rests on the principle that any repetitive complex waveform can be built up by a series of harmonically related sine waves of specified magnitude and phase relations. Figure 12.3*a* shows how such a signal can be analysed in terms of a series of sinusoids. To describe the signal fully it is necessary to specify both the amplitude and phase of each component and this information is not usually convenient for graphic display. A measure having amplitude and angle (phase) is called a vector and can be represented in terms of the amplitude of two components mutually at right angles. In the present case it is convenient to describe the hypothetical sinusoids making up the EEG by resolving each vector into two components, sine and cosine (often called 'imaginary' and 'real'), 90° apart. Hence the signal can be represented graphically by its *Fourier coefficients*, comprising sine and cosine components (Fig. 12.3*b*).

These coefficients, the Fourier transform of the signal, can be manipulated in various ways (Fig. 12.3*c*). The process can be reversed, restoring the original signal; various frequency com-

Fig. 12.2. The Cerebral
Function Monitor.
(*a*) Block diagram.
(*b*) Examples of write-
out: (left) abrupt re-
duction of cerebral
activity during cardiac
arrest and recovery
following defibrillation;
(right) impedance moni-
toring channel signalling
deteriorating electrode
contact. Note that
artefacts produce an
easily recognized cut-
out of the display
avoiding possible mis-
interpretation. (Repro-
duced with permission
of Dr D. Maynard.)

(*a*)

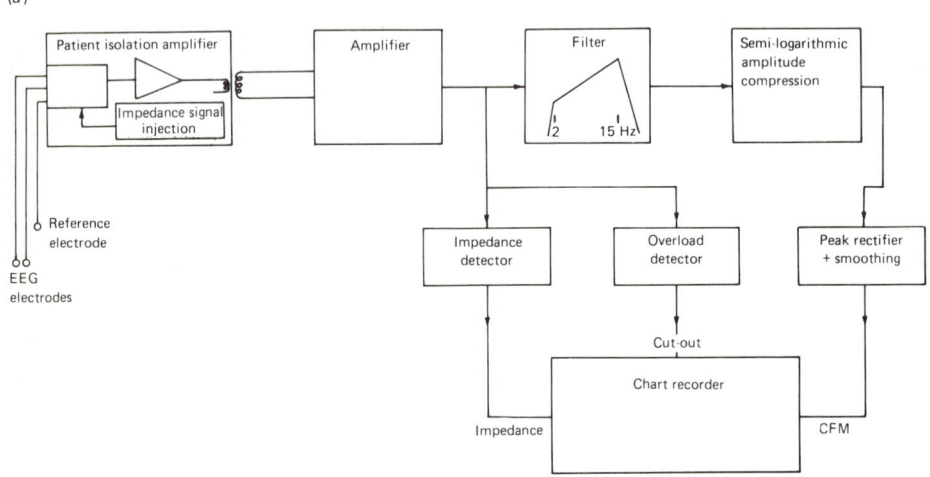

(*b*)

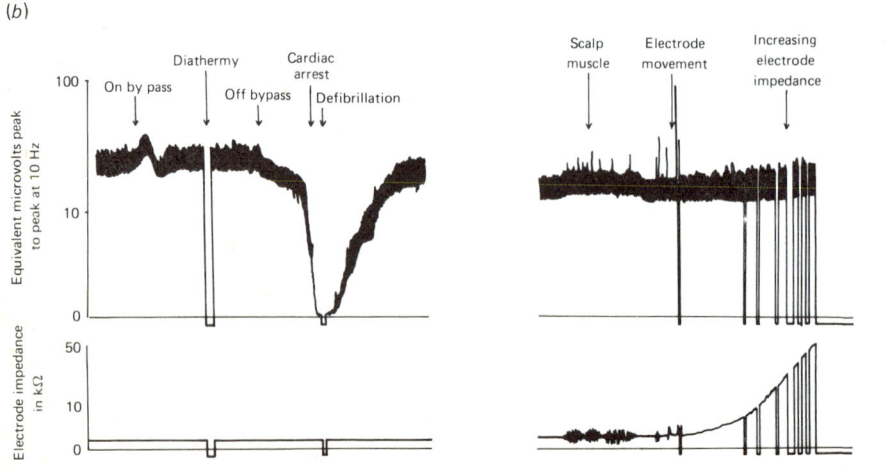

ponents can be removed before reverse transformation, achieving a highly selective filtration; the relationship between phase and frequency may be plotted as a *phase spectrum*; more usually the phase information is neglected and power alone is plotted as a *power spectrum*. There are a number of alternatives to Fourier analysis, for instance resolving the signal into square waves instead of sinusoids and these methods may have some computational advantages.

Related techniques allow the frequency and phase relationship between two different EEG channels to be studied (*cross-spectrum*) and inferences about common generating mechanisms to be made (*coherence*). These methods can be used to study the topography of the EEG and the transmission of evoked potentials or epileptic discharges (Brazier, 1972; Gotman, Ives and Gloor, 1977; Lopes da Silva *et al.*, 1979; Shaw and Ongley, 1972).

The above account skirted round some difficult theoretical problems of power spectra and the reader to whom these are of no interest may prefer to skip the remainder of this section.

It may not have escaped the notice that a fundamental assumption of Fourier analysis was that the signal should be repetitive. More strictly it should be 'stationary', that is to say that its statistical properties should not change with time. Very clearly the EEG does not satisfy this requirement, it changes from second to second with alterations of mental activity or opening and closing of the eyes, it changes over a time scale of 24 hours with the rhythms of waking and sleeping, and changes progressively from infancy to old age. Nevertheless, by choosing on the one hand to analyse epochs which are long enough to give reliable estimates of the average properties of the EEG but not so long that the subject's mental state is likely to change, and on the other hand contriving that during each epoch the state of the subject is kept as stable as possible, a tolerable approximation to stationarity can be achieved. The extent to which this endeavour is successful will influence the usefulness of the results obtained.

The Fourier transform also requires a random signal to be of infinite length. For an epoch with a finite length T s, it is impossible to measure the power at any specific discrete frequency; one can only *estimate* the power within frequency bands, with a width of $1/T$ Hz. Thus an 8-s epoch of EEG can be analysed to give estimates of the true *power spectral density* (PSD) curve at intervals of 1/8 Hz. Moreover, these estimates are themselves subject to a large variability which can be reduced by averaging

Fig. 12.3. (a) Principle
of Fourier analysis. The
repetitive signal above
can be resolved into
three component sinus-
oids of differing fre-
quency, amplitude and
phase. Phase and ampli-
tude can be represented
as vectors (right of fig.)
and each vector can it-
self be resolved into
two components,
mutually at right angles.
In (b) (facing page)
these are plotted
against frequency.

(a)

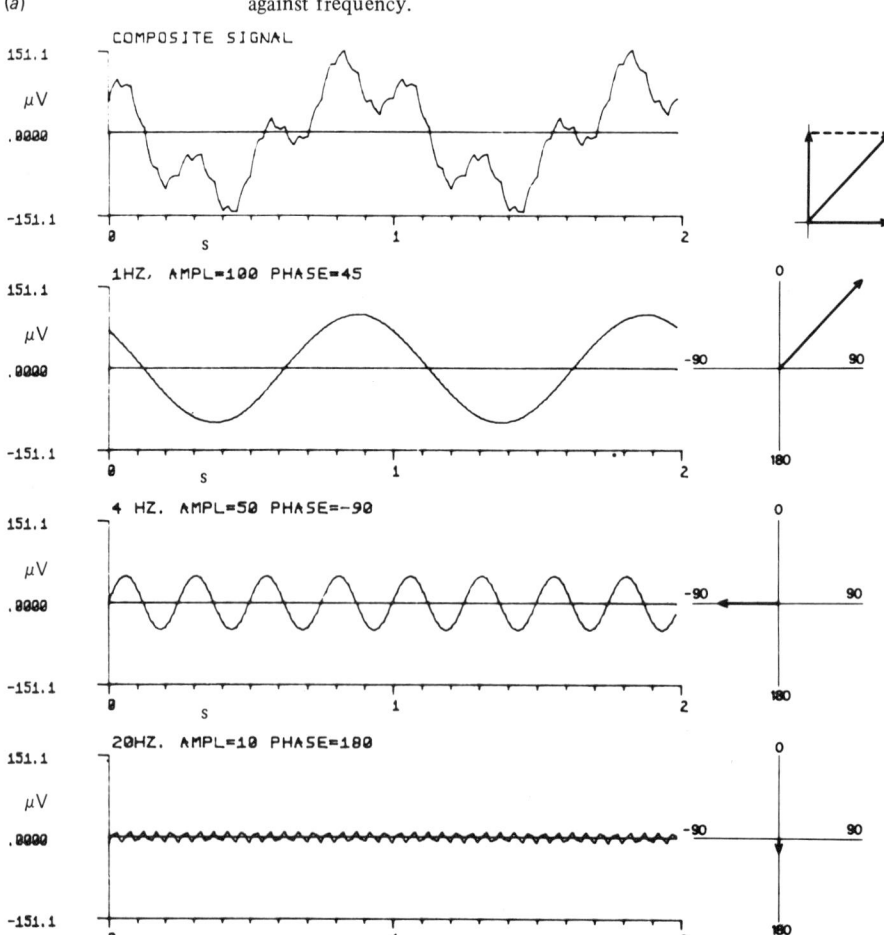

the values from many epochs and from adjacent frequency bands
(Fig. 12.3d).

Our problems are not yet over, for the analysis of short epochs
of abrupt beginning and end gives artefacts: a non-zero value at
the start of the epoch introduces a square wave, containing a wide
range of frequencies which will appear as spurious components in
the spectrum. This effect is called 'leakage' and may be minimized
by 'tapering' the signal by means of a 'cosine bell', as shown in
Fig. 12.4, but analysis of epochs shorter than about 4 s will be
rather inaccurate.

Fig. 12.3. (cont.)
(b) The same signal as
in (a), with its Fourier
coefficients ('real' and
'imaginary') and ampli-
tude and phase spectra.

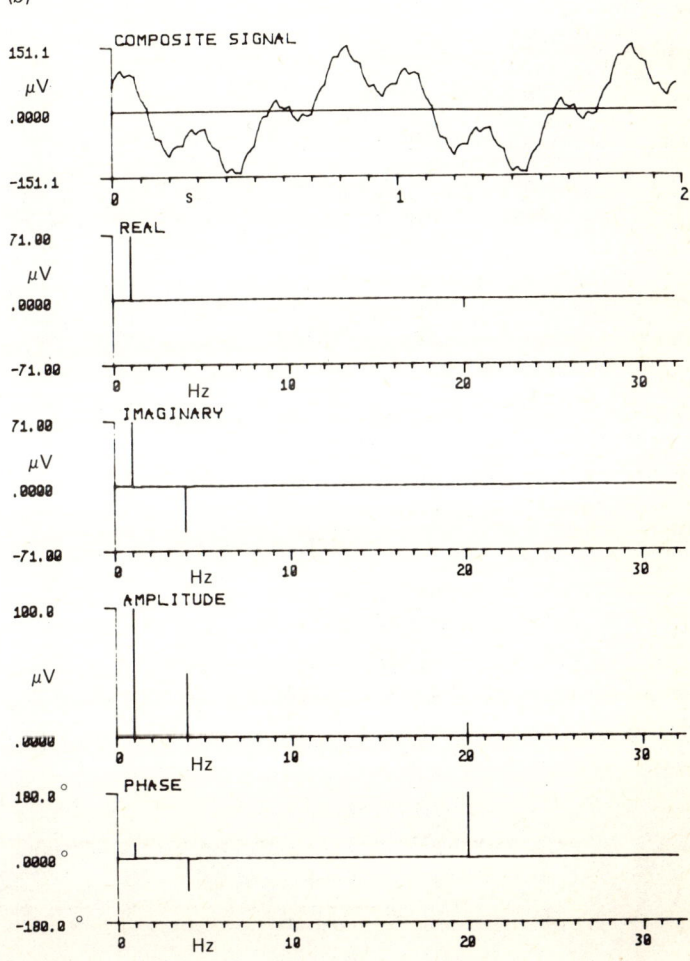

Fig. 12.3 (cont.)
(*c*) Spectral analysis of 1 s
sample of EEG. The
signal (above) is first
tapered and any DC
trend removed (see
also Fig. 12.4). From
the Fourier coefficients
(not shown) the discrete
power spectrum is ob-
tained; this gives an
estimate of the power
at intervals of 1 Hz. To
obtain a more accurate
estimate of the spec-
trum this is smoothed
(below), either by
averaging adjacent
points (continuous
curve) or by banding
into frequency ranges
(histogram).

The concept and use of coherence also present difficulties,
partly because this measure was developed for studying the transmission properties of systems, an application different from that
for which it is generally used in EEG analysis. If we compare
power spectral densities of the input and output of a system we
may find them to be similar; that is, both signals may contain a
large amount of energy in the same frequency bands. However,
before concluding that the common frequency components have
simply been transmitted through the system, one must consider
another possibility, that the output peaks were generated by
some other, unknown source. We would have stronger grounds
for inferring that the common frequency components had been
transmitted through the system if we could show that their phase

(*c*)

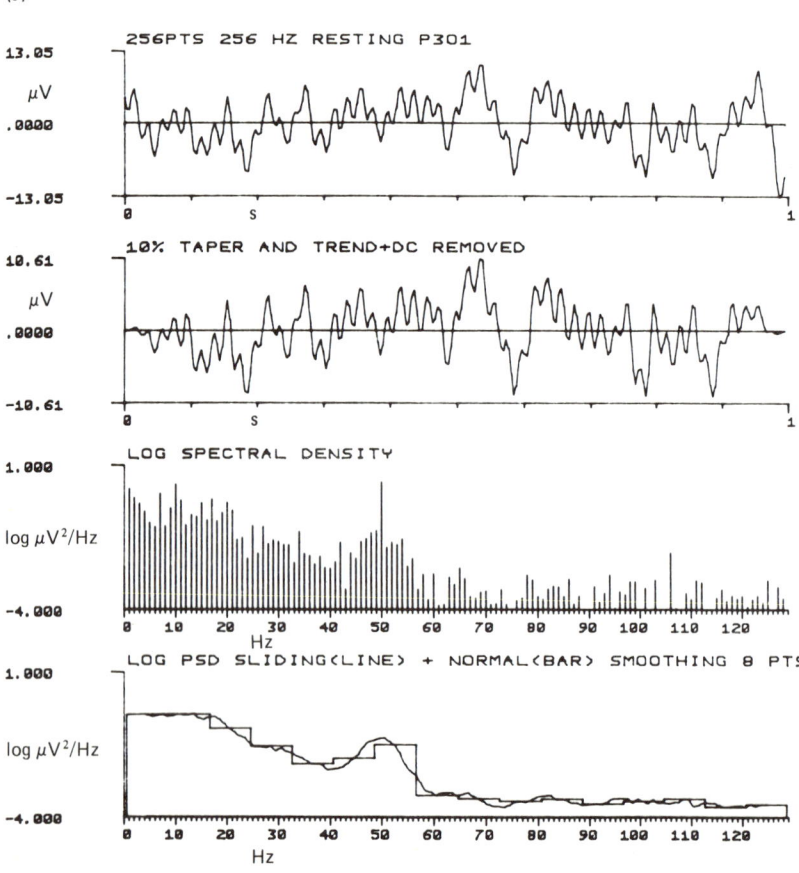

Fig. 12.3. (cont.)
(*d*) The EEG signal above is heavily contaminated with 50 Hz interference, which is reflected by a peak at 50 Hz in the amplitude spectrum. Removal of all Fourier components above 45 Hz gives the spectrum shown in the third line. Reverse transformation of the band-limited coefficients gives the filtered EEG signal below, uncontaminated by 50 Hz interference.

relations between input and output were constant and frequency dependent.*

The cross-spectrum measures the similarity of two signals in terms of the frequency and amplitude of common components with constant phase relations. By comparing this cross-spectrum with the power spectral densities of the two signals one can deduce to what extent the coincidence between them of energy in a particular frequency band reflects a common source. Coherence is a measure of this relationship and has a value of 1 for identical and 0 for unrelated signals. Formally:

$$C = \frac{|X|^2}{P1 \cdot P2}$$

where C is coherence, X is the cross-spectral density and $P1$ and $P2$ are the PSDs of the signals.

* If there is a constant transmission time then the phase shift will be frequency dependent: $360 \, D \cdot f$ degrees, where D is the delay in s and f the frequency in Hz.

(*d*)

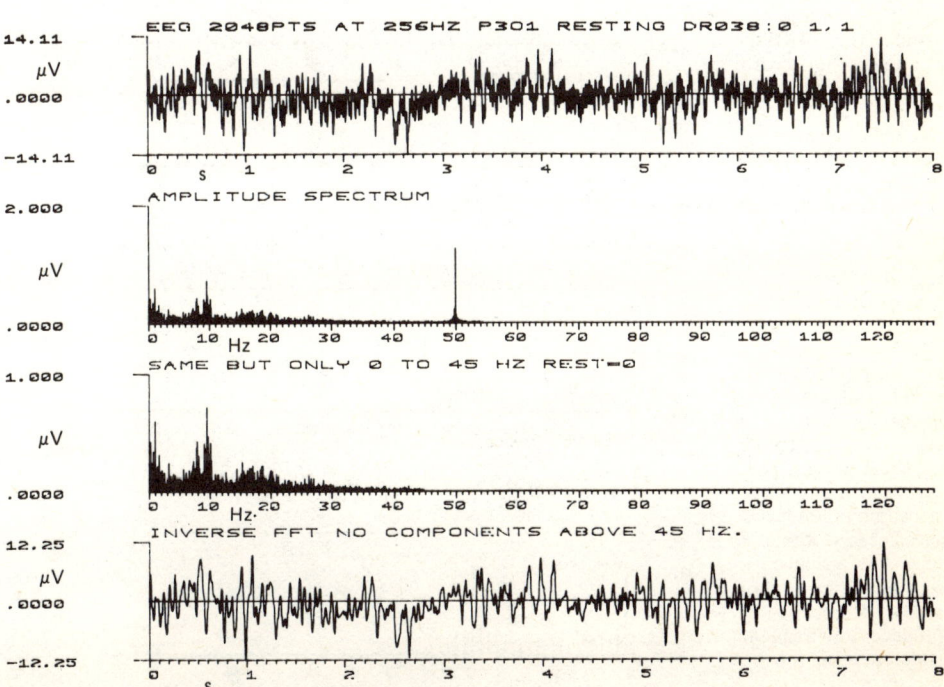

12.2.3. Time-domain analysis

Mathematicians and engineers may be accustomed to consider signals in terms of frequency, but the electroencephalographer sees the paper tracing as a series of waves of varying duration. Although frequency and period are obviously closely related, there are methods of EEG analysis which take as a starting point the measurement of the durations of individual waves ('period', 'interval' or 'wave duration' analysis). Possibly because these so-called *time-domain* techniques have a less formal mathematical basis, a multiplicity of different methods has been devised. The individual waves may be defined either by peaks and troughs or by the points at which the signal passes through a base-line or near zero threshold. In general, this family of techniques suffers

Fig. 12.4. Leakage and effects of DC trend. The signal above is a 20.5 Hz sinusoid sampled at 128 Hz. It will be seen that, although the sampling frequency is far higher than the minimum required to avoid aliasing (41 Hz) the waveform is slightly distorted. Note also that the values at the start and end of epoch are unequal. The spectrum shows not only a peak split between the two discrete frequencies (20 and 21 Hz) adjacent to the true value, but also spurious components due to leakage. If the signal is multiplied by a 10% cosine bell (third line) its ends are tapered so that the values at the start and end of epoch are equal to zero. The spectrum of this tapered signal shows less leakage. The lowest two lines show a similar signal superimposed on a slow DC trend which produces low-frequency components in the spectrum.

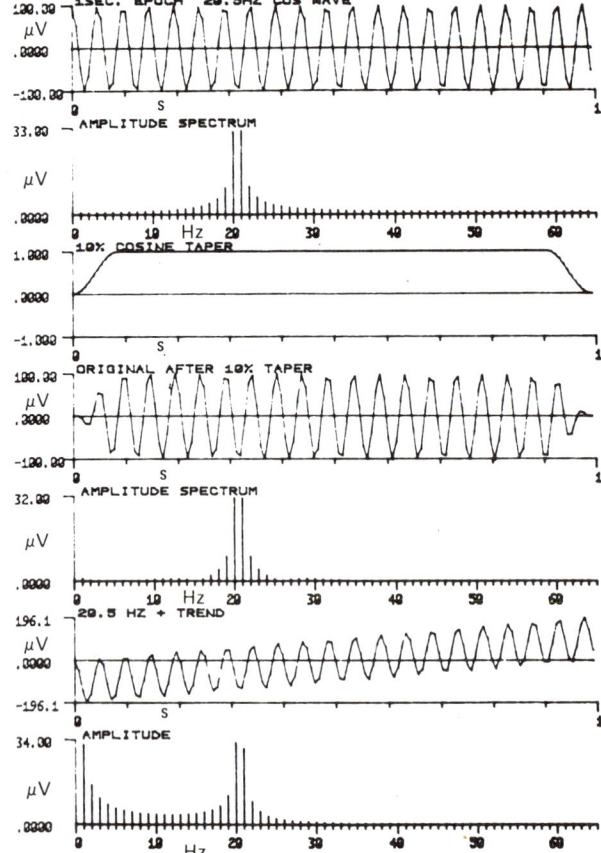

from the deficiency that interactions occur between components of different frequencies (Fig. 12.5).

When low-amplitude fast activity is superimposed on larger slow waves, the fast components will rarely produce a base crossing and may therefore be underestimated. Conversely, high-amplitude

Fig. 12.5. Wave duration analysis. (*a*) Zero cross analysis. Recognition of zero crossings (above) allows the duration of each half wave to be recognized. (centre) Slow activity may be masked by faster components and relatively low-amplitude fast activity may be underestimated in the presence of slow waves. (below) When faster and slower components of similar amplitudes are present the duration of the slow waves (L) will be under-estimated and the amplitude (A) over-estimated.
(*b*) Wave duration analysis by recognition of peaks: a simple algorithm will recognize either the wave ABC or the two waves Ade and eBC; to obtain an approximation to the power spectrum it is necessary to recognize all three waves Ade, eBC and AeC.

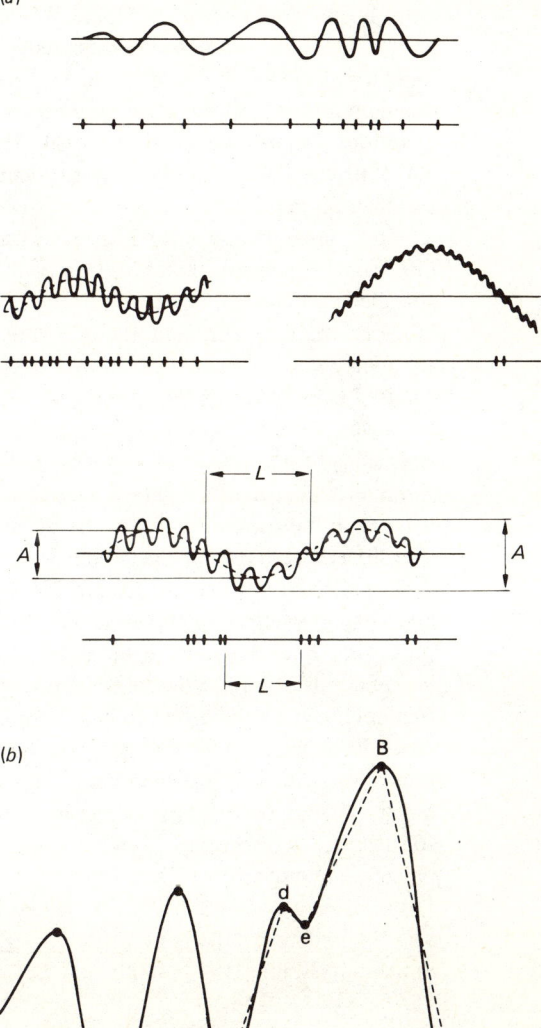

fast activity superimposed upon slow components may cause frequent base-line crossings so that the slow activity cannot be detected. When slow and faster activities are mixed in roughly equal amounts there is a tendency for the peak-to-peak amplitude of the slow components to be overestimated and for the period to be underestimated. Various solutions have been suggested, some imposing arbitrary constraints which at least ensure some consistency in the results (Leader, Cohn, Weihner and Caceres, 1967; Burch, Edwards, Nettleton and Sweeney, 1964; Stigsby, Obrist and Sulg, 1973). Other workers have come closer to solving the problem but only at the price of complex, time-consuming computations (Benoit *et al.*, 1973; Schenk, 1973; Monakhov *et al.*, 1974; Binnie, 1975), successively segmenting the curve into waves of different periods.

An interesting and novel approach was described by Hjorth (1970), who proposed a description of the EEG in terms of three so-called *normalized slope descriptors*. These three measures, 'activity, mobility and complexity' relate to the magnitude, mean frequency and frequency range of the signal. Activity is mean squared amplitude, measured therefore in μV^2 and closely related to power; mobility is root mean squared slope (first derivative) normalized for activity and its units are Hz; complexity compares the rate of change of slope (second derivative) with that of a sine wave with the same mobility as the signal and is measured in Hz. The difference between the mobility and the complexity of a signal reflects the scatter of frequencies present. The descriptors are comparatively simple* to calculate and take much less computer time than the power spectrum, yet bear a formal mathematical relationship to it. Whether or not they are useful for a particular clinical application can be determined only by trial and error. Experience so far suggests that they are of some value for monitoring biochemical disorders (Binnie, Bown, Lloyd and Smith, 1973a), can usefully be employed for detecting artefacts, for instance in recordings of evoked potentials, and for identifying paroxysmal discharges (Binnie, Fee, Lloyd and Roberts, 1973b; Lloyd, Binnie and Fee, 1973; Binnie and Lloyd, 1973), and can also be used to characterize different stages of sleep (Layzell, Smith and Binnie, 1973; Caille and Bassano, 1975). In routine

---

* The mathematical operations involved are simple but, for technical reasons, calculating Hjorth's descriptors accurately on a small computer requires quite sophisticated programming.

clinical EEG work, this method may be of less value than power spectral analysis (Binnie *et al.*, 1978a).

12.2.4. Applications of time-series analysis

Most methods for analysing background activity produce more information than can conveniently be interpreted. One solution is to use the results of analysis as the input to a further interpretative pattern-recognition process (see Section 12.7. below). Another method is to present the numerical values graphically and hence exploit the pattern-recognition capability of the human observer (Fig. 12.6). For some purposes the power spectrum can be summarized by a comparatively small number of parameters (Wennberg and Zetterberg, 1971).

What then has time-series analysis of the EEG achieved to date? In routine clinical work it has been little used but some groups of workers (Storm van Leeuwen, Arntz, Spoelstra and Wieneke, 1976, Magnus *et al.*, 1977) claim that the presentation of a power spectrum together with the conventional EEG assists interpretation of the latter. At the least, in a majority of subjects the power spectra support the conclusions from visual analysis concerning such features as dominant frequency, background asymmetry, etc. and in a small proportion of patients, new information is obtained which may be of diagnostic value. Other workers have used further processing of the power spectrum to permit computer-aided decision making (Section 12.7.). Otherwise, practical evalu-

Fig. 12.6. Hidden line display of power spectra during photic stimulation: as the flicker frequency is swept from 1 to 10 Hz, a fundamental following component is clearly seen, together with a second harmonic at some frequencies. This display presents very concisely the large amount of information contained in an experiment of several minutes' duration. (Reproduced with permission from Bickford, 1973 in Kellaway and Petersén, *Automation of Clinical Electroencephalography*, Raven Press, New York.)

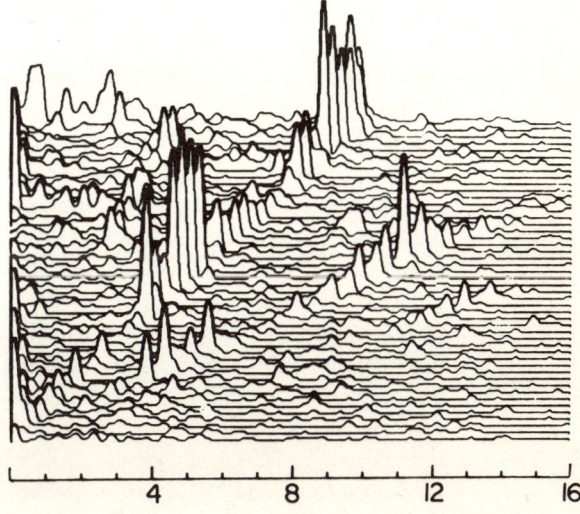

ation of the use of spectral or period analysis for clinical purposes has been restricted to a few biochemical applications, notably hepatic or renal failure (Kardel *et al.*, 1972; Bourne *et al.*, 1975). However, in a research context much more has been achieved. Just two different types of applications will be considered as examples. Using spectral EEG analysis, Sklar, Hanley and Simmons (1973) were able to differentiate between dyslexic children and normal controls matched for age and sex, and Montagu (1975) used similar measures to distinguish hyper-kinetic from normal children. Much more work has been carried out in the field of psychopharmacology and several groups of workers have now confirmed the findings of Itil (1974) that different types of psychotropic drugs may be identified by their effects on the EEG as assessed by power spectra or time-domain analysis. This is a development of great practical importance, for there are no very satisfactory animal models of human psychiatric disorders and the assessment of possible new psychotropic drugs presents considerable practical and ethical problems. A preliminary screening by measuring the EEG effects in normal volunteers could allow new agents of possible therapeutic value to be identified and then subjected to clinical trials in appropriate groups of patients.

12.3. Evoked responses

The simplest method of detecting evoked responses in the presence of background EEG activity is to superimpose a number of tracings each immediately following a stimulus (Fig. 12.7). The typical waveform of the evoked potential following the stimulus shows up against a confused background due to the random elements. This method is generally usable only if the amplitude of the evoked response is not less than that of the background activity, a condition which is rarely satisfied except by responses to flashes of light. More usually, *signal averaging* is necessary.

As the evoked potential follows a constant time course after stimulation, the average of several sections of EEG, each recorded immediately following stimulus presentation, shows the typical waveform of the evoked response. If, by contrast, the on-going EEG activity following the stimulus has a random time course and an amplitude randomly distributed about zero, its mean value must itself be zero and this component of the EEG will be reduced in the average. Thus averaging diminishes the unwanted 'noise' or random activity and highlights the evoked response. The process can be carried out by hand or by various ingenious optical techniques but for all practical purposes a computer is used.

Orthodox methods of signal averaging give a reduction of noise relative to the signal (*signal/noise ratio*) proportional to $\sqrt{n}$, where n is the number of responses averaged (Fig. 12.8). It will be seen that if the signal is not too noisy a fairly clear response emerges after about a dozen samples have been averaged. However, because the signal/noise ratio increases only as the square root of the number of samples averaged, if the amount of noise is large, the number of presentations of the stimulus required to produce a readable evoked response becomes prohibitive. With repeated, and particularly with regular, presentation of the stimulus, the responses become much smaller due to habituation; for most purposes irregular stimulus presentations at intervals of 1–10 s are desirable. In addition, the averaging process will enhance the signal only if the evoked waveform is constant; however, changes in attention due to boredom or drowsiness produce changes in

Fig. 12.7. Auditory evoked response displayed by superimposition of successive sweeps. Above: with a high stimulus intensity (80 dB) the response is clearly visible against the background of random activity. Below: at a lower stimulus intensity (20 dB) the response is no longer visible in the superimposed tracings though detectable by other methods. (From Binnie and McClelland, 1977.)

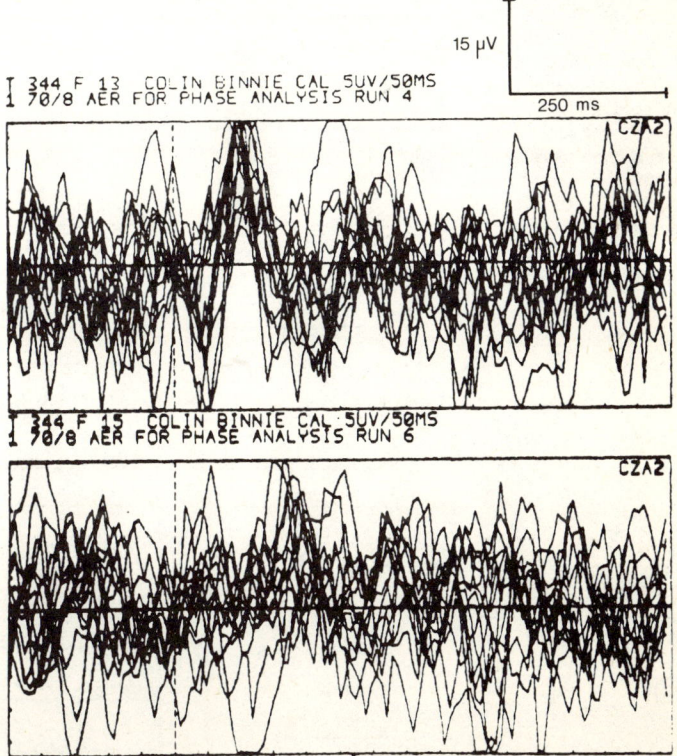

Fig. 12.8. (*a*) Auditory evoked responses displayed by signal averaging. With decreasing signal intensity (from above downwards) the amplitude of the response is less and the latency increases. The top and bottom tracings are averages of the signals in Fig. 12.7. (*b*) Effect of averaging increasing numbers of sweeps (from above downwards 1, 4, 16 and 32). The tracings on the left were obtained with eyes open and with a background EEG of low amplitude. Those on the right were recorded from the same subject with the eyes closed and the background EEG dominated by high-amplitude alpha activity. Note that in this case though the averaging of successive tracings produces progressive decrease in the amplitude of the average background activity no clear response emerges (From Binnie, 1976.)

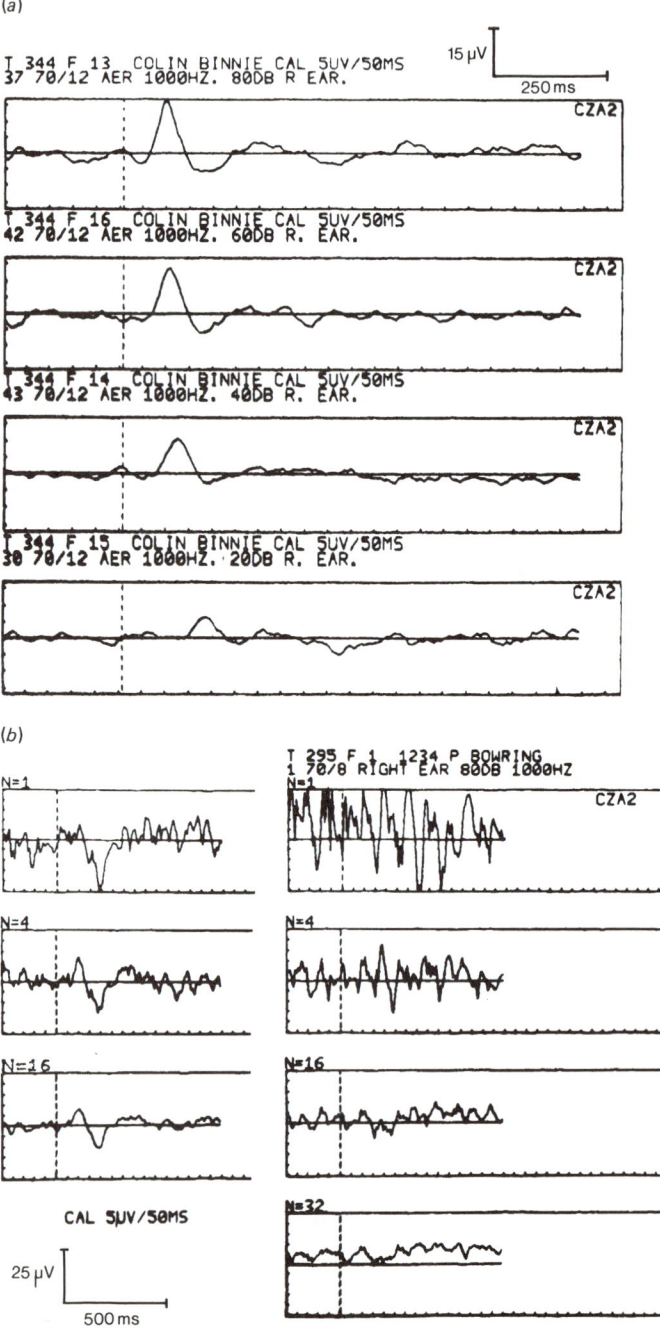

evoked responses. The consequence of all these factors is to impose a practical limit to the improvement of signal/noise ratio which can be obtained. If no satisfactory evoked potential can be seen after averaging the responses to some 30 stimulus presentations spread over a period of 2 minutes (signal/noise enhancement of $\sqrt{30}$, i.e. approximately five-fold), then to obtain a worthwhile, say two-fold further improvement of signal/noise ratio will involve continuing the stimulation for 8 minutes. During this time, the attention of the subject is likely to wander and vigilance will not be maintained, changing the waveform of the evoked responses and thus defeating the whole exercise.

Various methods may be adopted to obtain evoked responses from EEGs with high-voltage background activity or many artefacts. Where the noise is intermittent, a combination of averaging and superimposition, i.e. superimposing averages of some five responses, can be surprisingly successful; the averages contaminated by artefacts are so obviously different from the others that they can be ignored (Fig. 12.9). Alternatively, epochs containing artefacts can be omitted from the average either by some method of on-line artefact detection (Binnie *et al.*, 1973b) or by selectively averaging artefact-free epochs from a magnetic tape-recording after the experiment has been completed. Another approach is to use a different type of average, not the mean, but the median, which is less affected by occasional extremely high voltages. Where the high-amplitude noise is continuous, for example in a subject who simply has a high-voltage EEG, there is often no satisfactory solution and it may be extremely difficult to obtain legible averaged evoked responses.

Fig. 12.9. Average of 35 responses (above) compared with 7 superimposed sub-averages of 5 below. On the left the ensemble average was distorted by the presence of one large eye movement artefact and this produces one sub-average which is clearly different from the others and which may be ignored. On the right the noise took the form, not of an isolated artefact but of continuous background EEG activity and the method of superimposing sub-averages is even less satisfactory than simple averaging. (From Binnie, 1976.)

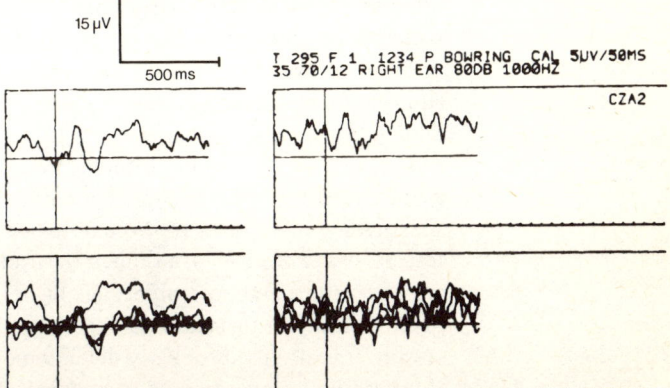

Some methods have been introduced to achieve detection of evoked potentials even where no readable average is obtainable. In Section 12.2.2. above it was explained how Fourier analysis can split the signals into series of harmonically related sine waves, each characterized by a particular amplitude and phase. In the absence of any stimulus the phases of the various frequency components within a series of short epochs should be randomly scattered. However, Sayers, Beagley and Hensall (1974) have shown that the non-random events in the EEG which follow a stimulus impose a phase constraint on the various frequency components so that the phase spectra become non-random and particular values of phase cluster at certain frequencies (Fig. 12.10). A method of detection which has perhaps been neglected is that of Krekule (1968). A zero-cross technique is used to give a histogram of intervals between the stimuli and base-line crossings. These may be expected to be randomly distributed if the stimulus has no effect upon the EEG, but a response produces an excess of crossings at particular intervals. Statistical methods are available for continuously testing the randomness of the intervals between the stimulus and base-line crossings so that the experiment can be terminated as soon as it has been shown with a specified level of confidence that the stimuli are having an effect upon the EEG.

One of the first practical applications of evoked responses was for evaluation of hearing (*evoked response audiometry*, ERA). There are a number of patients in whom conventional subjective hearing tests cannot be used. The majority are children presenting with speech difficulties where there is doubt as to whether the cause is deafness, or another disorder such as subnormality, a psychiatric illness or a social problem. Disturbed children will often not co-operate in conventional hearing tests and may show no behavioural reaction even to very loud noises. However, the presence of evoked responses to sound is evidence at least of auditory function, though not necessarily of perception. By determining the threshold stimulus intensity for obtaining an auditory evoked response at various different frequencies, it is possible to plot an audiogram, a curve relating sensitivity of hearing to pitch. This gives results similar to those obtained by subjective hearing tests (Davis *et al.*, 1967), although the evoked response thresholds are often some five to ten decibels higher. In co-operative but psychiatrically disturbed or malingering adults, ERA is very successful. It is also used for early detection of deafness in babies. However, in the largest group of patients who would seem suitable

Fig. 12.10. Evoked response detection by means of phase spectra. The results from 30 epochs have been superimposed, each point representing the phase (ordinate) at a particular frequency, values from each epoch being represented by a different letter or numeral.
(a) With a stimulus close to threshold the points are almost randomly scattered. (b) With a more intense stimulus there is clearly clustering at particular phase values at certain frequencies. (From Binnie, 1976.)

(a)

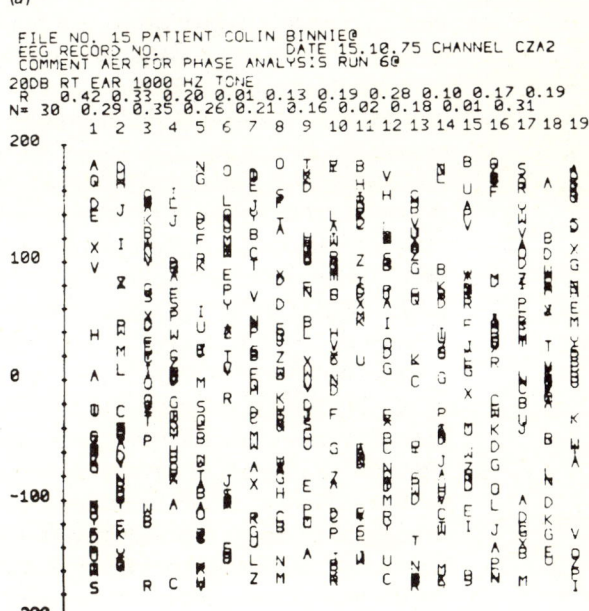

(b)

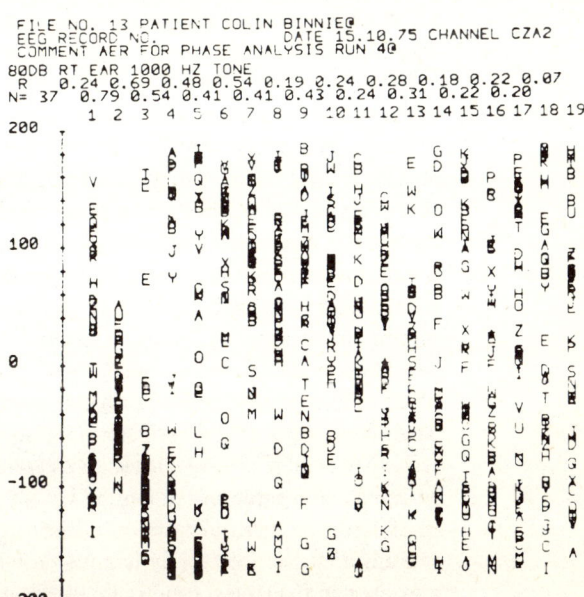

for this method of testing, namely children of an age at which speech disorders are likely to be first noticed and investigated, ERA can be extremely difficult. Children from one to four years are often extremely restless subjects for EEG recording, the more so if they are of subnormal intelligence or psychiatrically disturbed. The high-voltage EEG of a child further contaminated with movement and muscle artefacts may produce a signal/noise ratio so low that evoked responses cannot satisfactorily be demonstrated by averaging. Feasibility studies suggest that some limited form of evoked response audiometry is possible in most babies from 6 months to 2 years of age and in some 70% of subnormal children (Jones *et al.*, 1975, 1976). For quick audiometric screening in difficult children, the post-auricular myogenic response or the BAER (see below) may be more useful.

Evoked responses can similarly be used to test other sensory systems. The presence or absence of responses to flash is of course a somewhat crude test of visual function but pattern reversal allows more sensitive testing to be carried out. The pattern reversal stimulus typically consists of a black and white checker board in which the dark and light squares can abruptly be interchanged, usually by means of a mirror but sometimes by a television display (Arden *et al.*, 1977) or electronically (Evans *et al.*, 1974). By determining the size of squares necessary to elicit a response, visual acuity or refractive error can be measured (Regan, 1973).

More recently, clinical uses for evoked responses have been found, not so much in testing sensory function *per se* but as a means of detecting cerebral abnormality. For instance Laget *et al.* (1976) showed that asymmetries of somato-sensory evoked potentials in the newborn gave a more reliable prediction of subsequent hemiparesis than did either routine electroencephalography or conventional neurological examination. Pattern reversal evoked responses have particularly been used in investigation of patients with suspected multiple sclerosis which commonly produces delay in some components of the response, even where visual function is unaffected or has apparently returned to normal (Halliday, McDonald and Mushin, 1972).

A special class of evoked responses are the *event-related slow potentials*. If a subject is presented with paired stimuli about 1 s apart and is required to respond to the second, for instance by pressing a button, he rapidly learns to use the first stimulus as a warning cue that the second is about to occur. As he awaits the second stimulus there appears at the vertex a negative-going potential change, which disappears immediately after the response has been made (Fig. 12.11). This 'expectancy wave', more properly called the contingent negative variation (CNV) (Walter *et al.*, 1964) thus appears to be an electrophysiological correlate of a mental state. It is dependent upon the amount of attention that is directed to the task, is increased by high motivation and reduced by drowsiness or distraction. A similar negative potential change may be recorded over the contralateral central area about 1 s before a voluntary movement, the *Bereitschafts-potential* (Kornhuber and Deecke, 1965).

In addition to the classical evoked responses arising in the cerebral cortex, sensory stimuli produce a number of other bioelectrical phenomena. For instance, within 1–3 ms following an abrupt auditory stimulus a biphasic wave of about 1 μV amplitude may be recorded from an electrode located in or adjacent to the ear. This phenomenon, the electrocochleogram, permits considerably more precise testing of hearing than does the auditory evoked response. The cochleogram can be registered with an electrode over the mastoid process or on the ear-lobe, but a more satisfactory recording is obtained by means of a needle electrode passed through the eardrum into the promontory (a bony protuberance on the medial wall of the middle ear) and a reference on the ipsilateral ear-lobe. This procedure will therefore usually require the participation of an ENT surgeon and is more often

Fig. 12.11. Contingent negative variation. Note evoked responses elicited by the stimuli S_1 and S_2, the build-up of CNV during the intrastimulus interval and the abrupt collapse of the CNV in association with the response R.

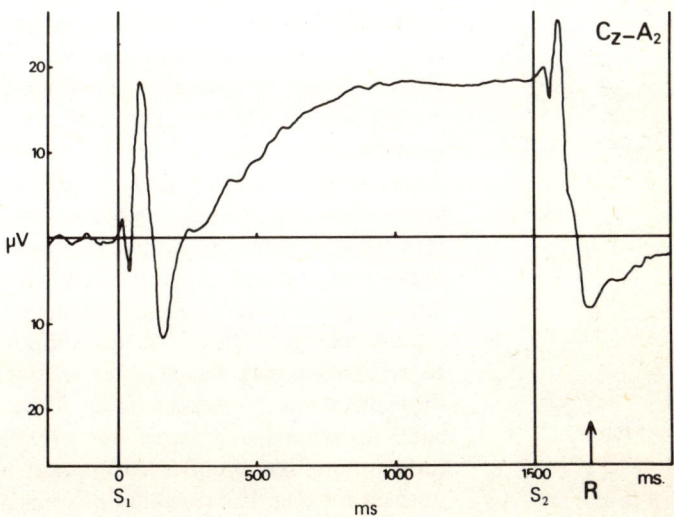

practised in audiological clinics than in EEG departments. Super-imposed upon the cochleogram which is generated by the VIIIth nerve, is a further potential change arising from the cochlea, the *cochlear microphonic*. The polarity of the microphonic is deter-mined by that of the sound pressure wave; an increase in pressure produces a positive microphonic and a decrease a negative re-sponse. It is therefore possible to separate the microphonic which is dependent upon the polarity of the sound wave from the cochleogram, which is not. The usual procedure is to present alternating positive and negative pressure waves and to average these separately; the sum of these two sub-averages gives the cochleogram (the positive and negative going microphonics cancelling each other out), whereas the difference cancels out the cochleogram and shows the microphonic (Fig. 12.12a). Some commercial evoked response systems incorporate facilities for this type of averaging.

With a remote electrode, a train of waves can be registered, forming a 'far-field' *brainstem auditory evoked response* (BAER). The topography of the BAER is complex and the waveform depends on the site of the electrodes. By recording from ear-lobe to vertex, six or seven waves (I–VII) may be detected over a period of 8–10 ms following the stimulus (Jewett, Bomans and Williston, 1970; Starr and Achor, 1975). As the origin of each of these waves is known (Lev and Sohmer, 1972), the absence of one of them may allow a lesion on the auditory pathway to be located with some precision (Fig. 12.12b). The technique is of diagnostic value in patients with a variety of neurological dis-orders, including multiple sclerosis, acoustic neuroma, and vascular lesions or tumours of the brain stem (Stockard and Rossiter, 1977). The potential changes are of much lower ampli-tude than the cortical evoked response (of the order of 1 μV). They are not affected by arousal level and do not exhibit habitu-ation during rapid stimulation to the same degree as the cortical response. It is therefore possible to present the stimuli at a much higher rate, for instance ten times per second, and to average responses to between one and four thousand stimulus presen-tations. At higher click frequencies (up to 70/s) the Vth wave persists, which may be adequate for audiometric purposes, but the earlier components are reduced. To record the BAER a band-width up to 2 kHz is essential, but for satisfactory registration of the waveform the amplifier must have an upper frequency limit of at least 5 kHz. The technique of stimulating with alternating

Fig. 12.12. (*a*) Cochlear microphonic displayed by subtracting sub-averages of responses to alternating compression and rarefaction clicks. (*b*) Brain stem evoked response obtained as a simple average of alternating compression and rarefaction clicks. The cochlear microphonic is no longer visible. (*c*) Early, medium and late auditory evoked potentials displayed upon a logarithmic time scale. (Reproduced with permission from Picton *et al.*, 1974.)

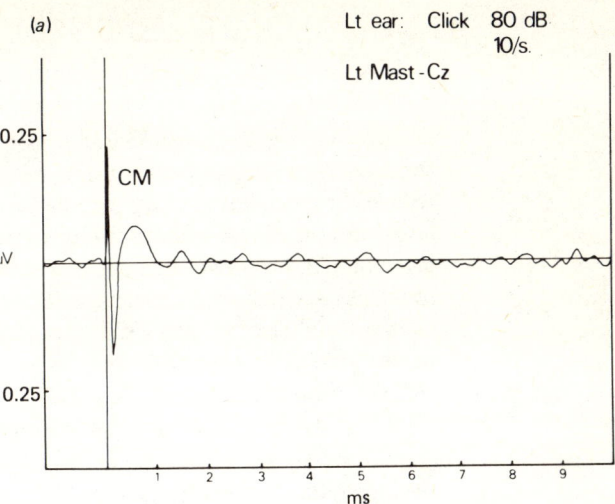

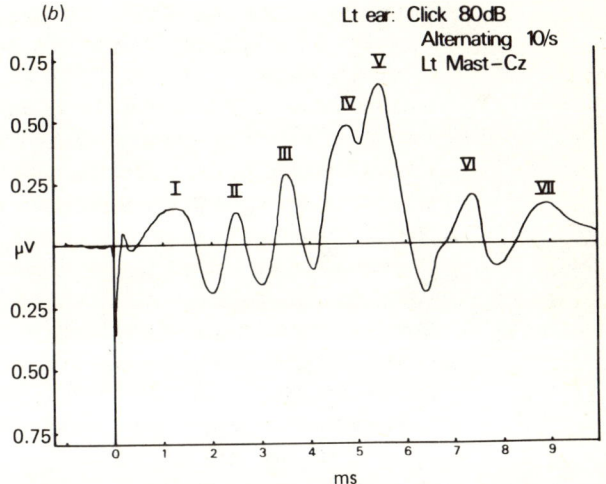

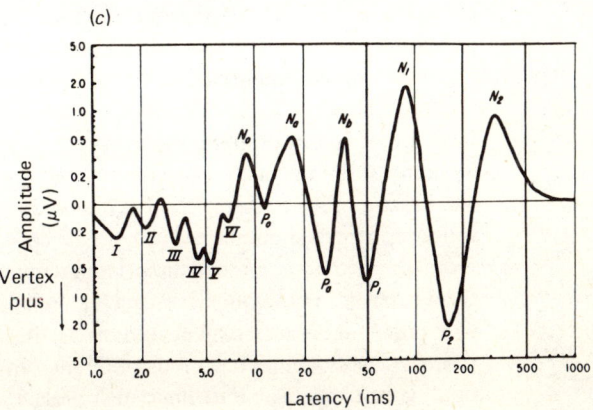

positive and negative pressure clicks may again be used to avoid
the cochlear microphonic obscuring wave I of the BAER and to
reduce the electrical artefact recorded from the headphones.
Some authors do not recommend this method for clinical BAER
investigations, as the latencies of responses to positive and negative clicks may differ in a patient with ear disease. See Stockard,
Stockard and Sharbrough (1978) for a detailed account of techniques for BAER registration and Chiappa, Gladstone and Young
(1979) for findings in normal controls.

If the auditory stimulus is an abrupt click, that is to say a
sound pressure wave with an abrupt rise time of not more than
50 μs, a reflex contraction of various muscles of the head, neck
and shoulders may take place. The resulting EMG signal may be
recorded most conveniently from an electrode placed behind the
ear over the post-auricular muscles (the *'post-auricular myogenic
response'*) (Cody and Bickford, 1969). This response is somewhat
inconstant and is influenced by pre-existing muscle tone; it can
for instance be enhanced by smiling and disappears if the subject
relaxes (Dùs and Wilson, 1975). Because of its variability it is not
satisfactory for audiometric testing. Nevertheless stimulation of
one ear produces post-auricular responses on both sides of the head
(paradoxically the contralateral or 'crossed acoustic response' is
larger than the ipsilateral potential); these phenomena can
therefore be used to test the integrity of the brain stem connections of the post-auricular muscle of one side to the contralateral
ear (Fig. 12.13) (Douek, Gibson and Humpfries, 1973).

Receptor responses can also be registered from the eye in
response to flash (the *electroretinogram*, or ERG). Electro-
retinography amounts to a subspeciality of ophthalmology and is
outside the scope of the present discussion; nevertheless the
techniques of recording and averaging are similar to those used
for other evoked potentials.

12.4. Detection of random transients
By contrast with evoked responses which have a constant temporal relationship to an external stimulus, some EEG transients
appear to occur spontaneously, notably epileptic discharges. In
some few instances these are associated with an easily detectable
event such as a myoclonic jerk which may be used as the reference point for an averaging procedure. In this case the signal of
interest usually comes before the reference and it is necessary to
employ 'back averaging' of the signals preceding the myoclonic

jerk. However, in the majority of instances the detection of random transients in the EEG depends upon identifying the electrophysiological event itself. The task may be approached in either of two ways. The most obvious is to attempt the recognition of the transient waveform. The second is to recognize simply that the EEG has undergone an abrupt change, regardless of its nature. In both cases the greatest difficulty lies in distinguishing the event of interest from other EEG changes or transients, such as myogenic or electrical artefacts. A large number of methods are available depending upon the phenomena to be detected, the circumstances of the recording, and the degree of reliability which is required.

A very simple approach might be just to recognize EEG waves above a certain specified amplitude. This is very adequate for detecting generalized spike-wave discharges (Ives, Thompson and Woods, 1973) but in its simplest form is also extremely sensitive to eye movement artefacts and a human operator is required to decide whether the events detected are in fact paroxysmal activity. Somewhat greater reliability can be achieved by first passing the EEG through a band-pass filter centered on 3 Hz. The slow wave component of the classical 3/s spike-wave discharge

Fig. 12.13. Post-auricular myogenic response (reproduced with permission from Dùs and Wilson, 1975).

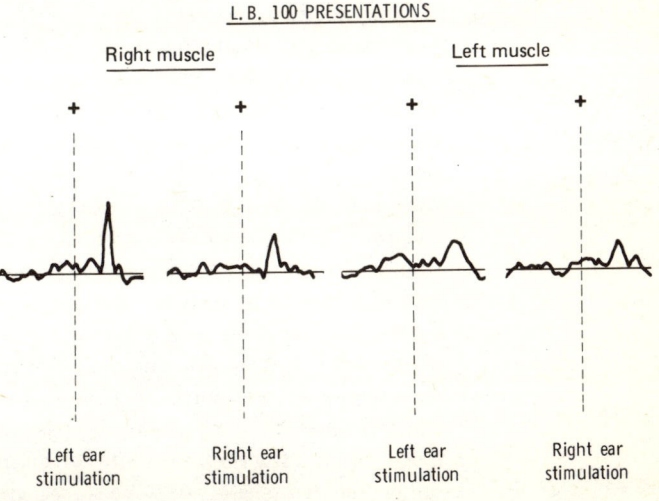

L.B. 100 PRESENTATIONS

Right muscle   Left muscle

+   +   +   +

Left ear   Right ear   Left ear   Right ear
stimulation   stimulation   stimulation   stimulation

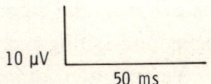

10 µV

50 ms

gives a high-amplitude output from the filter and the system is relatively insensitive to random eye movements or slow EEG waves unless these happen to be of the same frequency. A further improvement may be obtained by incorporating another filter to pass only the spikes and to regard a discharge as present only when a high-amplitude output is obtained from both filters simultaneously or in rapid succession. Unfortunately eye movements are often accompanied by spiky muscle potentials and therefore the system still fails to discriminate reliably against artefacts. Depending upon the application this state of affairs may be acceptable. For instance the authors have used such a device during 24-hour monitoring of patients with epilepsy. The system is used simply to identify sections of the EEG which may contain spike-wave discharges but a final decision is made by visual inspection. If the visual analysis of a 24-hour recording can be reduced to examination of only some 10 minutes of tracing, a very considerable saving in labour is achieved. In this particular application a high incidence of some 50% spurious identifications due to artefact is entirely acceptable. Such a system would not be suitable, of course, for recognizing other types of epileptic discharges, for instance isolated spikes, nor for a fully automatic analysis unchecked by visual inspection of a paper record.

Many methods have been described for spike recognition. The essential quality of spikiness is reflected in an abrupt change from ' a positive to a negative gradient of the waveform and this may be quantified by the mathematical operation of differentiation, which can be performed either with a digital computer or with a simple analogue device. Differentiation displays the gradient of the signal, and by repeating the operation one obtains the rate of change of gradient, which is maximal at the peak of the spike (Fig. 12.14). It may be sufficient to accept high values of this second derivative as evidence of a spike (Carrie, 1972) or, having detected a possible spike one may then measure the actual shape of the suspect wave. For this purpose suitable features are the duration between the preceding and succeeding minima, the rise and fall times, the height, and the peak angle or the ratio of height to duration (both measures of sharpness). Because of the rather rounded take-off of some spikes, greater reliability may be achieved by measuring, not only the shape of the entire wave, but also that of the section bounded by the steepest points of its rising and falling limbs (Ktonas and Smith, 1974).

Yet another approach to the recognition of clearly defined

transient waveforms, notably spike-wave complexes, is the use of a 'matched filter'. A matched filter may be implemented either in hardware or in a computer but is essentially a system tuned to recognize a particular waveform. Its impulse response (the response to the input of a very short pulse) is the time-inverse of the signal which it is set up to detect (Fig. 12.15). When the input signal has the waveform to which the system is tuned a maximum output is obtained. Spike-wave matched filters tend to discriminate rather poorly between spike-wave complexes and isolated slow waves. However, when a good match is obtained the output not only achieves a high value but also climbs to and falls away from this maximum very steeply: the output is itself a spike. If one therefore applies the simple spike-detection technique of double differentiation to the output of a matched filter it becomes more selective (Lloyd *et al.*, 1973). Further improvement can be achieved by preliminary manipulation of the EEG to give it a flat power spectrum ('pre-whitening'). This system discriminates well between spike-wave complexes and artefacts but has to be set up individually for the particular waveform of the paroxysmal activity found in a given patient. It is not suitable if the shape of the complexes is variable.

Fig. 12.14. Use of first and second derivatives to recognize spike. (*a*) Sinusoidal activity. (*b*) Triangular wave: the rising limb is steep giving a high value of the first derivative. (*c*) Spike: both rising and falling limbs are steep, therefore there is a high rate of change of gradient at the peak. This is reflected in a large negative value of the second derivative.

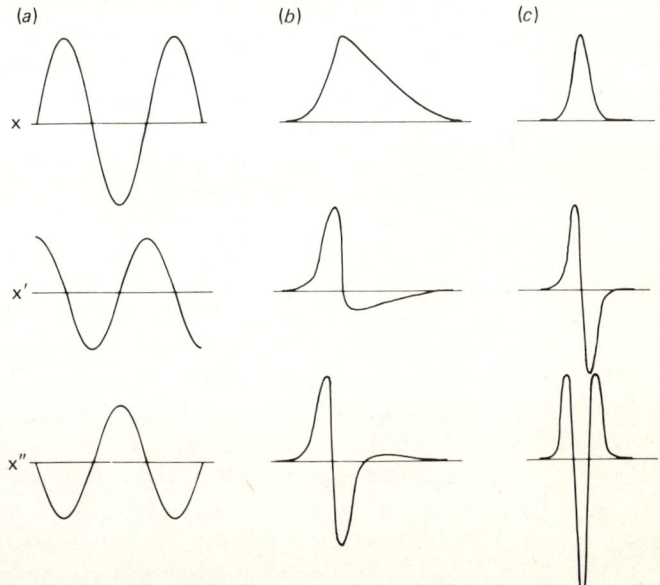

The empirical approach of simply detecting any change in the EEG has been developed by Lopes da Silva *et al.* (1977). By means of a so-called autoregressive function they measure the constancy of the spectral properties of the EEG; an abrupt 'non-stationarity' is taken to be evidence of a paroxysmal change. This method on its own is clearly inadequate for detecting epileptiform activity in long-term EEG recordings in which many sudden changes occur, for instance on opening and closing the eyes. It is, however, suitable for analysis of records obtained during seizures in which the timing of the onset of paroxysmal activity is already known to within a few seconds and the objective is to determine in which recording channel the change first occurs. This technique has been used very successfully in experimental epilepsy and may prove to be particularly valuable for localizing the origin of seizures in patients undergoing depth electrode recordings prior to surgical treatment of partial epilepsies. It has also been used as a preliminary screening method to detect non-stationarities which are then further analysed by more complex and time-consuming procedures designed to identify specific types of epileptiform discharges.

A compromise between identifying a particular waveform and simply recognizing a change is achieved by those workers who measure properties of the EEG which might reasonably be expected to have different values for background activity and for epileptiform discharges. For instance in a scatter diagram showing the amplitude and duration of each individual half wave (the excursion from a peak to a trough, or from a trough to a peak),

Fig. 12.15. The use of a matched filter to detect spike-wave complexes. (*a*) The response of the filter to a pulse input is a time-reversed spike-wave complex. (*b*) First line: raw EEG-tracing containing spike-wave complexes. Second line: output of matched filter. Third line: second derivative of filter output. Fourth: second derivative values passing through a specified threshold indicate the occurrence of a spike-wave complex. Below: the template used for this particular filter. (From Binnie, 1976.)

(a)

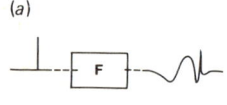

(b)

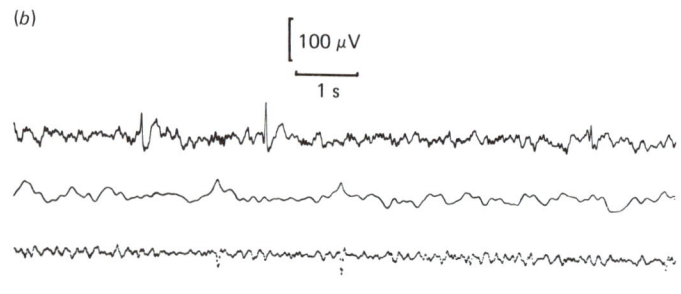

spike-wave complexes are seen as fast and slow components of higher amplitude relative to their duration than the background rhythms (Fig. 12.16). This method has been employed successfully by Harner (1978). Similarly it might be expected that the normalized slope descriptors of Hjorth (1970) (see Section 12.2) would change during a spike-wave discharge, reflecting the increased amplitude and the broadening of the power spectrum due to the increase in slow and fast components. This is indeed the case, and slope descriptor analysis based on short epochs of about a second is reasonably sensitive to paroxysmal activity of various types and also discriminates quite satisfactorily against common artefacts (Lloyd *et al.*, 1973).

Automatic recognition of epileptic activity has yet to realize its full potential in helping to solve practical clinical problems. Nevertheless, progress is being made, and there are indications that the following clinical areas may benefit from the application of these techniques:

(1) Quantification of paroxysmal activity in long-term recordings as a guide to adjusting anticonvulsant medication.

(2) Detection of the site of origin of discharges in suspected partial epilepsies.

(3) Monitoring systems to warn a patient of an impending seizure or to alert others to the occurrence of a seizure.

(4) Controlling psychological test procedures intended to detect impairment of cognitive function during epileptiform discharges (Binnie and Lloyd, 1973; Browne, Penry, Porter and Dreifuss, 1974).

Fig. 12.16. Plots of amplitude against period of individual waves in different regions of the head. (*a*) Normal background activity. (*b*) Characteristic patterns produced by spike-wave discharges. Mark on Y axis is 50 μV calibration; X axis is frequency equivalent of period. (Reproduced with permission from Harner and Ostergren, 1978.)

(a)

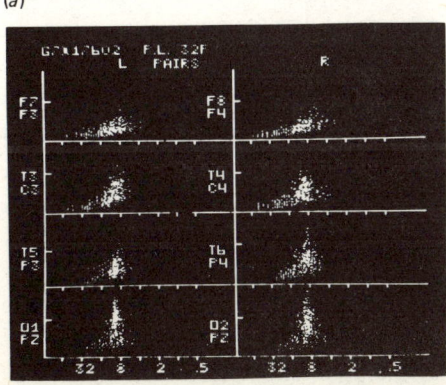

(b)

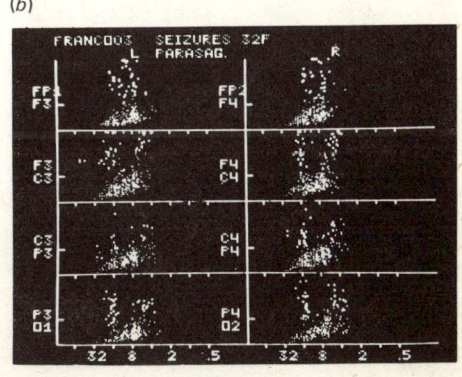

(5) Triggering EEG data acquisition systems intended to register selectively the EEG during seizures or epileptiform discharges (see Section 12.5 below).

For most of these possibilities to become a practical reality it will be necessary to develop considerably more reliable methods of discriminating between epileptic activities and artefacts 'on-line' in freely moving subjects.

12.5. EEG monitoring

A somewhat specialized use of computers which appears already to have an important practical clinical application is in long-term seizure monitoring. There is a substantial number of patients with suspected seizure disorders in whom interictal EEGs offer little diagnostic guidance and in whom, despite repeated recordings and prolonged clinical observation, uncertainty remains as to whether the attacks are in fact epileptic. A recording during a seizure offers the best chance of obtaining diagnostic EEG findings in these patients. There is also a need for seizure registrations in subjects being assessed for possible neurosurgical treatment of partial epilepsies. In these patients a solution is offered by the development of techniques for monitoring the EEG continuously over a period of several days. As noted in Section 9.3, the practical difficulty then arises that continuous recording results in the collection of great amounts of irrelevant data. It would be preferable to record selectively the EEG events immediately preceding, during and following a seizure or other clinical event of interest. It is too late to commence recording after a clinical change has already been recognized, as the initial EEG events in the seizure are often of the greatest diagnostic importance. However, by means of a digital computer, the EEG can be continually sampled and stored on a magnetic disc for a period of a few minutes after which it is over-written by more recent data. When a seizure is observed, a permanent record can be made of the signals already stored on the disc together with those obtained during and immediately after the seizure (Ives *et al.*, 1976; Lopes da Silva *et al.*, 1980; Binnie *et al.*, 1980). The trigger signal, which causes the computer to make a permanent record, may be provided by the patient himself, or by nursing personnel with the press of a button, by transducers to detect abnormal movements of the bed (Geursen, Terlouw and Wisman, 1978), or by detecting the occurrence of epileptiform discharges in the EEG itself. The numbers of patients to whom these monitoring techniques are applicable is sufficient to justify their use in units specializing in epilepsy (Stålberg, 1976; Binnie *et al.*, 1981).

12.6. Topographic displays

In Chapter 4 we discussed the problems of extracting topographical information from multichannel tracings showing the changes in potential difference between pairs of electrodes as a function of time. For most practical clinical purposes a good understanding of derivation technique on the part of both the recordist and the interpreter of the EEG will ensure that the distribution of activities over the surface of the scalp can be determined with no great difficulty. Nevertheless, it is sometimes instructive to present this information graphically, for instance as a contour-map, showing the potential distribution produced by a particular phenomenon. For instance, the map in Fig. 12.17 taken from a study of posterior slow activity in normal young adults gives a much clearer impression than does a conventional tracing. Plotting a contour-map of the potential distribution, for instance at the peak of a spike discharge, is a use-

Fig. 12.17. The topography of posterior temporal slow activity. (*a*) EEG from a 22-year-old subject showing posterior slow activity of maturational type.

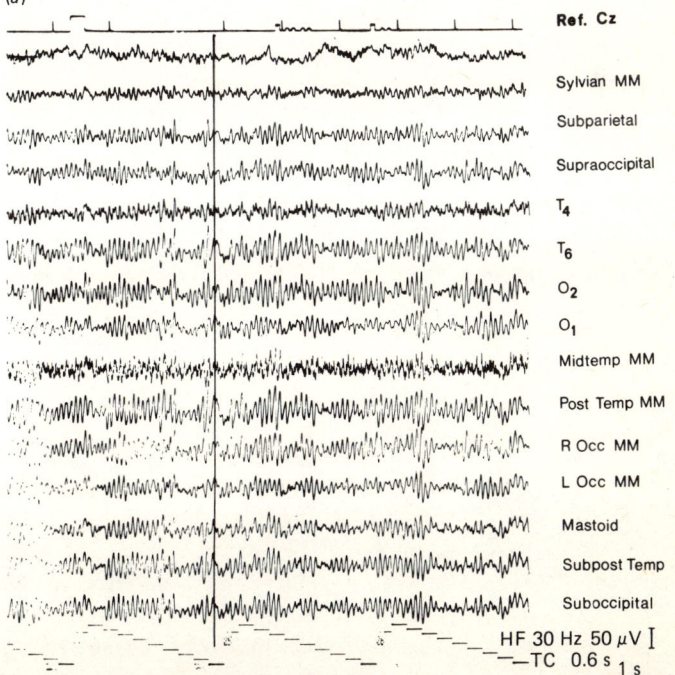

ful educational exercise which may improve one's understanding of derivation. It is necessary to begin with a common reference recording, so that the potential difference between any two electrodes on the head can be easily determined. The potential distribution over the scalp lying between the electrodes can then be calculated provided that certain assumptions are made concerning the potential gradients. Hence, by joining up points at the same potential the contours can be plotted, although the operation is not always so simple as might be supposed (Binnie, Ward and Heywood, 1971). If one wishes to produce a substantial number of EEG maps the process can easily be automated.

Fig. 12.17. (cont.)
(b) Topographic display
of the posterior slow
wave indicated in (a);
contour interval
3 μV. (Reproduced
with permission from
Lloyd and Wilson,
1973.)

(b)

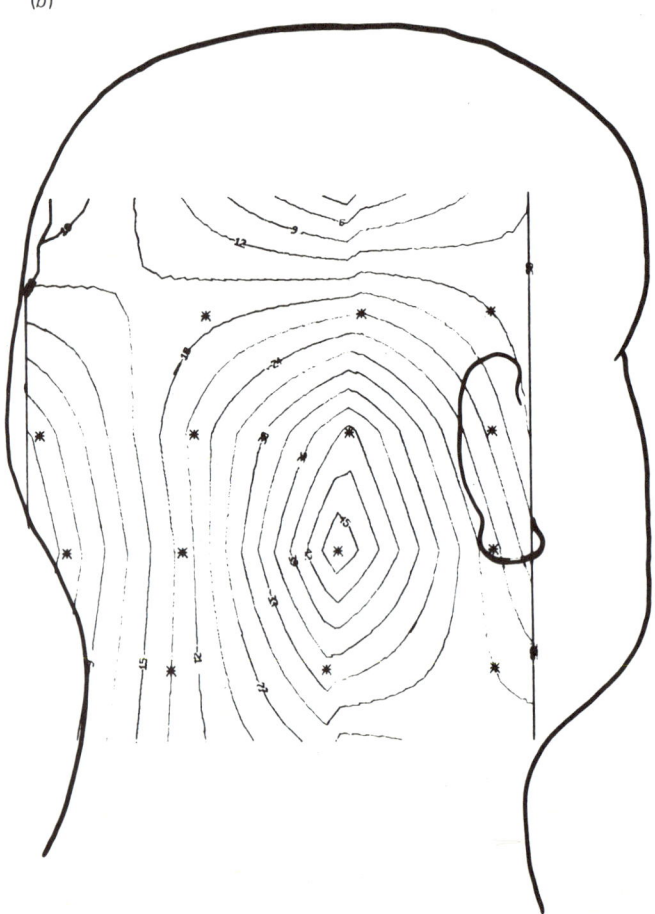

The results of EEG analysis can also be presented topographically as shown in Fig. 12.18. Such displays readily arouse the interest of the clinical users of an EEG service who may find them more easily understood and possibly more objective than verbal descriptions. However, their use to supplement or even to replace the conventional EEG report may be inadvisable: a graphic display on the outline of a head in a form which invites comparison with isotope scans or computer tomograms can encourage the clinical user wrongly to assume a direct topographic relationship between the distribution of EEG phenomena and that of underlying pathology (Binnie *et al.*, 1978a).

Of greater practical value is the use of topographic displays to show functional relationships between the electrical activities of different parts of the brain. The scheme shown in Fig. 12.19 from a study by Lopes da Silva *et al.* (1977) indicates how often spikes appeared simultaneously at various different recording sites during depth recording from an animal with experimental

Fig. 12.18. Topographic displays of the results of EEG analysis. (*a*) Normalized slope descriptors, local values indicated by the radii of the circles. Left parieto-temporal EEG abnormality overlying a tumour (reproduced from Binnie, 1976).

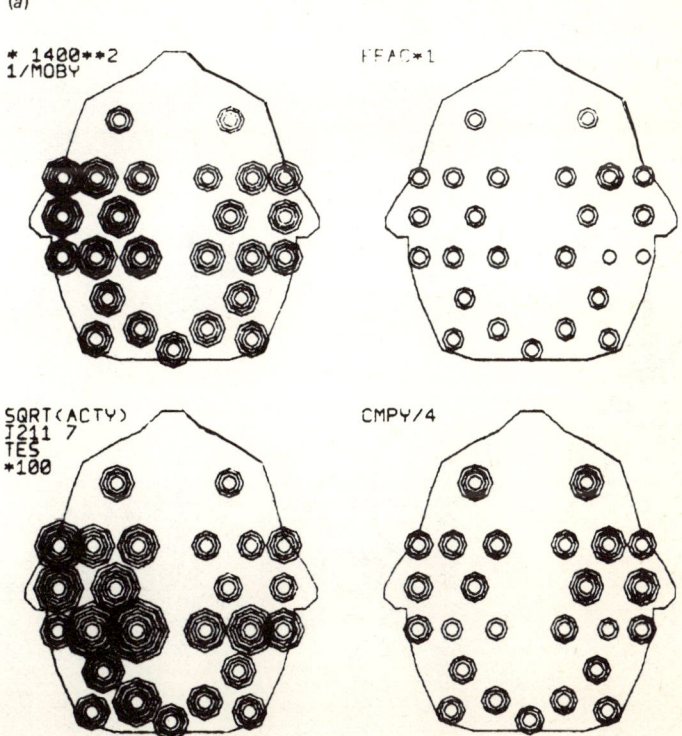

Fig. 12.18. (cont.) (b) Display indicating amounts of different frequency components compared with an original EEG: gross right-sided abnormality with depression of alpha and beta activity and gross excess of delta (reproduced with permission from Maulsby et al., 1973 in Kellaway and Petersén, *Automation of Clinical Electro-* *encephalography*, Raven Press, New York). (c) Compressed spectral arrays (see Fig. 12.6) superimposed upon a stylized head outline (reproduced with permission from Bickford, 1973 in Kellaway and Petersén, *Automation of Clinical Electro-* *encephalography*, Raven Press, New York).

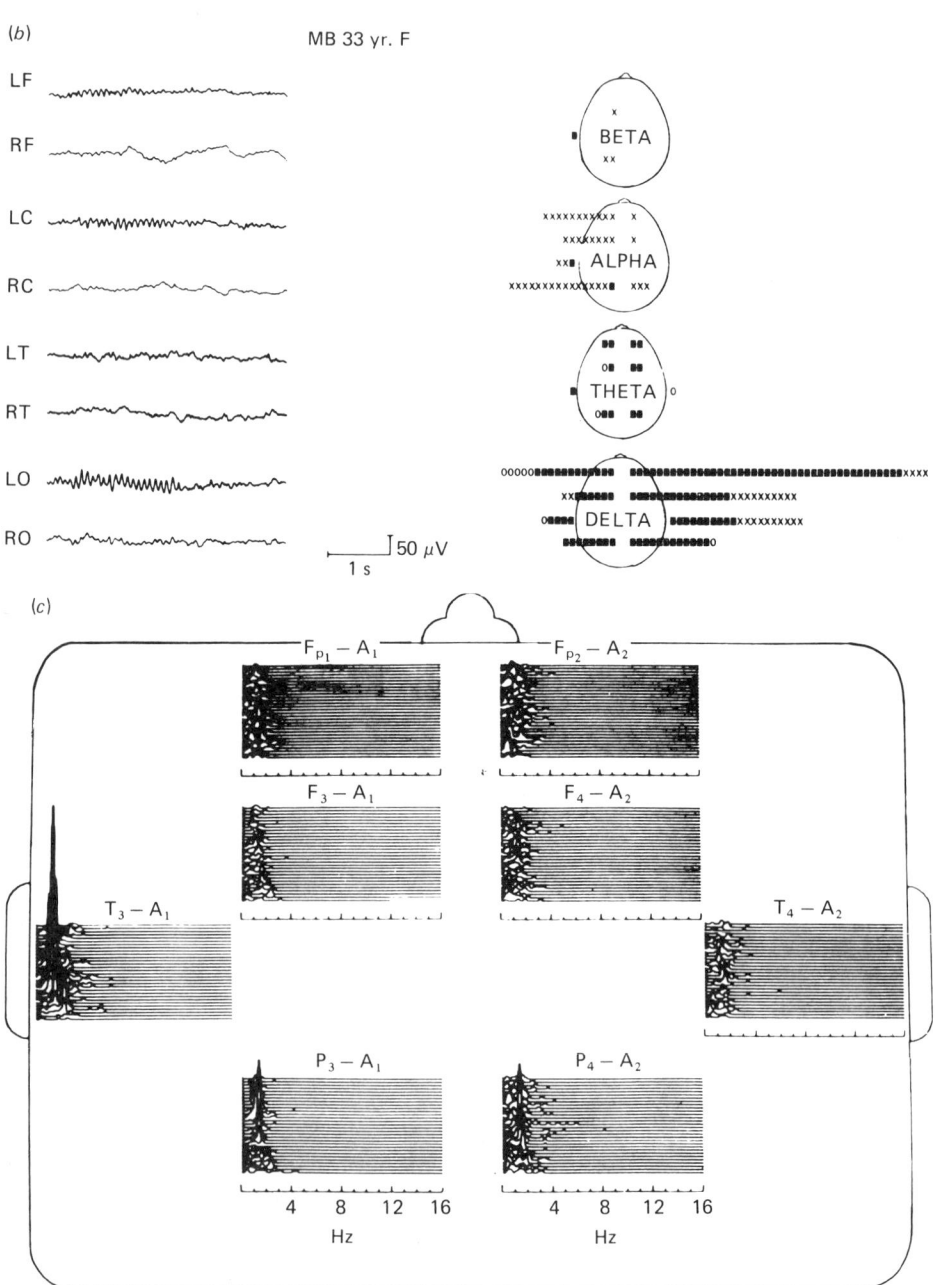

(b)

MB 33 yr. F

LF

RF

LC

RC

LT

RT

LO

RO

50 μV

1 s

BETA

ALPHA

THETA

DELTA

(c)

$F_{P_1} - A_1$

$F_{P_2} - A_2$

$F_3 - A_1$

$F_4 - A_2$

$T_3 - A_1$

$T_4 - A_2$

$P_3 - A_1$

$P_4 - A_2$

4   8   12   16
Hz

4   8   12   16
Hz

epilepsy. From such displays conclusions may be drawn about the functional interdependence of different cerebral regions and the mechanisms underlying transmission of epileptic discharges.

The topography of EEG phenomena can also be studied by means of the coherence function (Section 12.2). This indicates the extent to which particular frequency components in different regions of the head are functionally interdependent, arising from a common generator or spreading from one area to another. Such topographic relationships are also found to change with variations in state of awareness (Walter, Rhodes and Adey, 1967).

12.7. Computer-assisted EEG interpretation and pattern recognition

Clinical EEG interpretation involves two stages: first the visual analysis and description of the signals displayed on the chart, and then the formulation of the clinical decision based on the EEG phenomena together with information about the patient. A number of workers have attempted to automate either or both of these procedures. It might be expected that computers would excel at the preliminary quantification of the electrical signals and that decision making could better be performed by a human observer. Neither of these assumptions is necessarily correct. Though automatic methods provide simple, quantitative and objective measurements of the EEG, as soon as it becomes

Fig. 12.19. Display of functional interrelation-ships between different depth recording sites. The areas of the circles indicate the incidence of paroxysmal events at each site (depth electrodes L23–34) and the black inner discs, the number of maximum amplitudes at each. The widths of the lines joining them indicate how often events occurred at any pair of sites simultaneously. (Reproduced with permission from Lopes da Silva et al., 1977.)

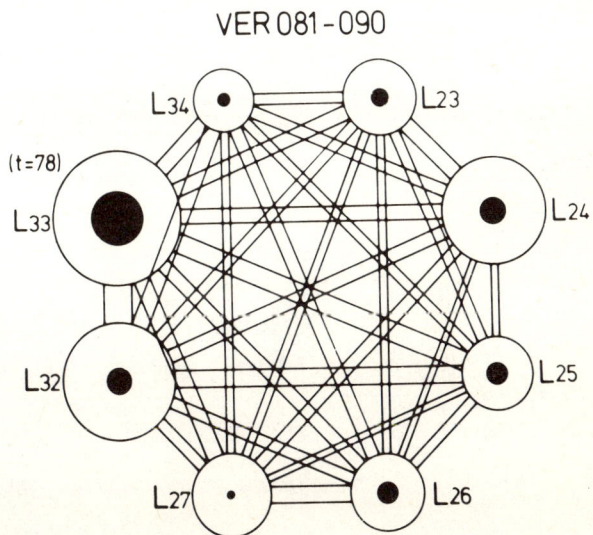

VER 081 - 090

necessary to distinguish between the wanted signals and artefacts, or to take account of the behavioural state or level of vigilance of the subject, a human observer may be much more effective at extracting the relevant features of the record. Conversely, human beings are considerably less competent than they may suppose at making objective decisions on the basis of more than about four different variables, which is in fact the strength of computer-based pattern recognition. Various combinations of human or computerized feature-extraction and decision making have been tried in clinical electroencephalography (Fig. 12.20).

The combination of a preliminary visual analysis of the EEG together with automatic decision making has the great advantage that it requires no special data processing facilities in the EEG laboratory, but merely off-line access to a system with standard statistical programs as are available in any university computer centre. Such an approach was found considerably to improve the reliability of EEG prediction of death or survival following cerebral anoxia (Binnie *et al.*, 1970).

Fig. 12.20. EEG interpretation: whether manual or automated, this generally involves the two stages of feature extraction and decision making. (From Binnie, 1976.)

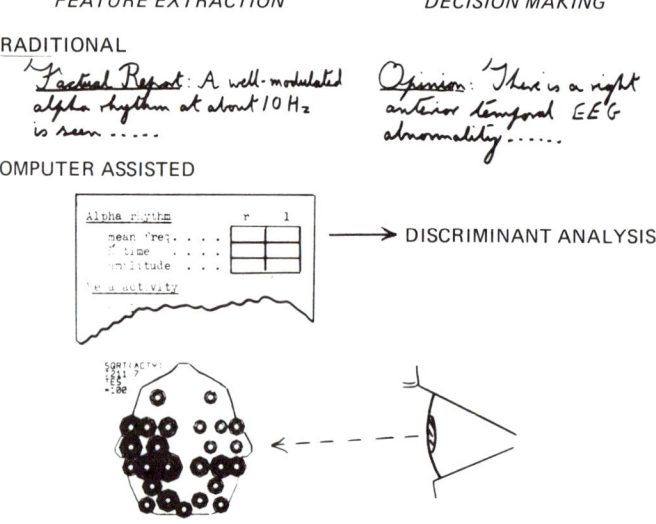

FEATURE EXTRACTION   *DECISION MAKING*

TRADITIONAL

COMPUTER ASSISTED

→ DISCRIMINANT ANALYSIS

AUTOMATED

SPECTRAL ANALYSIS   DISCRIMINANT ANALYSIS
PERIOD ANALYSIS   DECISION TREES
SLOPE DESCRIPTOR ANALYSIS   NON-LINEAR CLASSIFIERS
etc   FEATURE SPACE MAPPING
     etc

Many workers seeking to use computers to assist clinical EEG interpretation have nevertheless chosen the opposite approach of presenting the results of, for instance, power spectral analysis, to an electroencephalographer for subjective interpretation. For this purpose topographic displays as illustrated in Fig. 12.18 may be appropriate. Magnus *et al.* (1977) and Storm van Leeuwen *et al.* (1976) claim that this approach can usefully augment visual interpretation in routine clinical EEG practice, but a detailed study by Gotman, Gloor and Ray (1975) does not support this view.

Others (MacGillivray and Wadbrook, 1975; Harner, 1978) set themselves the task of a computer simulation of conventional EEG reporting. Yet others have used computer-based methods for detecting cerebral abnormality, thus automating both feature extraction and decision making. Matoušek and Petersén (1973) developed criteria for predicting the ages of children from the spectral characteristics of the EEGs. In the clinical application, a prediction of age is made from each recording channel of the EEG. A discrepancy between the predicted and the actual age may be regarded as evidence of abnormality and the results are presented both as a topographical display and as a verbal report (Fig. 12.21a). Similarly Gotman *et al.* (1975) based indices of abnormality on the ratio in each recording channel of alpha plus beta to theta plus delta activity after applying weighting factors related to the amounts of these activities in each region in normal subjects. Again the results were presented as a topographic display (Fig. 12.21b). Prediction of pathology from these diagrams compared favourably with interpretation of the primary tracings or of power spectra. Binnie *et al.* (1978a, 1979) employed a pattern-recognition technique to determine the probability of findings in a particular recording channel arising in a reference population of volunteers. 'Abnormality' was thus empirically defined as any pattern which did not commonly occur in healthy people. Here again a topographic display was available indicating the degree and distribution of cerebral electrical abnormality (Fig. 12.21c). Their method too was found to be more reliable than visual interpretation in detecting pathology.

Barlow (1979) in a recent comprehensive review of computerized clinical electroencephalography asks 'would it be worthwhile if it were possible?' and 'is it or will it be possible?'. An important consideration is the world-wide shortage of qualified electroencephalographers. A system which reliably performed the

(a)

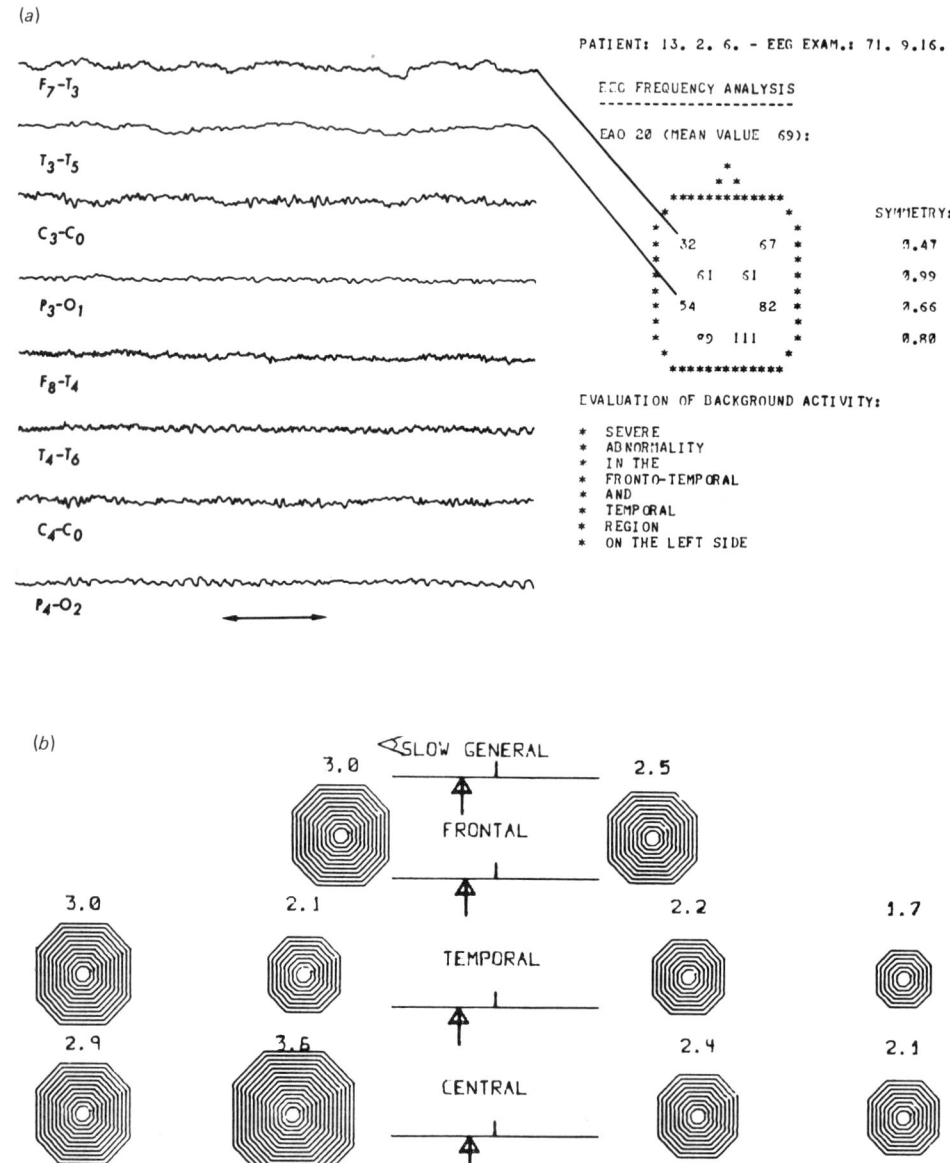

F₇-T₃

T₃-T₅

C₃-C₀

P₃-O₁

F₈-T₄

T₄-T₆

C₄-C₀

P₄-O₂

```
PATIENT: 13. 2. 6. - EEG EXAM.: 71. 9.16.

EEG FREQUENCY ANALYSIS
----------------------

EAO 20 (MEAN VALUE  69):

                   *
                 * *
         ***************
        *                *          SYMMETRY:
        *  32        67  *
        *                *           3.47
        *    61    51    *
        *                *           3.99
        *  54        82  *
        *                *           3.66
        *    09   111    *
        *                *           0.80
         ***************

EVALUATION OF BACKGROUND ACTIVITY:

    *  SEVERE
    *  ABNORMALITY
    *  IN THE
    *  FRONTO-TEMPORAL
    *  AND
    *  TEMPORAL
    *  REGION
    *  ON THE LEFT SIDE
```

(b)

SLOW GENERAL

3.0   2.5

FRONTAL

3.0   2.1   2.2   1.7

TEMPORAL

2.9   3.6   2.4   2.1

CENTRAL

3.4   4.6   2.0   2.0

SLOW PARIETAL

3.0   2.2

OCCIPITAL

fairly modest task of identifying abnormal EEGs could be cost-effective if it allowed trained personnel to devote their attention to records requiring expert interpretation. On the other hand, the emphasis of clinical EEG practice is shifting away from the detection of cerebral pathology towards the study of cerebral function. A clinically useful system will probably need to address specific problems such as quantifying epileptiform activity, monitoring cerebral function in metabolic disorders or during anaesthesia and testing the integrity of sensory systems. There is good evidence that such goals are attainable with present techniques and in the near future they may appear more worthwhile than computer-assisted interpretation of 'routine' EEGs.

The analysis of all-night sleep recordings, a tedious and time consuming procedure, appears to be a particularly worthwhile application for automation. Some workers have adopted quite simple approaches; for instance base-cross analysis is sensitive to the average frequency of the EEG and can discriminate with tolerable reliability between the non-REM stages of sleep (Frost, 1970). More complex systems involving a variety of methods of

Fig. 12.21. Topographic displays of indices of EEG abnormality. (a) Age-dependent quotients (reproduced with permission from Matoušek and Petersén, 1973). (b) Cannon-ograms, weighted ratios of faster to slower EEG components (repro-duced with permission from Gotman et al., 1975). (c) 'Deviance' measure of abnormality based on a pattern-recognition technique (Binnie et al., 1978). Note that all these dis-plays differ from those in Fig. 12.18 in that the information presented is not the primary result of EEG analysis but an interpretation in terms of normative data.

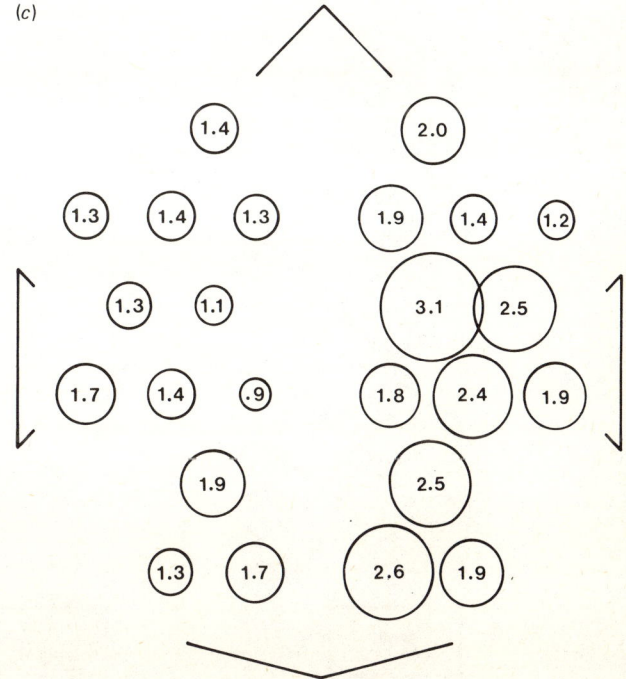

feature extraction together with pattern recognition achieve a reliability approaching that of the human observer (Martin *et al.*, 1972).

Pattern recognition is a rapidly expanding field of data processing which finds application in areas as diverse as automation of industrial plant, counting of chromosomes in microphotographs,

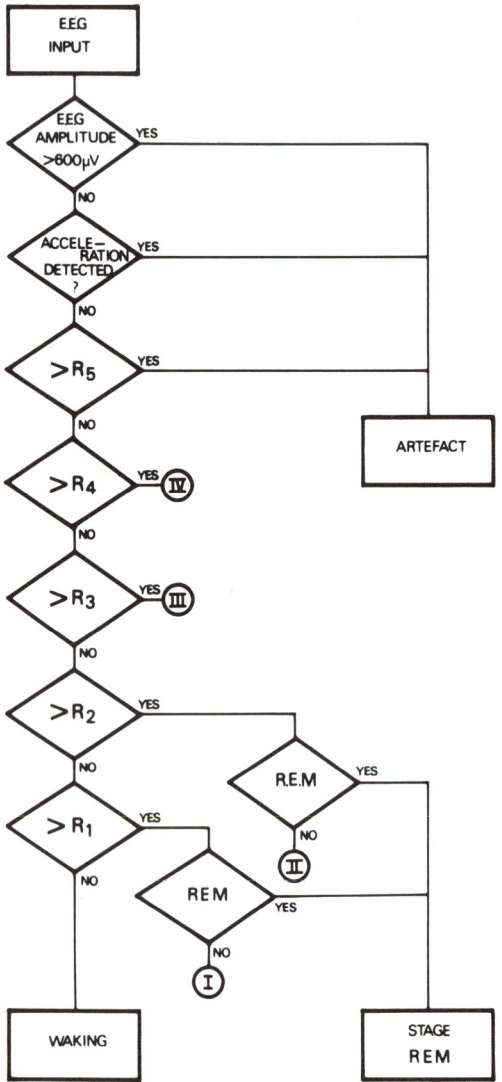

Fig. 12.22. Decision tree approach to sleep staging based on the method of Frost (1973). After preliminary recognition of artefacts by high amplitude or the detection of movement by means of an accelerometer, a measure of mean frequency based on a form of base cross analysis is compared with various thresholds. Where the EEG frequency is compatible with stages I, II or REM a further decision is based on the presence or absence of REM on an oculographic channel.

or the identification of aircraft by their radar echoes. For a non-technical introduction to pattern recognition in various fields, including EEG, see Batchelor (1978). The term 'pattern recognition' has somewhat different meanings to different users. In the present context it implies recognizing, from observations on a large number of EEG features, combinations of values characteristic of particular diagnoses, psychological states, sleep stages, etc. In the case of sleep staging, the classification is itself based upon particular EEG features and a simple sequence of logical steps, a 'decision tree', leads from the primary analysis to a conclusion about sleep stage (Fig. 12.22). In other cases no *a priori* criteria for the decision are known and they must be developed from experimental data. This is usually achieved by a so-called 'feature space' approach. Fig. 12.23 represents a simple hypothetical case: two variables or 'features', are plotted as a scatter-diagram. Let us suppose that V_1 is alpha frequency, V_2 alpha amplitude, and that the dots represent observations of normal EEGs and the circles observations on records from patients. If it so happened that all the dots fell above the dividing line in the figure and all the circles below it (a situation which unfortunately does not exist in reality) we could classify any unknown EEG by plotting the corresponding point on the graph. If it fell above the line then the

Fig. 12.23. Principle of linear discriminant analysis (see text).

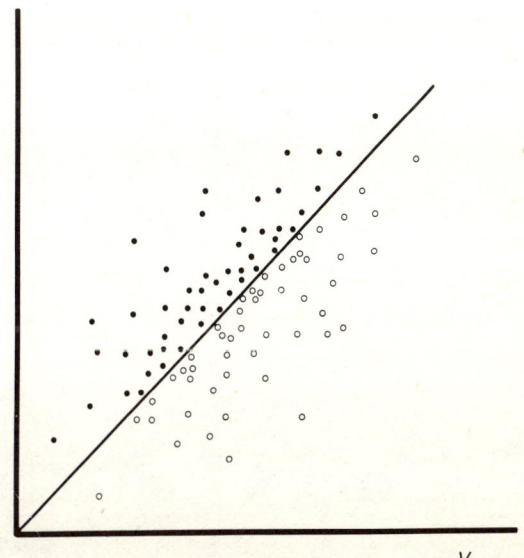

record would be considered normal, and if below then abnormal. If the method is extended to three dimensions (Fig. 12.24), the boundary between the two groups is not a line but a surface. The same principle can be applied to larger numbers of features; feature spaces of more than three dimensions cannot easily be illustrated but can be modelled mathematically. Where the categories can be separated by a flat surface, this mathematical modelling is achieved by a standard statistical technique called 'linear discriminant analysis', programs for which are available on most large computers. Where a curved or discontinuous boundary is required a number of methods are available; some can be implemented on special purpose machines, others involve complex computer programs and come within the field of 'machine intelligence'.

Fig. 12.24. (*a*) Division of a three-dimensional space by decision surface. (*b*) Non-linear pattern recognition: here the two classes, dots and circles, are divided by surfaces which are non-linear or even discontinuous.

(*a*)

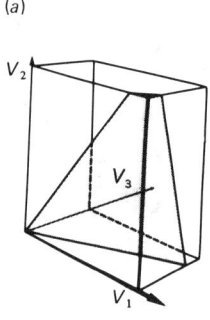

(*b*)

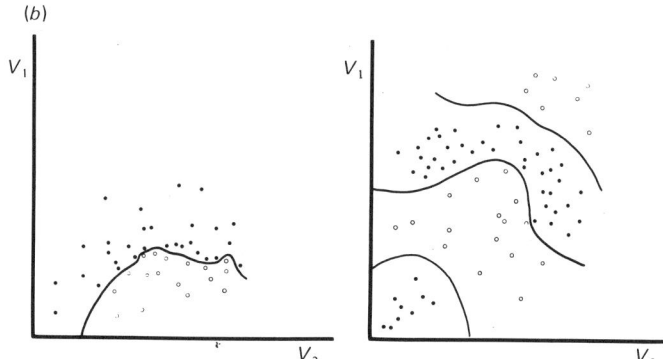

13. Practical aspects of EEG data processing

13.1. Computers

There are two main philosophies regarding the training of technicians to carry out EEG recording in general and to work with computers in particular. The 'black box' approach requires that the technicians perform complex procedures without knowledge of their theoretical backgrounds. Learning 'how' but not 'why' can produce successful results but in the end is self-defeating; people with intellectual curiosity, presumably including the readers of this book, soon become bored and their work inevitably suffers. Far preferable is the approach in which the practical aspects of a procedure flow naturally from an understanding of basic principles. This is the underlying philosophy of the following introduction to computers.

Information about measurements can be communicated in two ways, by the use of models, or by means of numbers. To find out whether a table will pass through a doorway one can take a piece of string, measure off the width of the table and then test the string against the doorposts: this is the use of *analogue* measurement. Alternatively one can take a tape measure, determine the size of the table in centimetres or inches and then measure the doorway in the same units: this is *digital* measurement. EEG signals may be regarded as analogue measurements of brain activity, and they can be processed by electronic circuits which change the signals in ways which may be described mathematically, such as squaring, integrating and differentiating. The low-frequency wave analyser (Section 12.2) was a special-purpose analogue device for EEG analysis. Analogue computers consist of a number of circuits for performing mathematical and logical operations which can be linked together to carry out a sequence, or program, of procedures. They are therefore more flexible than special-purpose analysers. Intermediate in complexity and flexibility is such equipment as the 'Devices Neurolog', a modular system of circuits for performing simple operations on neurophysiological signals, such as filtration, spike detection, etc. Analogue data-processing systems are comparatively inexpensive and fast but often somewhat inaccurate. One great drawback is that the end result of the processing is still an electrical signal which must usually be displayed on an oscilloscope, written out on a chart, or measured with a meter.

Digital computers, by contrast, handle numerical data and before they can process EEG signals these must be converted from analogue to digital form. The operation of *analogue-to-digital*

Fig. 13.1. Signals of different frequencies sampled at a constant digitization rate. In each case the original signal and the sampling points are shown below and the digitized representation above. Note that when the sampling rate falls below five times the signal frequency severe waveform distortion occurs. In the bottom example aliasing has occurred and the digitized signal contains a spurious low-frequency component.

Sampling/signal frequency

18 / 1

6 / 1

4.5 / 1

1.06 / 1

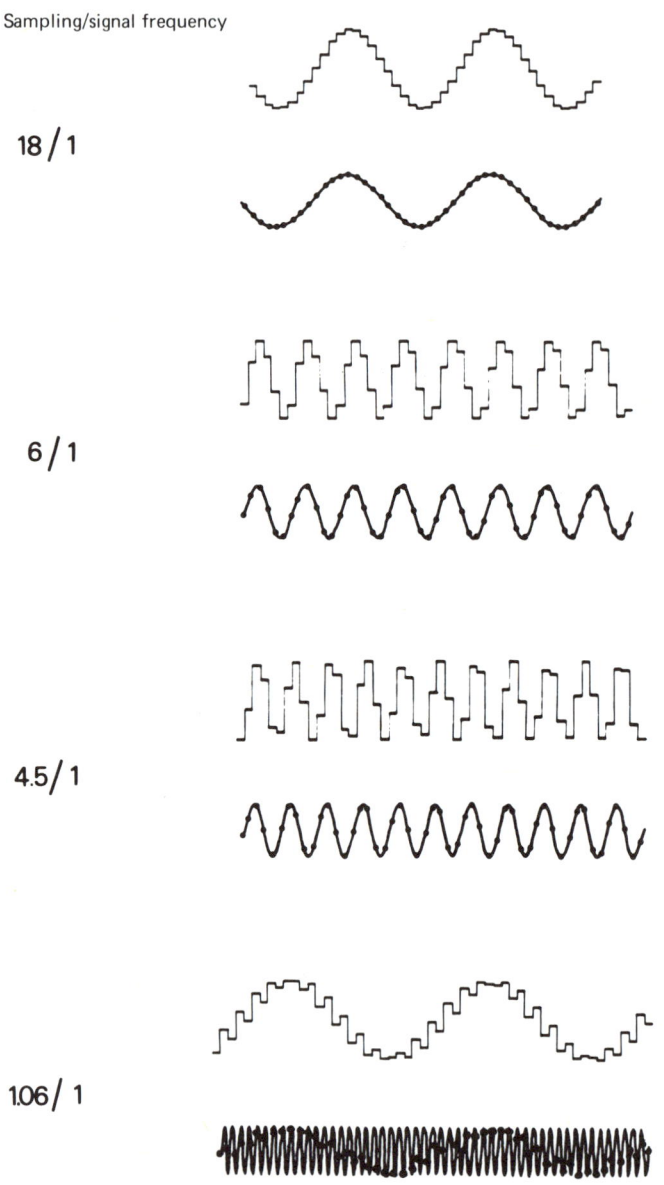

conversion involves sampling the voltage of each EEG channel at frequent intervals; thus a series of numbers replaces the continuously varying signal as input to the computer. The frequency resolution of analogue-to-digital conversion is dependent on the sampling rate. To reproduce a sine wave with tolerable accuracy at least five samples per cycle are needed (Fig. 13.1). To detect correctly the frequency components of a signal (for instance for power spectral analysis) without reproducing the waveform, a sampling rate of more than twice the maximum frequency in the signal is essential. Sampling too slowly results in *aliasing*, the appearance of spurious low-frequency components (Fig. 13.1). Note that this criterion is based on the maximum frequency present in the signal, not the maximum frequency of interest. If one wishes to study only the alpha rhythm with a digital computer one must not suppose that a sampling frequency of 50 Hz will be adequate; if the EEG is also contaminated with EMG artefact of up to 40 Hz a sampling frequency of 80 Hz will be required. The analogue-to-digital converter for the input to the computer may have a special anti-aliasing filter. If not, care must be taken to match the bandwidth of the signals and the filters of the EEG machine to the sampling frequency. It should also be noted that the cut-off of the high-frequency filters on the standard EEG

Fig. 13.2. A schematic representation of the operation of a digital computer. (1) The contents of the program counter (PC) indicates the memory address of the next instruction to be executed. (2) The next instruction is fetched from the specified memory address and stored in the instruction register (IR). This particular instruction is of the 'memory reference type' and comprises a numerical code indicating the operation to be performed (in this case to store the A register) and the memory address on which it should act. (3 and 4) Execution of the instruction causes the contents of the A register to be stored at the specified memory address. (5) Execution of this instruction also causes the contents of the program counter to be incremented by one so that when the sequence is repeated, starting at step (1), the following instruction of the program will be fetched from memory.

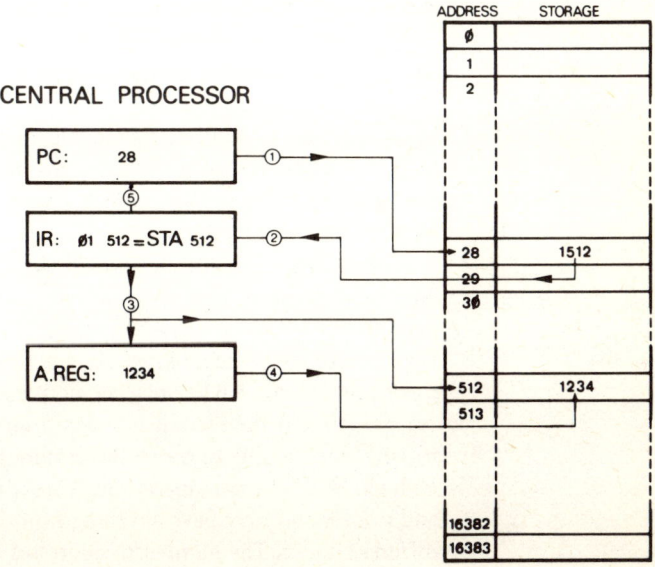

machine is very gradual; if one records at an HF setting of 30 Hz it does not follow that one can always safely sample the EEG at 70 or even at 100 Hz.

The digital computer itself consists of two main parts, the *memory* and the *central processor* (Fig. 13.2). The memory may be thought of as a series of 'pigeon-holes' in which numbers can be stored. Each pigeon-hole can accommodate one number and is itself identifiable by a unique *address*, also a number. Thus the central processor can store a number at a particular address in memory and can subsequently retrieve it from the same memory location. The central processor also contains 'pigeon-holes' for temporary storage of numbers, in this case called *registers*. The central processor can carry out various mathematical or logical operations on the contents of the registers and of specified memory addresses. It can, for instance, add together the contents of a register and of a memory location and place the result back in the register; alternatively it may test the number in a register to determine whether it is positive, negative, zero, odd or even and take various different actions depending upon the result. The repertoire of operations varies from one computer to another. The instructions which determine the operations performed by the central processor are numerical codes placed in a special register (the *instruction register*). Following the execution of each instruction a further operation code is automatically fetched from the memory. The address of the next instruction to be fetched is itself contained in another register called the *program counter*. The execution of most instructions also causes the value in the program counter to be increased by one so that instructions are brought from consecutive memory addresses and executed in sequence. However, some instructions may themselves change the program counter to some other value causing a 'jump' to another part of the program.

The individual operations which the computer can perform are so rudimentary that the simplest mathematical calculation may involve several steps. For instance just to add two numbers together it may be necessary to instruct the computer to fetch one of them from a particular memory address, to place it in a register, to add the second number from the memory into the register and finally to store the results in another memory address. Each of these operations is specified by a particular code and a computer may have anything from forty to four hundred different codes. The number of addresses in the memory is also considerable, ranging typically from 4000 to nearly 130 000, It may be imagined therefore that creating a program in the computer's own internal code, or *machine language*, is a complex and extremely tedious task. Fortunately it is possible for the user to write programs in a so-called *assembler language* which consists of abbreviations which are easily remembered, such as 'SUB' for subtract, 'JMP' for jump, and so on. The manufacturer of a computer provides an assembler program which translates this mnemonic code into the machine language and which also organizes the storage of instructions and data within the memory. Nevertheless, in assembler language there is generally a one-to-one relationship between the codes and central processor operations and thus the user is required to understand every detailed step involved in performing some simple procedure on a particular computer. This difficulty is overcome by the use of *high level languages* which consist of a sequence of instructions in a mixture of very simple English and mathematical notation. Fig. 13.3 shows a simple program to add two numbers together. Above is shown the coding in a high level language ('FORTRAN') and beneath is a version of the same program in assembler language together with a translation by the assembler program into the actual machine language codes and a list of the memory addresses in which they will be stored.

Although a memory capacity of some tens of thousands of numbers may seem very considerable, computers are often required to handle enormous amounts of data; indeed a 16-channel EEG sampled only one hundred times per second generates numbers at the rate of 1600 per second and would fill a large computer memory in less than one minute's recording time. Various bulk storage devices are therefore commonly linked to the computer for storing greater quantities of information. These include *magnetic disc units* with a capacity of several million numbers, *floppy discs* which are smaller, very much cheaper and will usually store only a few hundred thousand numbers, and *magnetic tape units*. Tape offers a greater storage capacity at a lower price than disc but has the disadvantage that it may take several minutes winding the tape in order to reach some particular information that is required. By contrast any data on the disc can be reached within some tens of milliseconds. Other apparatus is used for communication between the computer and the outside world. If one wishes to present the results of digital processing as an analogue signal, for instance to write out an evoked response on an EEG chart, *digital-to-analogue* conversion may be performed. A *teleprinter* or *visual display unit* (VDU) is commonly provided to allow the user to type messages or programs into the computer and for the computer to output messages, questions or results to the user. The maximum speed of a teleprinter is somewhat higher than that of a good typist, ten to thirty characters per second. A VDU is much faster but the display is on a TV screen and no hard copy is produced. To print large quantities of data, at hundreds of lines per minute, devices called *lineprinters* are available. Information may also sometimes be output or read into a computer by means of punched paper tape. To output diagrams, evoked responses, or topographic displays as discussed in Section 12.6 special display devices are available.

Fig. 13.3. Programming languages. A program to add two numbers together: (above) the coding in a high level language, FORTRAN; (below) the same encoded in mnemonic assembler language together with the numeric machine code instructions.

FORTRAN

I = 1 + 2

STOP

END

ASSEMBLER

Address, relative to first instruction	Machine Code	Mnemonic Language	Comment
		REL	This is a directive to instruct the assembler that the program must be encoded in such a way that it can be stored anywhere in memory
0	02 004	LDA X	Load register A with contents of address X
1	03 005	ADD Y	Add contents of address Y to A register
2	01 006	STA I	Store contents of A register in address I
3	00000	HLT	Stop the computer
4	00001	X DATA 1	Define a memory location as X and store value of 1 in it
5	00002	Y DATA 2	Define location Y and store 2 in it
6	00000	I DAC	Define address I, do not store any value in it
		END	Directive to instruct assembler that this is end of program

Throughout this discussion it is been taken for granted that numbers can somehow be represented inside the computer. The physical form in which they are represented in registers, memory, disc, magnetic tape, etc. varies but the method of coding is constant. Each store contains a number of electrical or magnetic elements which can exist in either of two states: for instance transistor switches which are either ON or OFF. These two states can be used to represent the digits, 0 and 1. Numbers inside the computer are made up only of these two digits, 0 and 1, or are in other words 'binary'. The convention followed is similar to that used in decimal notation, which employs ten different characters, but instead of each place in the number representing powers of ten (1, 10, 100, 1000 . . .), each place is a power of two (1,2,4, 8 . . .). Thus in binary one is 1, two is 10, three is 11, four is 100, five is 101, etc. (Fig. 13.4). This convention is of no consequence to the computer user who is not required to write programs, except for purposes of communication. For instance it may be necessary to enter the address of the first instruction into the program counter before starting the computer. This is usually done by means of illuminated switches on the front of the machine which are used to represent binary numbers. These are difficult to read or remember, but as the binary numbers nought (0) to seven (111) are easily recognized the simplest way of reading a large binary number is to split it into blocks of three characters and translate these into the eight digits nought to seven. This results in so-called octal notation (Fig. 13.4). These different number systems may be irritating to those who are not mathematically inclined but unfortunately designers of computers and of programs frequently require the user to communicate with machines in binary, octal or even hexadecimal (16 characters) notation.

13.2. EEG data acquisition and processing systems

It will be appreciated by the technician, more perhaps than by anyone else, that the requirement to make tape-recordings or perform computer analysis during EEG registration can only add to the complexity of what is already a difficult task. It is essential therefore that the whole system be planned with particular attention to the ergonomic aspects which will determine whether or not it is in fact usable in practice. For instance the decision to link an EEG machine to a data recording or processing system has important consequences for the choice of EEG apparatus. Some machines have a convenient multiway connector for output and

Fig. 13.4. Number systems. (a) Decimal, binary, octal and hexadecimal notation. (b) Binary to octal conversion. The binary number is divided into blocks of three digits each of which gives one octal digit.

(a)   **NUMBER SYSTEMS**

	DECIMAL		BINARY					OCTAL		HEXADECIMAL	
Base	10		2					8		16	
Digits	0–9		0 and 1					0–7		0–F	
	Tens	Units	Sixteens	Eights	Fours	Twos	Units	Eights	Units	Sixteens	Units
		0					0		0		0
		1					1		1		1
		2				1	0		2		2
		3				1	1		3		3
		4			1	0	0		4		4
		5			1	0	1		5		5
		6			1	1	0		6		6
		7			1	1	1		7		7
		8		1	0	0	0	1	0		8
		9		1	0	0	1	1	1		9
	1	0		1	0	1	0	1	2		A
	1	1		1	0	1	1	1	3		B
	1	2		1	1	0	0	1	4		C
	1	3		1	1	0	1	1	5		D
	1	4		1	1	1	0	1	6		E
	1	5		1	1	1	1	1	7		F
	1	6	1	0	0	0	0	2	0	1	0
	1	7	1	0	0	0	1	2	1	1	1
	2	4	1	1	0	0	0	3	0	1	8
	3	1	1	1	1	1	1	3	7	1	F

(b)   BINARY TO OCTAL CONVERSION

BINARY	111	010	111	110	100	001
OCTAL	1	6	5	7	2	1

input at a voltage compatible with most tape-recorders, and with independent controls for gain and DC level. If the EEG machine does not have these facilities a good deal of time may need to be expended on the construction of special amplifiers and attenuators for connecting the apparatus to the data processing system, and even more technician time may be expended in calibrating the apparatus whenever it is used.

Some manufacturers of EEG machines have recently experimented with special facilities for signalling to a computer the settings of all the operational controls, or conversely, allowing these to be set up remotely by the computer itself. A consideration which may lead some users to select an EEG machine with jet galvanometers for data processing applications is the fact that with these it is possible to write out alpha-numeric characters as a matrix of dots (Lloyd *et al.*, 1972b). This allows the computer to annotate the chart with information about the recording conditions, convey messages to the technician, or write out the results of an on-line analysis directly upon the record to which it relates (Fig. 13.5).

Ergonomic considerations will also influence the choice of computer peripherals. For instance, if communication between technician and computer is necessary during recording, a chattering teleprinter may disturb the patient; if so a silent VDU may be

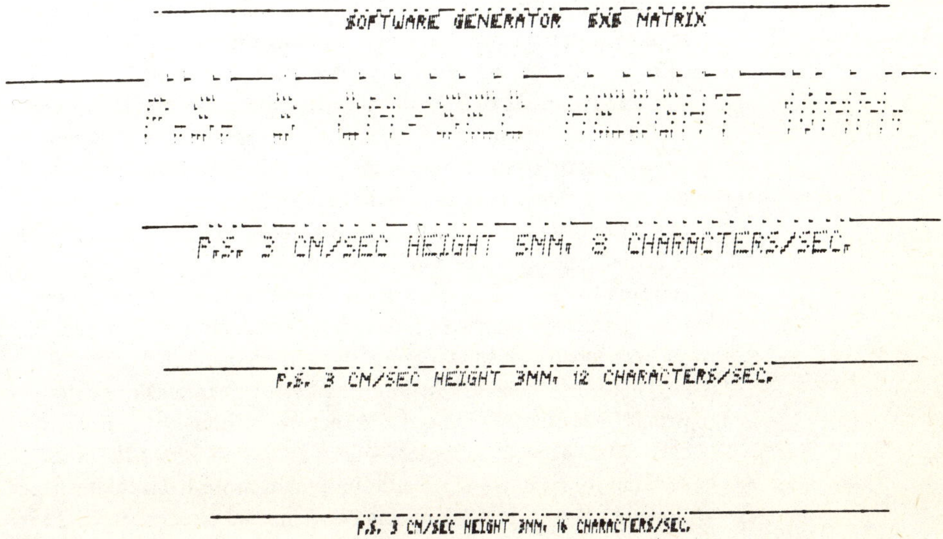

Fig. 13.5. Character generation on a moving chart recorder (reproduced with permission from Lloyd *et al.*, 1972b). The original tracing was in light-blue ink and there has been some loss of definition in the course of photographic reproduction.

SOFTWARE GENERATOR 6X6 MATRIX

P.S. 3 CM/SEC HEIGHT 7MM

P.S. 3 CM/SEC HEIGHT 5MM, 8 CHARACTERS/SEC.

P.S. 3 CM/SEC HEIGHT 3MM, 12 CHARACTERS/SEC.

P.S. 3 CM/SEC HEIGHT 3MM, 16 CHARACTERS/SEC.

appropriate. If the system is to be used for evoked response work, the graphic displays must be adequate and fast. It is extremely irritating when attempting an evoked response audiogram on a difficult child to have to wait repeatedly for a minute or two whilst a slow-moving plotter writes out the response. An oscilloscope will give an almost instantaneous display and if the data are temporarily stored on disc or tape hard copies for archival purposes can be made off-line when the experiment is over and the child has, to everyone's relief, gone home.

13.3. Tape-recording

For many purposes it may be more satisfactory to make a tape-recording of the EEG than to attempt to transmit it directly on-line to the computer. The need for direct cable connections from the EEG machine to the computer is eliminated and the data may be analysed in a different building or even in another country. Costly computer time is saved, as one may choose to analyse only those sections of the recording which are technically satisfactory and contain the relevant data. Some methods of EEG analysis by digital computer may be too slow to be carried out in real time and this problem is overcome by playing back the tape-recording slowly. Conversely (but less commonly, except in the case of analogue computers) the analysis can sometimes be carried out much faster than the signals are generated and computer time can therefore be saved by an accelerated play-back of the tape. This is an important consideration in the choice of a tape-recorder because the range, and more importantly the ratio, of tape speeds available on any machine is limited. Until recently the tape-recording of EEG signals presented considerable technical difficulties. Commonly a multi-channel recording is required, sometimes of 16 or more channels, and the frequency range of interest is below that of conventional hi-fi equipment. It was therefore usually necessary to make use of 'instrumentation tape-recorders' using wide, sometimes one inch, tape and carrier systems for recording the signals. These machines were costly, large, and the capacity of a reel of tape at a speed which gave the necessary bandwidth was rarely more than one hour.

There have recently been a number of new developments which have totally changed the picture, although it is not yet clear what type of recorders will in the event prove the most suitable for EEG work. One development arose from the realization that the difficulty of using conventional direct recorders for low-frequency signals such as the EEG arose, not during recording, but in play-back, as the slow changes in the magnetic flux of the tape passing the play-back head did not induce a sufficient e.m.f. to give a reasonable output signal. For those applications where an accelerated play-back is acceptable, or indeed desirable, a conventional direct recorder using no carrier system may be used. This principle has found a particular application in a development of very small portable cassette units which use a low tape speed during recording, allowing registrations of up to 24 hours on a single cassette. At play-back the tape is speeded up by a factor of 16 to 60. Such devices are presently limited to four to eight channels. Direct recording is very sensitive to defects in the tape and playback may be 'noisy'. A new system of 'flux-responsive' direct recording has been developed which is capable of reproducing low-frequency or even DC signals without accelerated play-back and this may prove ideal for EEG work. Another technical development which solves the difficulties due to the low frequency of the EEG and meets the need for many channels is multiplexing the signals. By switching the recorder input rapidly between a succession of EEG channels a composite signal is built up consisting of a succession of samples of each channel in turn. The effective frequency of the signal for purposes of tape-recording is not that of the EEG but that of the switching frequency. Thus by sampling sequentially 16 channels 200 times a second, one produces effectively a signal of a frequency of 3200 Hz, and this is suitable for registration on a conventional hi-fi tape-recorder or cassette unit. Facilities must of course be provided for demultiplexing the signals after play-back and various other pulses are inserted to identify the interlaced channels and possibly to control for defects in the tape (Barlow, 1975; Poortvliet, personal communication). The same principle may be taken a step further and the signals not only multiplexed but also digitized, the numeric values being represented by a sequence of pulses. This raises the effective frequency even further and at the same time offers a high degree of protection against interference and distortion. If an analogue recording is degraded by interference, variations in signal strength, or irregularities in the tape transport system, little can be done to restore the situation. By contrast, the pulses which make up a digital recording remain readable up to the point where they are so corrupted as to disappear altogether. Multi-channel tape-recorders employing this type of encoding of data (Pulse Code Modulation or PCM) are commercially available; alternatively it may be preferable to include the PCM encoder in the EEG registration system. One then may choose between recording on a hi-fi tape-recorder or cassette unit or on the audio channel of a video recorder, single channel radio telemetry, or transmission by cable to a remote computer, depending upon the application in question. Digital recorders carry out analogue-to-digital conversion and store the data in a format which may be directly readable by the magnetic tape unit of a computer. At least two EEG machines now incorporate an analogue-to-digital converter or PCM encoder as an optional feature.

Because of the long duration of many EEG recordings and the absence often of any distinctive features in the tracing, it is sometimes extremely difficult to locate the wanted data on analogue tape. To copy the readings of a tape counter on to the chart or to use an audio channel for voice annotation of a record is a partial but not very satisfactory solution. It may be possible to use a special code system of tone pulses on an audio channel which can be easily detected by ear, or displayed on a chart recorder at play-back. It is more satisfactory to have a complete time index on both the paper record and the tape. One system (Byford and Goddard, 1972) employs a pre-recorded time marker of pulse codes on one track. During EEG registration these codes are written out on to the chart (the method presupposes an advanced type of recorder, capable of recording on some channels while playing back simultaneously on another). During transcription an automatic system controls the tape transport, moving it to selected time codes at high speed, switching to normal play-back speed, and when appropriate giving signals to the computer to commence and terminate analysis. A simplified version of this system is incorporated in at least one commercial tape-recorder.

Another method which is more convenient for manual operation but does not readily permit automation is to record together with the EEG, both on the chart and on the tape, alphanumeric characters which can be written out by jet galvanometers. A microprocessor can readily be programmed to generate the necessary signals, and to annotate the chart and tape with information about date, time, recording conditions, etc. (Fig. 13.5). * Digital recordings can include data about elapsed time, together with the

* For complex but standardized procedures this information can be pre-recorded on the tape, together with instructions to the technician and used both to annotate the record and to control the experiment.

signals, and this information can easily be read back by the computer.

The technical specification of a tape-recorder for EEG use depends very much on the application envisaged. For instance if one is particularly concerned with the precise frequency characteristics of the EEG a minimum of flutter and wow (irregularities in tape speed) may be demanded. If one is moreover concerned with precise time relations between events in different channels, a multiplexed system which ordinarily samples the channels sequentially and not simultaneously may not be ideal. Conversely, if the object was to measure the amount of REM sleep during the night or to count the spike-wave discharges over 24 hours, a very poor frequency response, and even quite severe distortion of the signals would seem a reasonable price to pay for the ability to get the entire recording on one tape without manual intervention and to play it back considerably speeded up. One particular feature which should be checked carefully when a tape-recorder is selected is the signal/noise ratio. This is dependent on tape speed but is rarely greater than 40 dB for a direct recorder or 46 dB with a carrier system. It should be noted that the noise is usually specified as r.m.s. and the signal is assumed to be at the limits of the dynamic range of the system. At a recording sensitivity sufficiently low to enable high-voltage epileptiform discharges to be registered without distortion, low-voltage beta activity will generally be obscured by noise.

There is an international standard, 'IRIG', for tape recorders of 7, or 14 or 28 tracks and other apparatus, including EEG machines, is often equipped with inputs and outputs which are compatible with this standard. The choice of an IRIG recorder may therefore avoid the need to build special amplifiers or attenuators to link other devices to the system in the future.

It should be noted that some tape-recorders are extremely easy to set up and use, while others are daunting to anyone not familiar with electronic test equipment. Thus it is important to select a recorder which can without difficulty be operated by the available personnel.

When recording the EEG on tape it is necessary to match the amplitude of the signal to the dynamic range of the recorder. If the output of the EEG machine is too small the signal/noise ratio will be low. If the signal is too large the recording will be distorted. The form of the distortion depends on the type of recorder; if the signals merely become flattened at the peak amplitude, the fault is usually obvious at play-back; however, some systems invert over-large signals, producing bizarre spiky waveforms which may be mistaken for epileptiform activity.

In addition to the variable sensitivity of the EEG machine, the record and replay electronics also often have variable gain controls. It is unwise to rely simply on trying to set these up accurately; one should always record a calibration signal on the tape so that the sensitivity of the entire system can be checked at play-back. Generally the most appropriate calibration signal is a sine wave of a frequency at the middle of the bandwidth of interest (10 Hz for most EEG purposes) and with an amplitude near the limit of the linear dynamic range of the system.* Square waves and other frequencies may be added if one wishes to check the recording characteristics more fully.

Some recorders allow immediate play-back of the signals as they are recorded, and this allows one to obtain a simultaneous paper tracing of the data actually on the tape – a valuable check on faults or possible errors in connecting up the system.

13.4. Recording the EEG for analysis

The applications of EEG data processing are so varied that only some very general advice can be offered concerning the recording techniques likely to be appropriate. The two most common applications are the analysis of background activity and the registration of evoked potentials.

As discussed in Section 12.2, one of the major problems in obtaining reliable quantitative measurements on background activity is ensuring stability of the state of the subject. Various solutions have been adopted. One is to give him a task to perform which it is hoped will ensure a constant mental state. This is difficult in practice: for instance, we once used a reaction time task which was recommended by one author as suitable for stabilizing the state of the subject during psychopharmacological experiments, but it was so boring that almost everyone fell asleep. Nevertheless, tasks can be designed which are neither so tedious as to cause drowsiness nor so difficult or energetic as to produce artefacts. Another possibility is simply to record for a long time

---

* There are few commercially available oscillators with microvolt outputs and in any event they are often inaccurate in this range. For calibrating EEG equipment it may be advisable to run the oscillator at an output of about 1 V and reduce the signal with a precision attenuator.

and hope by averaging the results to compensate for statistical variation. There are some considerable theoretical objections to doing this, particularly if the analytical method used is Fourier analysis. An alternative is to collect comparatively short samples of the EEG but to try to ensure that the subject is in the same state during each epoch. For instance the patient may be asked to open or shut the eyes every 20 s, and 10 s sections of record may be taken for analysis, commencing 5 s after each eye closure, to allow the immediate transient effects of shutting the eyes to disappear (Lettich and Margerison, 1960). Hawkes and Prescott (1973) were, it must be admitted, unable to demonstrate that the sampling strategy under the circumstances of their recordings made a great deal of difference to the result. However, Cohen and Sances (1977) found that in the resting, eyes-closed state stationarity could be maintained for about 12 s but rapidly declined over longer epochs. If quantitative analysis is to be carried out on background activity it is of course necessary to have agreed protocols concerning the choice of control settings of the apparatus. To ensure reproducibility of results a number of other considerations should influence the experimental design, and depending upon the purpose of the study it may be necessary to standardize any or all of the following:

(1) Time of day.

(2) Time since, and size of, last meal (these will affect responses to hyperventilation and liability to drowsiness).

(3) Activities of the previous evening (if the patient went to bed late or over-indulged in alcohol it will affect his state on the following day).

(4) Phase of menstrual cycle (there is evidence of cyclic changes in the EEG – Margerison *et al.*, 1964).

(5) Medication, including not only obvious centrally acting drugs, but also remedies for hay fever, dysmenorrhoea, etc., and oral contraceptives.

(6) Smoking habit (the EEGs of smokers differ from those of non-smokers (Brown, 1963; Comer *et al.*, 1979) and the EEGs of smokers who have been required to abstain for some hours differ from those of smokers who have recently had a cigarette (Knott and Venables, 1977)).

(7) The identity of the technician recording the EEG (the interpersonal relationship may well affect the arousal level of the subject).

The procedure to be followed during evoked response experiments will depend chiefly on whether the purpose is to study the response or to determine a sensory threshold. For research, or where responses are being recorded for latency measurements (for example in the diagnosis of multiple sclerosis) a standardized procedure of recording and of stimulation may be appropriate. However, if the technique is being used for threshold measurements, particularly for evoked response audiometry (ERA), it will be necessary to monitor the results as the experiment proceeds and make rapid decisions concerning the next type of stimulus to be delivered. One might for instance begin by stimulating both ears simultaneously with loud tone pulses in the middle of the frequency range necessary for comprehension of speech, say 80 dB at 1000 Hz. Having established that an evoked response can in fact be obtained and observed its waveform, one may then choose to stimulate one ear at a time, masking the other with white noise in the headphones. Successively weaker stimuli are applied first to one ear and then to the other until no response is obtained from either. Other frequencies may then be similarly tested. The patients in whom ERA is performed are often unable to co-operate for very long and one may therefore have to adopt the strategy of trying to obtain as much useful information as possible in the limited time available. For example if one can demonstrate an evoked response to simultaneous stimulation of both ears at a stimulus intensity of 40 dB and frequencies of 500, 1000 and 2000 Hz, the patient probably has enough hearing function to understand speech. Alternatively if time and the co-operation of the subject permit, one may choose to plot accurate thresholds at many frequencies separately for each ear. Children requiring evoked response audiometry may sometimes need sedation or even anaesthesia which in turn produce interpretive difficulties as they change the amplitude of evoked responses; in any event it is useful to have the help of a nurse or colleague to manage the patient. Jones *et al.*, (1975, 1976) give some idea of the possibilities and practical limitations of ERA in babies and subnormal children.

Conventional cortical evoked responses can be recorded at the bandwidth normally used for the EEG. Slow event-related potentials, such as the CNV, require a longer time constant of the order of 5 to 10 s. If DC recording is attempted special preparation of the electrodes may be necessary (see Chapter 3). The post-auricular myogenic response, cochleogram, and brain stem responses are made up of components in the 100–2000 Hz range.

With the HF-filters switched out, the amplifiers of some modern EEG machines may provide an adequate bandwidth; otherwise it will be necessary to use special purpose ERA equipment or an EMG machine.

Finally it should be noted that when interpreting the results of EEG data processing it is generally advisable to have the conventional paper record to hand, not least to allow one to check for artefacts or unwanted changes in vigilance of the subject. Careful documentation of computer tapes and print-outs of the EEG itself are essential if errors are to be avoided. Ideally this is achieved by using the computer itself to annotate the chart by means of a character generation facility (see Section 13.2).

Appendix I

I.1. Preparation of bentonite paste
This formulation, described by Taylor and Abraham (1969) is slightly more prone to drying than preparations containing calcium chloride which is used for its hygroscopic properties but is less likely to give skin reactions.

Bentonite 100 g
Normal saline 130 ml
Glycerine 10 ml

Stir the bentonite gradually into the saline breaking up any lumps. Add glycerine until a paste of suitable consistency is formed. The preparation should be rather softer than plasticine and sticky. It keeps for a week or two in a closed container.

Appendix II

II.1. The 10-20 system
(Reprinted with permission, from Jasper, 1958.)

Method of measurement

The anterior-posterior measurements are based upon the distance between the nasion and the inion over the vertex in the mid-line. Five points are then marked along this line, designated Frontal pole (F_p), Frontal (F), Central (C), Parietal (P), and Occipital (O). The first point (F_p) is 10% of the nasion-inion distance above the nasion; the second point (F) is 20% of this distance back from the point F_p, and so on in 20% steps back for the Central, Parietal and Occipital mid-line points (hence the name 10-20 system). These divisions are illustrated in Fig. II.1. It will be noted that this places the Central line of electrodes just one half the distance between nasion and inion.

For example, if the nasion-inion distance is 30 cm for a given patient, the F_p line will be 3 cm above the nasion, the F line 6 cm back of the F_p line (or 9 cm from the nasion), the C line 6 cm back of the F line (or 15 cm from the nasion). There will also be 6 cm between the C and P lines, and 6 cm between P and O. The occipital points are then 3 cm above the inion.

Fig. II.1. Lateral view of the skull to show methods of measurement from nasion to inion at the mid-line. F_p is frontal pole position, F is the frontal line of electrodes, C is the central line of electrodes, P is the parietal line of electrodes and 0 is the occipital line. Percentages indicated represent proportions of the measured distance from the nasion to the inion. Note that the central line is 50% of this distance. The frontal pole and occipital electrodes are 10% from the nasion and inion respectively. Twice this distance, or 20%, separates the outer line of electrodes.

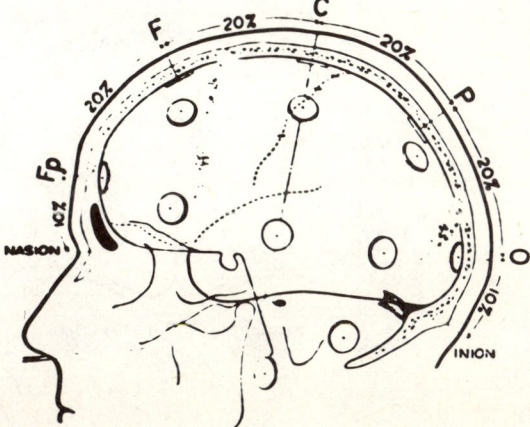

Lateral measurements are based upon the Central coronal plane. The distance is first measured from left to right preauricular points (felt as depressions at the root of the zygoma just anterior to the tragus). These points were selected because they seemed easier to determine with accuracy than the external auditory meati. Be sure the tape is passing through the pre-determined Central point at the vertex when making this measurement. 10% of this distance is then taken for the temporal point up from the preauricular point on either side. The Central points are then marked 20% of the distance above the temporal points, as shown in Fig. II.2.

The A–P line of electrodes over the temporal lobe, frontal to occipital, is determined by measuring the distance between the F_p mid-line point (as determined above), through the T position of the Central line, and back to the mid occipital point. The Fp electrode position is then marked 10% of this distance from the mid-line in front, and the occipital electrode position 10% of the distance from the mid-line in back. The inferior Frontal and posterior temporal positions then fall 20% of the distance from the F_p and O electrodes respectively along this line, as shown in Fig. II.3.

The remaining mid-Frontal (F_3 and F_4) and mid-Parietal (P_3 and P_4) electrodes are then placed along the Frontal and Parietal coronal lines respectively, equidistant between the mid-line and temporal line of electrodes on either side, as shown in Fig. II.4.

Fig. II.2. Frontal view of the skull showing the method of measurement for the central line of electrodes as described in the text.

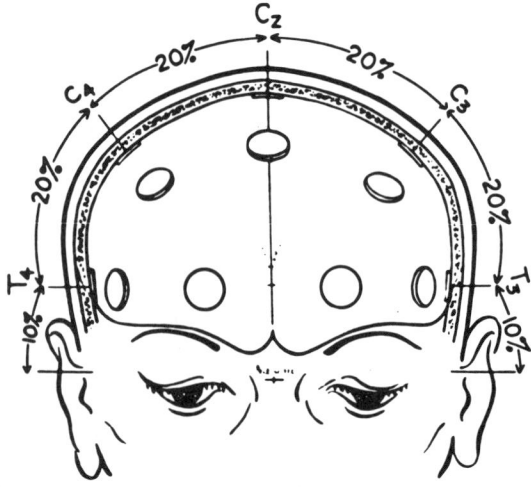

This provides a total of 21 standard electrode positions, including mid-line electrodes in Frontal, Central and Parietal regions, and the two auricular electrodes. Electrode separations are approximately the same for all pairs in the A-P direction. Coronal lines of electrodes are also approximately equally spaced, with the exception of the shorter distance between the auricular and mid-temporal points. Additional electrodes may be placed between any of these principal standard positions for especially refined localization studies (with numbers provided for these special positions as well, as indicated below).

Designations of electrode positions
Traditional anatomical terms have been employed to designate electrode positions over the various lobes of the brain, with the exception of the Central region which is, strictly speaking, partly frontal and partly parietal. It represents the cortex in the vicinity of the Central Sulcus, both pre and post-central. It is sometimes called the *sensori-motor area.*

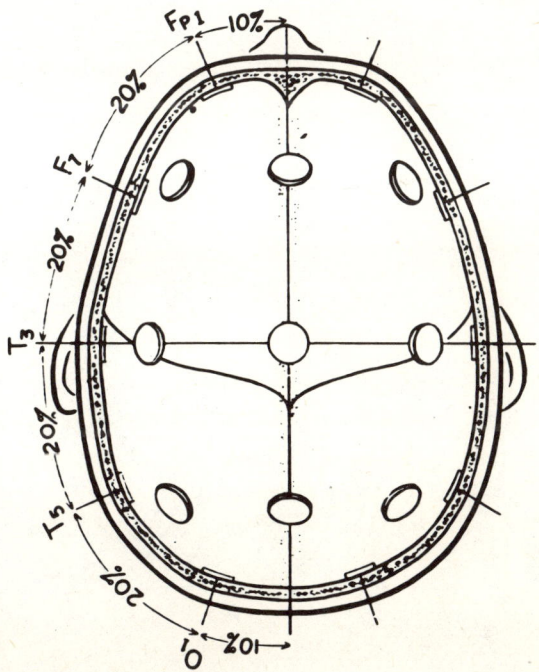

Fig. II.3. Superior view with cross-section of skull through the temporal line of electrodes illustrating the 10-20 system applied in this direction and described in the text.

Fig. II.4. The lateral view of left and right hemispheres showing all standard electrode positions, omitting intermediate positions (such as C_5 and C_6) which are used only for special studies with more closely spaced electrodes. These drawings were made from a series of X-ray projections with true lateral views. The location of principal fissures was determined by silver clips placed at operation and by other anatomical studies described in the text. The location of pharyngeal electrodes (P_{g1} and P_{g2}) was also obtained from X-ray studies with these electrodes in place.

In order to differentiate between homologous positions over the left and right hemispheres it was decided to use even numbers as subscripts for the right hemisphere, and odd numbers for the left hemisphere. F_{p2}, F_4, F_8, C_4, P_4, T_4, T_6 and O_2 become standard positions on the lateral aspect of the right hemisphere, while F_{p1}, F_3, F_7, C_3, P_3, T_3, T_5 and O_1 become standard lateral positions over the left hemisphere. These numbers were selected to allow for intermediate positions (e.g. F_2, C_2, C_6, etc.) for special localization studies.

Electrodes at the mid-line in Frontal, Central and Parietal regions were originally designated F_o, C_o and P_o but this led to some confusion since P_o, for example, might be interpreted as parieto-occipital. Consequently the mid-line positions have been changed to F_z, C_z and P_z (z for zero!). The complete system of placements with designations is shown in Figs. II.4, II.5 and II.6.

In addition to the positions described above pharyngeal electrodes are designated P_{g1} or P_{g2} for the left and right side respectively. Additional electrode positions over the posterior fossa are also shown, designated C_{b1} and C_{b2} (Cerebellar) for the left and right sides respectively.

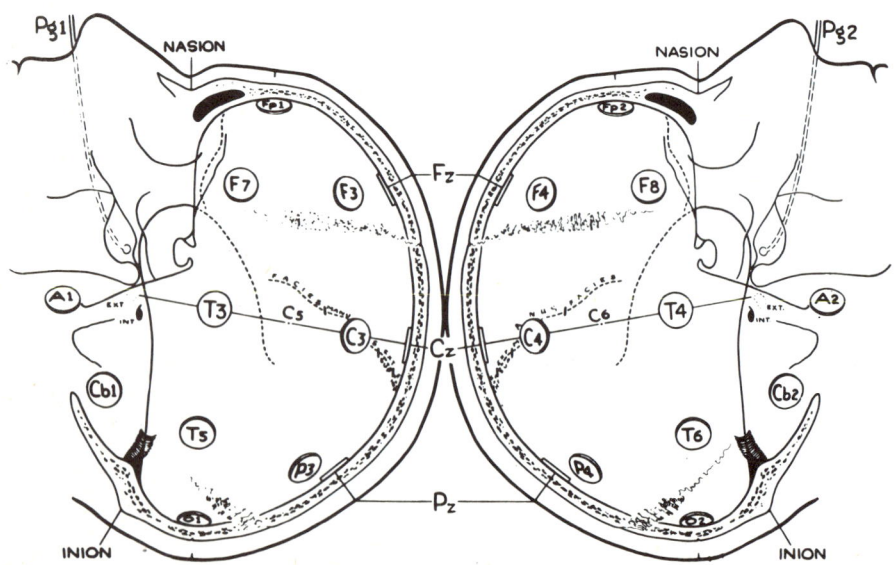

Fig. II.5. Frontal superior and posterior views showing all the standard electrode positions as described in the text.

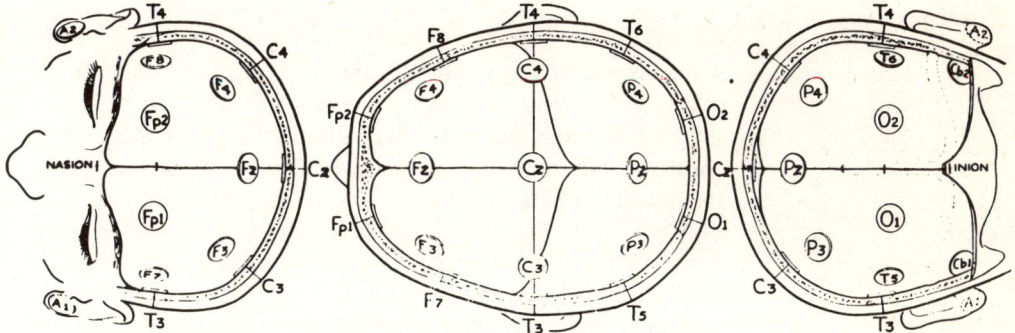

Fig. II.6. A single plane projection of the head, showing all standard positions and the location of the Rolandic and Sylvian fissures. The outer circle was drawn at the level of the nasion and inion.

The inner circle represents the temporal line of electrodes. This diagram provides a useful stamp for the indication of electrode placements in routine recording.

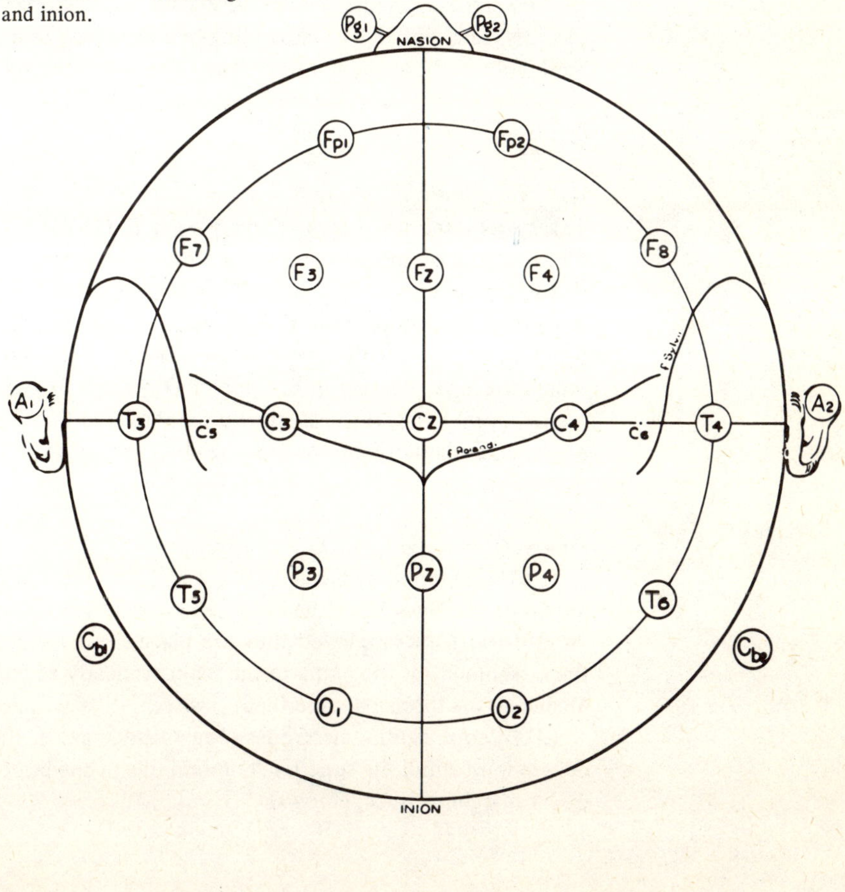

Anatomical studies

After these electrode positions were agreed upon, anatomical studies were carried out with the help of Dr Penfield, Dr McRae and Dr Caveness to determine the cortical areas over which each position would lie in the average brain. Two methods were employed: (1) metal clips placed along the Central and Sylvian fissures at operation were then used to identify these fissures in X-ray studies of the skull after the EEG electrodes had been applied, and (2) electrode positions were carefully marked in the head of cadavers, drill holes placed through the skull and the cortex marked with India ink in each position before removing the brain for examination. Brains with gross lesions or local atrophy were excluded.

Although some variability was found, and is to be expected, the position of the two principal fissures should be within plus or minus about 1 cm of that indicated on the drawings, provided the head measurements are carefully made and the brain is free of gross distortion due to expanding or contracting lesions. Due to the obliquity of the Central Fissure the upper central electrodes will usually lie pre-central while the lower ones will be post-central in most cases.

II.2. An alternative electrode system

This system, reprinted from Margerison *et al.* (1970) is favoured by a number of British departments usually having a special interest in epilepsy. It is based with minor modifications on that developed by Pampiglione (1956) at the Maudsley Hospital, London. It superficially resembles the 10-20 system, but provides more extensive coverage of the cerebral convexity particularly of the temporal lobes. It is also more closely related to bony landmarks and adapts therefore more readily to heads of different shapes.

Points determined by surface landmarks

(1) *Midtemporal* electrodes (Right and Left) in the upper portion of the concha of the ear when pads are used; when stick-on electrodes are employed they are placed above and behind the attachment of the pinna to the scalp, as nearly as possible medial to the locus just described.

(2) *Inferior frontal* electrodes (Right and Left) in the bony depression behind the superior temporal line at the level of the upper margin of the eyebrows.

(3) *Midoccipital* electrode (median) 2 cm above the external occipital protuberance.

Points determined by measurements

(1) *Prefrontal* electrodes (Right and Left) at the junction of the median and lateral thirds of a line from the right to the left inferior frontal electrode passing through a point 2 cm above the glabella.

(2) *Vertex* electrode (median) at the midpoint of a line passing in the sagittal plane from the glabella to the external occipital protuberance; on a symmetrical head this electrode should be equidistant from the two midtemporal electrodes.

(3) *Midfrontal* electrode (median) in the sagittal plane half-way between the vertex electrode and the midpoint of a line joining the prefrontal electrodes.

(4) *Midparietal* electrode (median) in the sagittal plane half-way between the vertex electrode and the midoccipital electrode.

(5) *Occipital* electrodes (Right and Left) 2 cm lateral to the midoccipital electrode.

(6) *Posterior temporal* electrodes (Right and Left) at the mid-point of a line joining the midtemporal to the occipital electrode.

(7) *Central electrodes* (Right and Left) at the junction of the medial with the intermediate third of a line joining the vertex electrode to the midtemporal electrode.

(8) *Sylvian* electrodes (Right and Left) at the junction of the lateral with the intermediate third of a line joining the vertex electrode to the midtemporal electrode.

(9) *Parietal* electrodes (Right and Left) at a point equidistant from the midparietal and posterior temporal electrodes and equidistant from the central and occipital electrodes.

(10) *Superior frontal* electrodes (Right and Left) at a point equidistant from the midfrontal and inferior frontal electrodes and equidistant from the prefrontal and central electrodes.

Appendix III

Calibration procedure for Elema-Schönander/Siemens Mingograph EEG Universal*

(1) *Paper and Ink:* check supplies.

(2) *Prepare for calibration:* sensitivity 500 μV/cm, time constant 0.3 s, high-frequency filter 700 Hz, paper speed 30 mm/s, calibration 1000 μV.

(3) *Line thickness:* turn machine on, check that the line thickness is acceptable and equal. Adjust if necessary, leave machine running.

(4) *Electrical centering:* (power amplifier EMT 7) press start button whilst machine is still running, paper drive will temporarily stop, trace deflection indicates DC offset and should be adjusted. (EMT 8-amplifiers) check that pairs of lamps on power amplifiers are of equal brightness or that the trace positions correspond to the markings on a ruler made when the machine was last set up by a service engineer – not very satisfactory! Leave the machine still running.

(5) *Alignment, hysteresis, and mechanical centering:* release drive capstan, depress calibration button and hold it depressed until the trace returns to baseline, momentarily re-engage drive and stop the paper again after it has moved a few millimetres, release calibrate button, re-engage drive capstan, release drives, depress and release calibrate button, re-engage drive. This produces the write-out shown in Fig. 6.2 and allows all functions listed above to be checked. If jets are not aligned, adjust; if upward or downward deflections are clearly unequal, replace galvanometer. Leave machine running.

(6) *Sensitivity and damping:* switch paper speed to 60 mm/s, deliver calibration pulse of about 3 s duration. Stop machine and measure tracing. Upward and downward deflections should have mean value of 20 mm on all channels, adjust to within 1 mm. Inspect tracing for evidence of overdamping or gross underdamping. If a channel appears overdamped check filter switch, if fault remains, replace galvanometer. If there is gross underdamping, more than 15% overshoot, replace galvanometer.

* Though this model has recently been superseded, it held a leading position in the market for over a decade and seems a suitable example of a machine combining a number of traditional and more advanced features.

(7) *Linearity:* switch machine on, inject calibration pulses of 500, 200, 100, 50 and 20 μV; in the last case press the calibrate button in and out as rapidly as possible for one second to check damping at low amplitudes.

(8) *Stepped attenuators:* switch to paper speed 15 mm/s, calibration 1000 μV, sensitivity 1000 μV, other controls unchanged. Using feature of mechanical coupling of calibration-amplitude and sensitivity controls, inject a calibration signal of 1000 μV at 1000 μV/cm, 200 μV at 200 μV/cm, 100 μV at 100 μV/cm, 70 μV at 70 μV/cm, 50 μV at 50 μV/cm, and 20 μV at 20 μV/cm. Leave machine running.

(9) *Noise and high-frequency filters:* sensitivity is still set at 20 μV/cm, calibration at 20 μV, and HF at 700. Increase paper speed to 30 mm/s. Observe noise level, inject calibration signal and observe overshoot or rounding of the peak. Repeat at HF settings 70, 30 and 15 Hz.

(10) *Paper speed and time marker:* switch channel 1 to open circuit. If there is not an adequate 50 Hz write-out, return HF setting to 70. If 50 Hz signal is too large, reduce sensitivity as necessary. Select paper speed 60 mm/s. Count 25 cycles of the mains signal and check that these correspond to 30 mm. Observe tracing for evidence of judder. Check that spacing of the time marker pulses is 60 mm (subject to any necessary correction if the paper speed was wrong). Select paper speed 30 and 15 mm/s and check against time marker.

(11) *Time constants:* select sensitivity 70 μV/cm, calibration 140 μV, HF filter 70, time constant 1.2, paper speed 60 mm/s. Deliver calibration pulse of about 5 s duration. Repeat with shorter calibration pulses as appropriate at time constant settings of 0.6, 0.3, 0.15, 0.015 s, observe decay of tracings and check that these are similar on all channels. Do not attempt to measure.

The above can be carried out without stopping the paper, except for purposes of measurement, in a total chart running time of 40 s. During all switching operations, except for paper speed, the deblocking switch should be depressed. Otherwise the procedure will be unnecessarily delayed by the need to wait for the tracing to return to baseline.

Appendix IV. Extended testing of EEG machines *By T. Wisman*

In Chapter 6 a battery of tests was described which should be performed before and after every EEG investigation. This Appendix describes a more extensive set of tests requiring special equipment and possibly the presence of an electronic engineer. These should be performed (together with the tests described in Chapter 6) on delivery of any new machine and at regular intervals thereafter. In general 6 monthly testing will be adequate but if the apparatus proves unreliable it may be found necessary to carry out checks and to correct faults at much shorter intervals.

IV.1. General

(1) Check casing, trim, wheels, brakes, carrying handles, etc. Obvious damage may indicate points to which extra attention should be directed during subsequent tests.

(2) Ensure that the machine is clean and in particular that there are no heavy ink deposits on and around the galvanometers, inkwells, etc.

(3) Check that all cables are intact and securely attached to their connectors.

(4) Check that the various control knobs are securely attached and that no switches are too stiff or loose.

(5) On those machines where a number of independent switches are mechanically interlinked, for instance to allow the time constants of all channels to be changed simultaneously, check that the linkages do not slip.

IV.2. Safety

(1) Check that correct fuses have been used.

(2) Check that resistance is not greater than 0.2 Ω from earth pin of mains lead to any conducting part of chassis or headbox.

(3) If possible, open mains plugs and check that the wires are securely attached.

(4) Check earth leak current. Test equipment for this purpose is commercially available. Basically it provides a facility for replacing the mains earth connection by a load representing a patient (a 1 kΩ resistor and a 0.15 μF capacitor in parallel). The voltage across this load divided by the impedance indicates the leakage current. A facility is also provided for reversing the live and neutral mains connections in view of the possibility of a socket outlet being incorrectly wired. Under both conditions the leakage current from chassis to earth must not exceed (according

to present day specifications) 100 μA. The test should also be repeated with the chassis earth disconnected and the 'patient leakage current' measured from each of the headbox sockets to mains earth. This should not exceed 50 μA. Increase mains supply voltage to 10% above normal value, by means of a variable transformer. Earth leak currents should remain within limits specified.

(5) Check total power consumption of the apparatus, a substantial change from the usual value may indicate malfunction.

IV.3. Inputs

(1) Check that the pre-selectors are wired according to specification (necessary only with a machine which is new or which has been extensively re-wired). This may be done by connecting a 10-Hz 1-mV signal to the appropriate channel.

(2) Common mode rejection ratio: by means of the input selector switches connect an oscillator giving a 1 mV signal of the required frequency across the inputs to one channel; select and if necessary adjust sensitivity so that a write-out of 1 cm is obtained. Now connect the 2 input leads of the channel together through a 4.7 kΩ resistor and connect the oscillator between one of the input leads and earth. Determine the amplitude of applied signal required to produce the same amplitude of write-out (1 cm). The ratio of the amplitude of this signal to 1 mV indicates the common mode rejection. It should be at least 10 000 to 1 at frequencies of 10 and 50 Hz. Note that a change in common mode rejection ratio often indicates an impending amplifier fault.

IV.4. Amplifiers

(1) Cross talk. Connect all channels but one to a source of a 10-Hz 1-mV signal; select a sensitivity on all channels of 500 μV/cm. That channel which has not been connected should not exhibit a write-out at 10 Hz greater than the trace thickness or 0.5 mm peak-to-peak.

(2) Time constants. With the help of an oscillator plot frequency characteristics at the various time constant settings. (Fig. 5.6) and check that these give 30% attenuation at a frequency equal to $1/2\pi T$/Hz, where T is the nominal time constant in seconds.

(3) HF filters. Check as for time constants by plotting a characteristic curve (Fig. 5.5).

(4) Noise and drift. Short circuit each channel through a 4.7 kΩ resistor, select maximum sensitivity, HF approximately

70 Hz, a time constant of about 1 s and the minimum paper
speed, run the machine for at least 5 minutes. The continuous
noise should not exceed 2 μV and pulses of more than 4 μV
amplitude should not occur more than once/minute. The base-
line should not drift by more than the equivalent of 1.5 μV
during the test. Repeat the test with the mains supply connected
through a variable transformer and check that the specifications
above are satisfied at mains voltage 10% above and 10% below the
normal values.

IV.5. Microphonics
With the machine set to maximum sensitivity and bandwidth
strike the casing vigorously with the hand to check that microphonic effects do not occur.

IV.6. Deblock
Abruptly connect a 1.5-V DC source across the input of each
channel at sensitivity 70 μV/cm and maximum time constant
setting. Immediately actuate deblock switch. Disconnect DC
source and repeat deblocking. In both instances the tracing
should return to baseline within 10 s.

IV.7. Oscillation of amplifiers
With all channels shorted through 4.7 kΩ resistors apply an oscilloscope to the power amplifier outputs (tape-recorder connection
for instance) to check that no oscillations are generated in the
amplifiers. Different machines tend to oscillate at different
frequencies, which may be from 200 to several 1000 Hz, depending on the design.

IV.8. Write-out system
(1) Paper transport. Repeat tests for time-marker and paper
transport as described in Chapter 6, but pull firmly on the paper
against the transport. The paper should start to tear before the
transport slips.

(2) Check that inkwells are in good repair and that capillary
tubes are intact and of approximately equal length.

(3) Perform tests of damping, pen alignment, centering,
hysteresis, etc. as in Chapter 6.

(4) Apply test signal such as to give 1-cm peak-to-peak pen
deflection. Now check total range of pen deflection and linearity
over that range either by applying a variable DC signal in series

with the AC component or by use of the electrical centering control. Check that linearity is maintained over the range specified and that this is symmetrical about the zero line.

On modern machines the maximum deflection is electrically limited and is less than that which may be obtained by displacing the pen lightly with the finger; in machines where this is applicable check that the range conforms to specification. Repeat this test with an applied signal expected to give only 1-mm deflection. In particular note any loss of sensitivity close to the zero position which may reflect either a faulty galvanometer bearing or an amplifier defect ('cross-over distortion').

(5) If a mechanical system is provided for lifting the pens and possibly for resting them on rubber pads when not in use check that this works correctly.

(6) Check and adjust sensitivity using the internal calibration facility. Re-check with an applied signal of the same type from the headbox. (Note that a square wave contains HF components which should be limited by the HF filters, if one sets up sensitivity with a square wave and then re-checks against a 10-Hz sine-wave the sensitivity setting will appear to be 10% too high – except on machines having an exceptionally wide bandwidth such as those using jet galvanometers.)

IV.9. Miscellaneous

(1) Check that switches for polygraphy, connecting and disconnecting ECG, selectable average reference, sindex, etc. work correctly. Ad hoc tests will have to be devised depending upon design of machine.

(2) Check that the event-marker works.

(3) Check resistance-measurement circuit with resistance network inserted into headbox (a suitable device is usually obtainable from the manufacturer of the machine).

(4) Suppressor amplifier: connect an oscillator between G1 (suppressor amplifier input) and earth. If no earth socket is available on the headbox, as is the case on some machines with active earth systems, use an earthing point on the machine chassis or mains socket outlet. Measure output of suppressor amplifier with an oscilloscope connected between G2 and earth. For applied signals of 1 mV from 1 to 70 Hz the output should be in the range 30–50 mV (or as specified by the manufacturer).

(5) Document test results and any remedial action taken.

Appendix V

Checklist for portable EEG
Trolley and papertray
Mains lead
Earth lead
Machine spares:
    Machine handbook
    Pens
    Galvanometer
    Fuses
    Spare amplifiers
Blotting Rollers (Siemens machines only)
Recording paper
Ink
Air-compressor pump
Air gun (and spare)
Silver-silver chloride stick-on electrodes
Short silver chloride stick-on electrodes
Leads for short silver chloride stick-on electrodes
Platinum needle electrodes (sterile)
Collodion
Ether-meths
Acetone
Head-rest (hard cylindrical pillow)
Sticky discs
Sticky tape
Jelly needles
Syringes 2 ml
Electrode jelly
Galley pot
Tape measure
Wax pencil
Cotton-wool
Paper towels
Rubber gloves
ECG leads, electrodes and straps
Steel combs, coarse and fine
Scissors
Thermocouple
Photic stimulator
Photo-electric cell
Montage stamp
Ink-pad

Pens
Pencils
Rubber
Ruler
Cursor
Binding tape for record
Request forms
Patient report forms
Special state of patient forms for ITU or unconscious patients
Blotting paper
Carbon paper (to make a copy of anything the EEGist writes in
    the patient's notes)
Screwdrivers (various)
Pliers
Wirecutters

CLINICAL CHECKLIST FOR EEG DURING INTENSIVE CARE

HOSP. NO.	NAME		REG. NO.	AGE	SEX
DAY	DATE	TIME	WHERE RECORDED		TECH'S NAME

STATE OF CONSCIOUSNESS: — ALERT, RESTLESS, DROWSY OR ASLEEP (ROUSABLE NOT
CONFUSED), CONFUSED OR STUPOROSE (NOT ROUSABLE), COMATOSE — LIGHT (RESPONDS
TO PAIN), COMATOSE — DEEP (NO RESPONSE TO PAIN), ANY OTHER DESCRIPTION.

STIMULATION — PATIENT'S RESPONSE

CALL NAME	CLAP	PAINFUL STIMULATION

RESPIRATIONS SPONTANEOUS	NORMAL	ABNORMAL	ON RESPIRATOR

GENERAL CLINICAL STATE OF PATIENT & OTHER INFORMATION

LAST ARREST	CARDIAC A.	RESP. A.

TEMPERATURE:	PULSE:	/MIN RESP:	B.P.

SEIZURES. (DESCRIPTION WITH TIME AND DATE)

MEDICATION	MACHINE CHECK		ELECTRODES
	SENSITIVITY	PEN ALIGNMENT	STICK ONS
	LINEARITY	PEN CENTRING	NEEDLES
		NOISE LEVEL	

METABOLIC STATE ETC.

CHLORIDE	BICARBONATE	SODIUM	POTASSIUM	UREA	Hb
BASE EXCESS	pCO_2	pO_2	SATURATION	pH	PCV
BARBITURATE	CALCIUM	OTHER:			WBC
BILIRUBIN	GLUCOSE				PLATELETS

References

Adrian, E.D. and Matthews, B.H.C. (1934). The Berger rhythm: potential changes from the occipital lobes in man. *Brain*, 57, 356–85.

Adrian, E.D. and Yamagiwa, K. (1935). The origin of the Berger rhythm. *Brain*, 58, 22.

Arden, G.B., Bodis-Wollner, I., Halliday, A.M., Jeffreys, A., Kulikovski, J. J., Spekreiijsse, H. and Regan, D, (1977). Methodology of patterned visual stimulation. In *Visual Evoked Potentials in Man*, ed. J.E. Desmedt, pp. 3–15. Clarendon Press, Oxford.

Arellano, A.P. (1949). A tympanic lead. *Electroencephalogr. Clin. Neurophysiol.*, 1, 112–13.

Babb, T.L., Mariani, E. and Grandall, P.H. (1974). An electronic circuit for detection of EEG seizures recorded with implanted electrodes. *Electroencephalogr. Clin. Neurophysiol.*, 37, 305–8.

Baker, R.N. and Klass, D.W. (1957). The Metrazol activated electroencephalogram in normal subjects. *Electroencephalogr. Clin. Neurophysiol.*, 9, 169.

Baldock, G.R. and Walter, W.G. (1946). A new electronic analyser. *Electron. Engng.*, 18, 339–42.

Bancaud, J. (1975). Stereoelectroencephalography. In *Handbook of Electroencephalography and Clinical Neurophysiology 10B*, ed. A. Rémond, pp. 1–65. Elsevier, Amsterdam.

Bancaud, J., Talairach, J., Waltregny, P., Bresson, M. and Morel, P. (1968). L'activation par le Mégimide dans la diagnostique topographique des épilepsies corticales focales (étude clinique, EEG et SEEG). *Rev. Neurol.*, 119, 320–5.

Barlow, J.S. (1975). A 16-channel cassette tape recorder system for clinical EEGs. *Electroencephalogr. Clin. Neurophysiol.*, 38, 183–6.

Barlow, J.S. (1979). Computerized clinical electroencephalography in perspective. *IEEE Trans. Biomed. Eng.*, 26, 377–91.

Batchelor, B.G. (Ed.) (1978). *Pattern Recognition: Ideas in Practice*. Plenum Publishing Co., London.

Bates, J.A.V. (1963). Special investigation techniques. Indwelling electrodes and electrocorticography. In *Electroencephalography*, ed. D. Hill and G. Parr, pp. 429–79. Macdonald, London.

Bechinger, D. and Kornhuber, H.H. (1976). The sleep deprivation EEG in childhood. *Electroencephalogr. Clin. Neurophysiol.*, 41, 654.

Bennett, D.R., Ziter, F.A. and Liske, E.A. (1969). Electroencephalographic study of sleep deprivation in flying personnel. *Neurology (Minneap.)*, 19, 375–7.

Benoit, J.P., Baillon, J.F., Findji, F., Renault, B. and Rémond, A. (1973). Une méthode informatique de traitement de l'électroencéphalogramme visant à reconnaitre et à quantifier les différents paramètres des graphoéléments usuels des électroencéphalographistes. In *Die Quantifizierung des Elektroencephalograms*, ed. G.K. Schenk, pp. 281–91. AEG Telefunken, Konstanz.

Berger, H. (1929). Uber das Elektroenkephalogramm des Menschen. *Arch. f. Psychiat.*, 87, 527–70.

Bickford, R.G., Brimm, J., Berger, L. and Aung, M. (1973). Application of compressed spectral array in clinical EEG. In *Automation of Clinical Electroencephalography*, ed. P. Kellaway and I. Petersén, pp. 55–64. Raven Press, New York.

Bickford, R.G., Sem-Jacobsen C.W., White, P.T. and Daley, D. (1952).
    Some observations on the mechanism of photic and photometrazol
    activation. *Electroencephalogr. Clin. Neurophysiol.*, **4**, 275–82.
Billinger, T.W. and Frank, G.S. (1969). Effect of posture on EEG slowing
    during hyperventilation. *Amer. J. EEG Technol.*, **9**, 22–7.
Binnie, C.D. (1975a). A comparison of different methods of period
    analysis. *Electroencephalogr. Clin. Neurophysiol.*, **38**, 662.
Binnie, C.D. (1975b). The EEG in intensive care: interpretation. *J. Electro-
    physiol. Technol.*, **1**, 5–18.
Binnie, C.D. (1976). Computers in neurophysiology: clinical applications.
    J. Electro-physiol. Technol., **2**, 2–28.
Binnie, C.D. (1980). The use of the EEG in the diagnosis of the epilepsies.
    In *Epilepsie en Praktijk*, ed. H. Meinardi and M. de Vlieger, pp. 61–82.
    Stafleu, Alphen.
Binnie, C.D., Batchelor, B.G., Bowring, P.A., Darby, C.E., Herbert, L.,
    Lloyd, D.S.L., Smith, D.M., Smith, G.F. and Smith, M. (1978a).
    Computer-assisted interpretation of clinical EEGs. *Electroencephalogr.
    Clin. Neurophysiol.*, **44**, 575–85.
Binnie, C.D., Batchelor, B.G., Gainsborough, A.J., Lloyd, D.S.L., Smith,
    D.M. and Smith, G.F. (1979). Visual and computer-assisted assessment
    of the EEG in epilepsy of late onset. *Electroencephalogr. Clin. Neuro-
    physiol.*, **47**, 102–7.
Binnie, C.D., Batchelor, B.G. and Smith, G.F. (1978b). Pattern recognition
    in electroencephalography. In *Pattern Recognition: Ideas in Practice*,
    ed. B.G. Batchelor, pp. 399–426. Plenum Publishing Co., London.
Binnie, C.D., Bown, R., Lloyd, D.S.L. and Smith, M. (1973a). Some
    electroencephalographic and psychological findings in minimal hepatic
    encephalopathy. *Electroencephalogr. Clin. Neurophysiol.*, **34**, 108.
Binnie, C.D., Coles, P.A. and Margerison, J.H. (1969). The influence of
    end-tidal carbon dioxide tension on EEG changes during routine
    hyperventilation in different age groups. *Electroencephalogr. Clin.
    Neurophysiol.*, **27**, 304–6.
Binnie, C.D., Fee, G.Y., Lloyd, D.S.L. and Roberts, J.R. (1973b). Reducing
    artefact in measurements of average evoked potentials. *Electro-
    encephalogr. Clin. Neurophysiol.*, **35**, 418.
Binnie, C.D. and Lloyd, D.S.L. (1973). A technique for measuring
    reaction times during paroxysmal discharges. *Electroencephalogr. Clin.
    Neurophysiol.*, **35**, 418.
Binnie, C.D. and McClelland, R.J. (1977). Electroencephalography: tech-
    niques, instrumentation and current methods of data processing. In
    Physical Techniques in Medicine, vol. 1, ed. J.T. McMullan, pp. 235–85.
    John Wiley and Sons, Chichester.
Binnie, C.D., Overweg, J. and Rowan, A.J. (1980). Long-term EEG and
    video monitoring in epilepsy. In *Proceedings of the Second European
    Congress of Electroencephalography and Clinical Neurophysiology*, ed.
    H. Lechner and A. Aranibar, Excerpta Medica, Amsterdam, pp. 83–8.
Binnie, C.D., Prior, P.F., Lloyd, D.S.L., Scott, D.F. and Margerison, J.H.
    (1970). Electroencephalographic prediction of fatal anoxic brain
    damage after resuscitation from cardiac arrest. *Br. Med. J.*, 1970, **4**,
    265–8.

Binnie, C.D., Rowan, A.J., Overweg, J., Meinardi, H., Wisman, T., Kamp, A. and Lopes da Silva, F. (1981). Telemetric EEG and video monitoring in epilepsy. *Neurology (Minneap.)*, **31**, 298–303.

Binnie, C.D., Ward, P.A. and Heywood, J. (1971). EEG contour mapping: 1. Theory and practice. *Proc. Electro-physiol. Technol. Assoc.*, **18**, 12.

Bourne, J.R., Ward, J.W., Teschan, P.E., Musso, M., Johnston, H.B. and Ginn, H.E. (1975). Quantitative assessment of the electroencephalogram in renal disease. *Electroencephalogr. Clin. Neurophysiol.*, **39**, 377–88.

Branthwaite, M.A. (1973). Detection of neurological damage during open heart surgery. *Thorax*, **28**, 464–72.

Brazier, M.A.B. (1972). Spread of seizure discharges in epilepsy: anatomical and electrophysiological considerations. *Exp. Neurol.*, **36**, 253–72.

Bremer, F. (1935). Cerveau isolé et physiologie du sommeil. *CR Soc. Biol. (Paris)*, **118**, 1235–41.

Brown, B.B. (1963). Some characteristic EEG differences between heavy smoker and non-smoker subjects. *Neurophyschologica*, **6**, 381–8.

Browne, T.R., Penry, S.K., Porter, R.J. and Dreifuss, F.E. (1974). Responsiveness before, during and after spike-wave paroxysms. *Neurology (Minneap.)*, **24**, 659–65.

Burch, N.R., Edwards, R.J., Nettleton, W.J. and Sweeney, J. (1964). Period analysis of the electroencephalogram on a general purpose digital computer. *Ann. NY Acad. Sci.*, **115**, 827–43.

Byford, G.H. and Goddard, C.R. (1972). A magnetic tape index, including facilities for controlling both the acquisition of data and its subsequent analysis. *J. Physiol.*, **224**, 13.

Caille, E.J. and Bassano, J.L. (1975). Value and limits of sleep statistical analysis: objective parameters and subjective evaluations. In *CEAN: Computerized EEG Analysis*, ed. G. Dolce and H. Künkel, pp. 227–35. Fischer, Stuttgart.

Carrie, J.R.G. (1972). Hybrid computer system for detecting and quantifying spike and wave EEG patterns. *Electroencephalogr. Clin. Neurophysiol.*, **33**, 339–41.

Caton, R. (1875). The electric currents of the brain. *Br. Med. J.*, 1875, **2**, 278.

Chatrian, G.E., Bergamini, L., Dondey, M., Klass, D.W., Lennox-Buchthal, M. and Petersén, I. (1974). A glossary of terms most commonly used by clinical electroencephalographers. *Electroencephalogr. Clin. Neurophysiol.*, **37**, 538–48.

Chiappa, K.H., Gladstone, K.J. and Young, R.R. (1979). Brain stem auditory evoked responses. Study of wave-form variations in 50 normal human subjects. *Arch. Neurol.*, **36**, 81–7.

Christian, W. (1975). *Klinische Electroencephalographie Lehrbuch und Atlas*. Georg Thieme, Stuttgart.

Christodoulou, G. (1967). Sphenoidal electrodes. *Acta Neurol. Scand.*, **43**, 587–93.

Clendenning, W.E. and Auerbach, R. (1964). Traumatic calcium deposition in skin. *Arch. Derm.*, **89**, 360–3.

Cody, D.T.R. and Bickford, R.G. (1969). Averaged evoked myogenic responses in normal man. *Laryngoscope*, **79**, 400–16.

Cohen, B.A. and Sances, A. (1977). Stationarity of the human electroencephalogram. *Med. Biol. Eng.*, **15**, 513–18.

Coles, P.A. and Binnie, C.D. (1968). An alternative method of chloriding EEG electrodes. *Proc. Electro-physiol. Technol. Assoc.*, 15, 195–201.

Comer, A.K., Binnie, C.D., Gainsborough, A.J., Lewis, P.H., Lloyd, D.S.L., Oldman, M. and Thornton, R.E. (1979). An electroencephalographic study of smokers and non-smokers with reference to age, sex and personality. In *Electrophysiological Effects of Nicotine*, ed. A. Rémond and C. Izard, pp. 117–31. Elsevier, Amsterdam.

Compes, P. (1977). *Grundlagen Sicherheits Technik*. Gesamthochschule, Wuppertal.

Cooper, R. (1956). Storage of silver chloride electrodes. *Electroencephalogr. Clin. Neurophysiol.*, 8, 692.

Cooper, R., and Walter, V.J. (1957). Suction cup electrodes. *Electroencephalogr. Clin. Neurophysiol.*, 9, 733.

Creutzfeldt, O.D., Watanabe, S. and Lux, H.D. (1966). Relations between EEG phenomena and potentials of single cortical cells. II Spontaneous and convulsoid activity. *Electroencephalogr. Clin. Neurophysiol.*, 20, 19–37.

Daly, D.D. (1968). The effect of sleep upon the electroencephalogram in patients with brain tumors. *Electroencephalogr. Clin. Neurophysiol.*, 25, 521–9.

Darby, C.E., de Korte, R.A., Binnie, C.D. and Wilkins, A.J. (1980b). The self-induction of epileptic seizures by eye-closure. *Epilepsia*, 21, 31–42.

Darby, C.E., Lettich, E. and Margerison, J.H. (1958). The placement of scalp electrodes with respect to underlying cerebral cortex. *Proc. Electro-physiol. Technol. Assoc.*, 7, 43–8.

Darby, C.E., Wilkins, A.J., Binnie, C.D. and de Korte, R. (1980a). Routine testing for pattern sensitivity. *J. Electro-physiol. Technol.*, 6, 202–10.

Davis, H. (1964). Enhancement of evoked cortical potentials in humans related to a task requiring a decision. *Science*, 145, 182–3.

Davis, H., Hirsh, S.K., Shelnutt, J. and Bowers, C. (1967). Further validation of evoked response audiometry (ERA). *J. Speech Hear. Res.*, 10, 717–32.

Day, J. and Lippitt, M. (1964). A long-term electrode system for electrocardiography and impedance pneumography. *Psychophysiology*, 1, 174–82.

Dement, W. and Kleitman, N. (1957). Cyclic variations in EEG during sleep and their relation to eye movements, body mobility, and dreaming. *Electroencephalogr. Clin. Neurophysiol.*, 9, 673–90.

Dempsey, E.W. and Morison, R.S. (1942). The production of rhythmically recurrent cortical potentials after localized thalamic stimulation. *Amer. J. Physiol.*, 135, 293–300.

Deonna, Th., Beaumanoir, A., Gaillard, F. and Assal, G. (1977). Acquired aphasia in childhood with seizure disorder: a heterogeneous syndrome. *Neuropädiatrie*, 8, 263–73.

Dietsch, G. (1932). Fourier-analyse von Elektrencephalogrammen des Menschen. *Pfluegers Arch.*, 230, 106–12.

Doenicke, A., Kügler, J., Schellenberger, A. and Gürtner, Th. (1966). The use of electroencephalography to measure recovery time after intravenous anaesthesia. *Br. J. Anaesth.*, 38, 580–90.

Douek, E., Gibson, W. and Humpfries, K. (1973). The crossed acoustic response. *J. Laryngol. Otol.*, 87, 771–26.

Drasdo, N. (1975). A discussion of the photometric method. In *Photosensitive Epilepsy*. P.M. Jeavons and G.F. Harding, Heinemann, London.

Driver, M.V. (1962). A study of the photosensitive threshold. *Electroencephalogr. Clin. Neurophysiol.*, 14, 359–67.

Drohocki, Z. (1969). Utilisation de l'analyseur statistique d'amplitudes ASA en pharmacodynamie cérébrale l'action de l'immenoctal (sécobarbital). *Rev. Neurol.*, 121, L. 357–61.

Dumermuth, G. (1976). *Elektroencephalographie in Kindesalter*. Georg Thieme, Stuttgart.

Dus. V. and Wilson, S.J. (1975). The click-evoked post-auricular myogenic response in normal subjects. *Electroencephalogr. Clin. Neurophysiol.*, 39, 523–5.

Edelberg. R. (1963). Personal communication. Cited by L.A. Geddes, *Electrodes and the Measurement of Bioelectric Events*, p. 364. Wiley-Interscience, New York, 1972.

Egmond, P. van., Binnie, C. D. and Veldhuizen, R. (1980). The effect of background illumination on sensitivity to intermittent photic stimulation. *Electroencephalogr. Clin. Neurophysiol.*, 48, 599–601.

Ehrenberg, B.L. and Penry, J.K. (1976). Computer recognition of generalized spike-wave discharges. *Electroencephalogr. Clin. Neurophysiol.*, 41, 25–36.

Evans, B.T., Binnie, C.D. and Lloyd, D.S.L. (1974). A simple visual pattern stimulator. *Electroencephalogr. Clin. Neurophysiol.*, 37, 403–6.

Frost, J.D. (1970). An automatic sleep analyser. *Electroencephalogr. Clin. Neurophysiol.*, 29, 88–92.

Frost, J.D. (1973). A sleep-analysis system as a model of automation of clinical electroencephalography. In *Automation of Clinical Electroencephalography*, ed. P. Kellaway and I. Petersén, pp. 31–43. Raven Press, New York.

Gatzke, R.D. (1974). The electrode: a measurement systems viewpoint. In *Biomedical Electrode Technology*, ed. H.A. Miller and D.C. Harrison, p. 447. Academic Press, New York.

Gay, P. and Muras, J.S. (1969). A device for promoting hyperventilation in children. *Proc. Electro-physiol. Technol. Assoc.*, 16, 270–2.

Geddes, L.A. (1972). *Electrodes and the Measurement of Bioelectric Events*. Wiley-Interscience, New York.

Geddes, L.A. and Baker, L.E. (1967). Chlorided silver electrodes. *Med. Res. Eng.*, 6, 33–4.

Geursen, J., Terlouw, W. and Wisman, T. (1978). Aanvalssignalering bij in bed liggende epilepsiepatienten. *Het Ziekenhuis*, 20, 526–8.

Gibbs, F.A. and Gibbs, E.L. (1950). *Atlas of Electroencephalography*, vol. I. Addison-Wesley Press, Cambridge, Mass.

Gloor, P. (1972). Generalized spike and wave discharge: a consideration of cortical and subcortical mechanisms of their genesis and synchronization. In *Synchronization of EEG Activity in Epilepsies*, ed. H. Petsche and M.A.B. Brazier, pp. 382–408., Springer Verlag, Berlin, Heidelberg and New York.

Gloor, P., Tsai, C. and Hadded, F. (1958). An assessment of the value of sleep-electroencephalography for the diagnosis of temporal lobe epilepsy. *Electroencephalogr. Clin. Neurophysiol.*, 10, 633–48.

Golla, F.L. and Winter, A.L. (1958). Analysis of cerebral responses to flicker in patients complaining of episodic headache. *Electro-encephalogr. Clin. Neurophysiol.*, 11, 539–49.

Gotman, J. and Gloor, P. (1976). Automatic recognition and quantification of interictal epileptic activity in the human scale EEG. *Electroencephalogr. Clin. Neurophysiol.*, 41, 513–29.

Gotman, J., Gloor, P. and Ray, W.F. (1975). A quantitative comparison of traditional reading of the EEG and interpretation of computer-extracted features in patients with supratentorial brain lesions. *Electroencephalogr. Clin. Neurophysiol.*, 38, 623–39.

Gotman, J., Gloor, P. and Schaul, N. (1978). Comparison of traditional reading of the EEG and automatic recognition of interictal epileptic activity. *Electroencephalogr. Clin. Neurophysiol.*, 44, 48–60.

Gotman, J., Ives, J.R. and Gloor, P. (1977). Relationships between different regions during epileptic seizures in humans. *Electroencephalogr. Clin. Neurophysiol.*, 43, 476.

Gurdjian, E.S., Webster, J.E., Hardy, W.G. and Lindner, D.W. (1958). Nonexistence of the so-called cerebral form of carotid sinus syncope. *Neurology (Minneap.)*, 8, 818–26.

Halliday, A.M., McDonald, W.I. and Mushin, J. (1972). Delayed visual evoked responses in optic neuritis. *Lancet*, 1972, 2, 982–5.

Hanley, J., Adey, W.R., Zweizig, J.R. and Kado, R.T. (1971) EEG electrode-amplifier harness. *Electroencephalogr. Clin. Neurophysiol.*, 30, 147–50.

Harner, R.N. (1978). Computer analysis and clinical EEG interpretation, perspective and application. In *CEAN Computerized EEG analysis*, ed. G. Dolce and H. Künkel, pp. 337–43. Fischer, Stuttgart.

Harner, R.N. and Ostergren, K.A. (1978). Computed EEG topography. In *Contemporary Clinical Neurophysiology.*, ed. W.A. Cobb and H. van Duijn, pp. 151–61. Elsevier, Amsterdam.

Hawkes, C.H. and Prescott, R.J. (1973). Clinical note: EEG variation in healthy subjects. *Electroencephalogr. Clin. Neurophysiol.*, 34, 197–9.

Heppenstall, M.E. (1944). The relation between the effects of the blood sugar levels and hyperventilation on the electroencephalogram. *J. Neurol. Neurosurg. Psychiat.*, 4, 112–18.

Hess, R. (1966). *EEG Handbook*. Sandoz, London.

Hjorth, B. (1970). EEG analysis based on time domain properties. *Electro-encephalogr. Clin. Neurophysiol.*, 29, 306–10.

Hjorth, B. (1975). An on-line transformation of EEG scalp potentials into orthogonal source derivations. *Electroencephalogr. Clin. Neurophysiol.*, 39, 526–30.

Hjorth, B. (1979). Multichannel EEG preprocessing: analogue matrix operations in the study of local effects. *Pharmakopsychiat.*, 12, 111–18.

International Electrotechnical Commission (1973). *Common Aspects of Electrical Equipment used in Medical Practice*. IEC Secretariat, Geneva.

Itil, T.M. (1974). *Modern Problems of Pharmacopsychiatry. 8: Psycho-tropic Drugs and the Human EEG*. S. Karger, Basel and München.

Ives, J.R. and Gloor, P. (1977). New sphenoidal electrode assembly to permit long-term monitoring of the patient's ictal or interictal EEG. *Electroencephalogr. Clin. Neurophysiol.*, 42, 575–80.

Ives, J.R. and Gloor, P. (1978). A long-term time-lapse video system to document the patient's spontaneous clinical seizure synchronized with the EEG. *Electroencephalogr. Clin. Neurophysiol.*, **45**, 412–16.

Ives, J.R., Thompson, C.J. and Gloor, P. (1976). Seizure monitoring: a new tool in electroencephalography. *Electroencephalogr. Clin. Neurophysiol.*, **41**, 422–7.

Ives, J.R., Thompson, C.J. and Woods, J.F. (1973). Acquisition by telemetry and computer analysis of 4 channel long-term EEG recordings from patients subject to "petit-mal" absence attacks. *Electroencephalogr. Clin. Neurophysiol.*, **34**, 665–8.

Ives, J.R. and Woods, J.F. (1975). 4-channel 24 hour cassette recorder for long-term EEG monitoring of ambulatory patients. *Electroencephalogr. Clin. Neurophysiol.*, **39**, 88–92.

Jasper, H.H. (1949). Personal communication. Cited by R.S. Schwab, *Electroencephalography in Clinical Practice*. Saunders, Philadelphia, 1951.

Jasper, H.H. (1958). Report of the committee on methods of clinical examination in electroencephalography. *Electroencephalogr. Clin. Neurophysiol.*, **10**, 370–5.

Jeavons, P.M. and Harding, G.F.A. (1975). *Photosensitive Epilepsy*. Heinemann, London.

Jeavons, P.M., Harding, G.F.A., Panayiotopoulos, C.P. and Drasdo, N. (1972). The effect of geometric patterns combined with intermittent photic stimulation in photosensitive epilepsy. *Electroencephalogr. Clin. Neurophysiol.*, **33**, 221–4.

Jewett, D.L., Bomans, M.N. and Williston, J.S. (1970). Human auditory evoked potentials: possible brainstem components detected on the scalp. *Science*, **167**, 1517–18.

Jones, B.N., Binnie, C.D., Cassidy, B. and Roberts, J.R. (1976). Feasibility studies of evoked response audiometry in the subnormal. *J. Ment. Def. Res.*, **20**, 1–8.

Jones, B.N., Scott, S.C., Binnie, C.D. and Roberts, J.R. (1975). Clinical and evoked response assessment of hearing in late infancy. *Dev. Med. Child Neurol.*, **17**, 726–31.

Jones, D.P. (1951). Recording of the basal EEG with sphenoidal electrodes. *Electroencephalogr. Clin. Neurophysiol.*, **3**, 100.

Kado, R.T. and Adey, W.R. (1968). Electrode problems in central nervous monitoring in performing subjects. *Ann. NY Acad. Sci.*, **148**, 263–78.

Kardel, T., Zander Olsen, P., Stigsby, B. and Tonnesan, K. (1972). Hepatic encephalopathy evaluated by automatic period analysis of the EEG during lactulose treatment. *Acta Med.*, **192**, 493–8.

Kiloh, L.G., McComas, A.J. and Osselton, J.W. (1972). *Clinical Electroencephalography*. Butterworths, London.

Klass, D.W. and Daly, D.D. (1979). *Current Practice of Clinical Electroencephalography*. Raven Press, New York.

Klass, D.W. and Fischer-Williams, M. (1976). Sensory stimulation, sleep and sleep deprivation. In *Handbook of Electroencephalography and Clinical Neurophysiology*, 3 D Section I, ed. A. Rémond, pp. 5–73. Elsevier, Amsterdam.

Knott, V.J. and Venables, P.H. (1977). EEG alpha correlates of non-smokers, smokers, smoking, and smoking deprivation. *Psychophysiology*, **14**, 150–6.

Kooi, K.A. (1971). *Fundamentals of Electroencephalography*. Harper and Row, New York.

Kooi, K.A., Eckman, G.H. and Thomas, M.H. (1957). Observations on the response to photic stimulation in organic cerebral dysfunction. *Electroencephalogr. Clin. Neurophysiol.*, **9**, 239–50.

Kooi, K.A., Tucker, R.P. and Marstall, R.E. (1978). *Fundamentals of Electroencephalography*. Harper and Row, Hagerstown.

Kornhuber, H.H. and Deecke, L. (1964). Hirnpotentialänderungen beim Menschen vor und nach Willkurbewegungen. *Pfluegers Arch.*, **281**, 52.

Kornhuber, H.H. and Deecke, L. (1965). Hirnpotentialänderungen bei Willkurbewegungen und Passiven Bewegungen des Menschen: Beretschaftspontential und reafferente Potentiale. *Pfluegers Arch.*, **284**, 1–17.

Krekule, I. (1968). Zero crossing detection of the presence of evoked responses. *Electroencephalogr. Clin. Neurophysiol.*, **25**, 175–6.

Kristensen, O. and Sindrup, E.H. (1978). Sphenoidal electrodes. *Acta Neurol. Scand.*, **58**, 157.

Ktonas, P.Y. and Smith, J.R. (1974). Quantification of abnormal EEG spike characteristics. *Comput. Biol. Med.*, **4**, 157–63.

Kuyer, A. (1978). Epilepsy and Exercise. Thesis: University of Amsterdam.

Laget, P., Salbreux, R., Raimbault, J., d'Allest, A.M. and Mariani, J. (1976). Relationship between changes in somesthetic evoked responses and electroencephalographic findings in the child with hemiplegia. *Dev. Med. Child Neurol.*, **18**, 620–31.

Laidlaw, J. and Read, A.E. (1963). The EEG in hepatic encephalopathy. *Clin. Sci.*, **24**, 109–20.

Lansing, R.W. and Thomas, H. (1964). The laterality of photic driving in normal adults. *Electroencephalogr. Clin. Neurophysiol.*, **16**, 290–4.

Layzell, J., Smith, D. and Binnie, C.D. (1973). Automatic staging of sleep by spectral descriptors. *Electroencephalogr. Clin. Neurophysiol.*, **35**, 418.

Leader, H.S., Cohn, R., Weihner, A.L. and Caceres, C.A. (1967). Pattern reading of the clinical electroencephalogram with a digital computer. *Electroencephalogr. Clin. Neurophysiol.*, **23**, 566–70.

Lehtinen, L.O.J. and Bergström, L. (1970). Naso-ethmoidal electrode for recording the electrical activity of the inferior surface of the frontal lobe. *Electroencephalogr. Clin. Neurophysiol.*, **29**, 303–5.

Letemendia, F. and Pampiglione, G. (1958). Clinical and electroencephalographic observations in Alzheimer's disease. *J. Neurol. Neurosurg. Psychiat.*, **21**, 167–72.

Lettich, E. and Margerison, J.H. (1960). The use of data from low frequency analysis to illustrate serial EEG in depressed patients during treatment with iproniazid. *J. Ment. Sci.*, **106**, 1111–4.

Lev, A. and Sohmer, H. (1972). Sources of averaged neural responses recorded in animal and human subjects during cochlear audiometry (electrocochleogram). *Arch. Klin. Exp. Ohren Nasen Kehlkopfheilkd.*, **201**, 79–90.

Liske, E. (1965). "H-response" in the electroencephalograms of aircrew personnel. *Aerospace Med.*, **36**, 884–7.

Lloyd, D.S.L., Binnie, C.D. and Batchelor, B.G. (1972a). Pattern recognition in EEG. *Adv. Behav. Biol.*, **5**, 153–66.

Lloyd, D.S.L., Binnie, C.D. and Fee, G.Y. (1973). Some applications of time domain descriptors. *Electroencephalogr. Clin. Neurophysiol.*, **34**, 749.

Lloyd, D.S.L., Binnie, C.D., Stenfors, S.G.B. and Roberts, J.R. (1972b). Character generation on a moving chart recorder. *Bio. Med. Eng.*, **7**, 274–7.

Lloyd, D.S.L. and Wilson, S. (1973). The distribution of posterior temporal slow waves: implications of electrode placement systems. *Proc. Electro-physiol. Technol. Assoc.*, **20**, 151–8.

Lopes da Silva, F.H., van Hulten, K., Lommen, J.G., Storm van Leeuwen, W., van Veelen, G.W.M. and Vliegenthart, W. (1977). Automatic detection and localization of epileptic foci. *Electroencephalogr. Clin. Neurophysiol.*, **43**, 1–13.

Lopes da Silva, F.H., Kamp, A., Mars, N.J.I., Bultstra, G., Lommen, J.G. and van Hulten, K. (1980). Quantitative analysis of EEGs in epileptics. In *Proceedings of Congress der Gesellschaft für Neuroelektrodiagnostik der DDR*, ed. G. Rabending.

MacGillivray, B.B. and Wadbrook, D.G. (1975). A system for extracting a diagnosis from the clinical EEG. In *CEAN Computerized EEG analysis*, ed. G. Dolce and H. Künkel, pp. 344–64, Fischer, Stuttgart.

MacInnes, D.A. (1961). *The Principles of Electrochemistry*. Reingold, New York.

Magnus, O., van der Wulf, C.J., van der Holst, M.J.C., van Huffelen, A.C. and Heimans, J. (1977). Application of computer analysis to EEG interpretation. *Electroencephalogr. Clin. Neurophysiol.*, **43**, 547.

Margerison, J.H., Anderson, W.Mc., Dawson, J. and Lettich, E. (1964). Plasma sodium and the EEG in the menstrual cycle. *Electroencephalogr. Clin. Neurophysiol.*, **17**, 339–41.

Margerison, J.H., Binnie, C.D. and McCaul, I.R. (1970). Electroencephalographic signs employed in the location of ruptured intracranial arterial aneurysms. *Electroencephalogr. Clin. Neurophysiol.*, **28**, 296–306.

Margerison, J.H., Binnie, C.D. and Venables, P.H. (1967). Physical principles. In *A Manual of Psychophysiological Methods*, ed. P.H. Venables and I. Martin, pp. 3–52. North Holland Publishing Co., Amsterdam.

Margerison, J.H., St. John-Loe, P. and Binnie, C.D. (1967). Electroencephalography. In *A Manual of Psychophysiological Methods*, ed. P.H. Venables and I. Martin, pp. 351–402. North Holland Publishing Co., Amsterdam.

Martin, W.B., Johnson, L.C., Viglione, S.S., Naitoh, P., Joseph, R.D. and Moses, J.D. (1972). Pattern recognition of EEG-EOG as a technique for all-night sleep stage scoring. *Electroencephalogr. Clin. Neurophysiol.*, **32**, 417–27.

Matoušek, M. (1967). *Automatic Analysis in Clinical Electroencephalography*. Psychiatric Research Institute, Prague.

Matoušek, M. and Petersén, I. (1973). Automatic evaluation of EEG background activity by means of age-dependant EEG quotients. *Electroencephalogr. Clin. Neurophysiol.*, **35**, 603–12.

Maulsby, R.L. and Markand, O.N. (1972). Use of activation procedures in routine EEG examinations. *Spike and Wave*, 5, 15–31.

Maulsby, R.L., Saltzberg, B. and Lustick, L.S. (1973). Towards an EEG screening test: a single system for analysis and display of clinical EEG data. In *Automation of Clinical Electroencephalography*, ed. P. Kellaway and I. Petersén, pp. 45–53. Raven Press, New York.

Mavor, H., Ajax, E.T. and Hellen, M.K. (1965). Personal communication. Cited by C.D. Binnie, B.B. MacGillivray and J.W. Osselton, (1974). In A. Rémond. (Ed.) *Handbook of Electroencephalography and Clinical Neurophysiology*, 3 C. Elsevier, Amsterdam.

Maynard, D.E., Prior, P.F. and Scott, D.F. (1969). Device for continuous monitoring of cerebral activity in resuscitated patients. *Brit. Med. J.*, 1969, 4, 545–6.

Merlis, J.K. (1970). Proposal for an international classification of the epilepsies. *Epilepsia*, 11, 114–19.

Merlis, J.K., Hendriksen, G.F. and Grossman, C. (1950). Metrazol activation of seizure discharges in epileptics with normal routine electro-encephalograms. *Electroencephalogr. Clin. Neurophysiol.*, 2, 17–22.

Meyer, J.R., Sakamoto, K., Akiyama, M., Yoshida, K. and Yoshitake. (1967). Monitoring cerebral blood flow, metabolism and EEG. *Electro-encephalogr. Clin. Neurophysiol.*, 23, 497–508.

Miller, J. (1977). *Bibliography on Electrical Hazards, Safety and Standards in Biomedical Engineering*. Beckman Instruments Inc., Fullerton.

Monakhov, K.K., Epstein, G. L., Nikiforov, A. I. and Bochkarev, V. K. (1974). Formalyu-matematicheskie metody izucheniya sootnosheniya elektricheskoi aktivnosti mosga i psikhicheskikh fenomenov. *Zh. Vyssh. Nerv. Delat.*, 24, 202–8.

Montagu, J.D. (1966). The application of electro-luminescence to photic stimulation. *Electroencephalogr. Clin. Neurophysiol.*, 21, 393–5.

Montagu, J.D. (1975). The hyperkinetic child: a behavioural, electro-dermal and EEG investigation. *Develop. Med. Child. Neurol.*, 17, 229–305.

Moruzzi, G. and Magoun, H.W. (1949). Brain stem reticular formation and activation of the EEG. *Electroencephalogr. Clin. Neurophysiol.*, 1, 455–73.

Mulholland, T. and Evans, C.R. (1966). Oculomotor function and the alpha activation cycle. *Nature*, 211, 1278–9.

Naquet, R. (Ed.) (1976). Activation and provocation methods in clinical electroencephalography. In *Handbook of Electroencephalography and Clinical Neurophysiology*, 3D, ed. A. Rémond, pp. 1–174. Elsevier, Amsterdam.

Nelligan, D.P. (1964). Eye movement artefacts and electrical recording of eye position. *Proc. Electro-physiol. Technol. Assoc.*, 11, 25–43.

O'Connell, D.N., Tursk, B. and Orne, M.T. (1960). Electrodes for recording skin potential. *Arch. Gen. Psychiat.*, 3, 252–8.

O'Kane, M.J. and Sauter, R. (1977). Long-term intensive monitoring of epileptic patients. In *Epilepsy. The Eighth International Symposium*, ed. J.K. Penry, pp. 125–9. Raven Press, New York.

Osselton, J.W. (1970). Techniques for data compression in the recording and analysis of prolonged EEG and other electrophysiological signals. *Am. J. EEG Technol.*, **10**, 97–116.

Pampiglione, G. (1952). Induced fast activity in cerebral lesions. *Electroencephalogr., Clin. Neurophysiol.*, **4**, 79–82.

Pampiglione, G. (1956). Some anatomical considerations upon electrode placement in routine EEG. *Proc. Electro-physiol. Technol. Assoc.*, **7, 1**, 20–30.

Pampiglione, G. and Harden, A. (1977). So-called neuronal ceroid lipofuscinosis. *J. Neurol. Neurosurg. Psychiat.*, **40**, 323–30.

Pampiglione, G. and Kerridge, J. (1956). EEG-abnormalities from the temporal lobe studied with sphenoidal electrodes. *J. Neurol. Neurosurg. Psychiat.*, **19**, 117.

Panayiotopoulos, C.P. (1974). Effectiveness of photic stimulation on various eye-states in photosensitive epilepsy. *J. Neurol. Sci.*, **23**, 165–73.

Papakostopoulos, D., Winter, A. and Newton, P. (1973). New techniques for the control of eye potential artefacts in multichannel CNV recordings. *Electroencephalogr. Clin. Neurophysiol.*, **34**, 651–3.

Penry, J.K. and Porter, R.J. (1977). Intensive monitoring of patients with intractable seizures. In *Epilepsy. The Eighth International Symposium*, ed. J.K. Penry, pp. 95–101. Raven Press, New York.

Picton, T.W., Hillyard, S.A., Krausz, H.I. and Galambos, R. (1974). Human auditory evoked potentials. *Electroencephalogr. Clin. Neurophysiol.*, **36**, 179–96.

Porter, R.J., Wolf, A.A. and Penry, J.K. (1971). Human electroencephalographic telemetry. *Amer. J. EEG. Technol.*, **11**, 145–59.

Pratt, K.L., Mattson, R.H., Welkers, N.J. and Williams, R. (1968). EEG-activation of epileptics following sleep deprivation: a prospective study of 114 cases. *Electroencephalogr. Clin. Neurophysiol.*, **24**, 11–15.

Prior, P.F. (1979). *Monitoring Cerebral Function*. Elsevier, Amsterdam.

Prior, P.F., Maynard, D.E., Sheaff, P.C., Simpson, B.R., Strunin, L., Weaver, E.J.M. and Scott, D.F. (1971). Monitoring cerebral function: clinical experience with new device for continuous recording of electrical activity of brain. *Br. Med. J.*, 1971, **2**, 736–8.

Radcliffe, H., Darby, C. and Tierney, P. (1969). An unusual fast activity. *Proc. Electro-physiol. Technol. Assoc.*, **16**, 263–9.

Rechtschaffen, A. and Kales, A. (1968). *A Manual of Standardized Terminology, Techniques and Scoring System for Sleep Stages of Human Subjects*. NIH Publications, no. 204, US Government Printing Office, Washington DC.

Regan, D. (1973). Rapid objective refraction using evoked brain potentials. *Investigative Opthalmology*, **12**, 669–79.

Rémond, A. and Torres, F. (1964). A method of electrode placement with a view to topographical research. I: basic concepts. *Electroencephalogr. Clin. Neurophysiol.*, **17**, 577–8.

Riehl, J.L. (1966). Analysis of the frequency/voltage ratio of the EEG in intracranial diseases. *Electroencephalogr. Clin. Neurophysiol.*, **21**, 325–34.

Ritter, W. and Vaughan, H.G. (1969). Average evoked responses in vigilance and discrimination: a reassessment. *Science*, **164**, 326–8.

Roberts, J.R., Hicks, B., Piper, R. and Binnie, C.D. (1974). An improved apparatus for slow chloriding of EEG electrodes. *Proc. Electro-physiol. Technol. Assoc.*, **21**, 62–5.

Robin, J.J., Tolan, G.D. and Arnold, J.W. (1978). Ten-year experience with abnormal EEGs in asymptomatic adult males. *Aviat. Space Environ. Med.*, **49**, 732–6.

Roth, B. (1976). Narcolepsy and hypersomnia: review and classification of 642 personally observed cases. *Arch. Suis. Neurol. Neurochir. Psych.*, **19**, 31–41.

Roubíček, J., Volavka, J., Matoušek, M. (1967). Elektroencefalogram u normalni populace. *Cesk. Psychiat.*, **63**, 1, 14–19.

Rowan, A.J., Binnie, C.D., Warfield, C.A., Meinardi, H. and Meyer J.W.A. (1979). The delayed effect of sodium valproate on the photosensitive response in man. *Epilepsia*, **20**, 61–8.

Sayers, B.M.A., Beagley, H.A. and Hensall, W.R. (1974). The mechanisms of the auditory evoked EEG responses. *Nature*, **247**, 481.

Schenk, G.K. (1973). Die Quantifizierung des EEG mittels vektorieller Iterationstechnik, einer Simulationsmethode der visuellen Analyse. In *Die Quantifizierung des Electroencephalogramms*, ed. G.K. Schenk, pp. 307–43. AEG Telefunken, Konstanz.

Schmidt, R.F. (1978). *Fundamentals of Neurophysiology*. Springer Verlag, New York.

Schoppenhorst, M. and Kubicki, St. (1973). Veränderungen organisch-bedingter EEG-Herde im Schlaf. *Z. EEG.EMG*, **4**, 22–9.

Schwamb, H.H., Clausen, R.E. and Summer, J.W. (1956). Pentylenetetrazol (Metrazol) activation of the electroencephalogram. *Arch. Neurol.*, **75**, 198–202.

Scollo-Lavizzari, G., Pralle, W. and de la Cruz. N. (1975). Activation effects of sleep deprivation and sleep in seizure patients. *Eur. Neurol.*, **13**, 1–5.

Shackel, B. (1958). A rubber suction cup surface electrode with high electrical stability. *J. Appl. Physiol.*, **13**, 153–8.

Shackel, B. (1959). Skin drilling: a method of diminishing galvanic skin-potentials. *Am. J. Psychol.*, **72**, 114–21.

Shaw, J.C. and Ongley, C. (1972). The measurement of synchronization. In *Synchronization of EEG Activity in Epilepsies*, ed. H. Petsche and M.A.B. Brazier, pp. 204–16. Springer Verlag, Berlin, Heidelberg and New York.

Sherwin, I. and Hooge, J.P. (1973). Comparative effectiveness of natural sleep and methohexital. Provocative tests in electroencephalography. *Neurology (Minneap.)*, **23**, 9, 973–6.

Sherwood, S.L. (1970). A system designed to extract information on seizures. *Electroencephalogr. Clin. Neurophysiol.*, **28**, 100–1.

Silverman, D. (1956). Sleep as a general activation procedure in electro-encephalography. *Electroencephalogr. Clin. Neurophysiol.*, **8**, 317–24.

Silverman, D. (1960). The anterior temporal electrode and the 10-20 system. *Electroencephalogr. Clin. Neurophysiol.*, **12**, 735–7.

Silverman, D. and Groff, R.A. (1957). Brain tumor depth determination by electrographic recordings during sleep. *Arch. Neurol.*, **78**, 15–28.

Silverman, D., Masland, R.L., Saunders, M.G. and Schwab, R.S. (1969). Minimal electroencephalographic recording techniques in suspected cerebral death. *Electroencephalogr. Clin. Neurophysiol.*, **27**, 731.

Sima, H. (1966). Flussiskeitsstrahl-Oszillografen. *Elektronik*, 6, 179–82.

Sklar, B., Hanley, J. and Simmons, W.W. (1973). A computer analysis of EEG spectral signatures from normal and dyslexic children. *IEEE Trans. Biomed. Eng.*, 20, 20–26.

Spadetta, V. (1971). La privazione di sonno nella diagnosi elettroencefalografica di epilessia. *Acta Neurol. (Napoli)*, 26, 7–13.

Stålberg, E. (1976). Experiences with long-term telemetry in routine diagnostic work. In *Quantitative Analytic Studies in Epilepsy*, ed. P. Kellaway and I. Petersén, pp. 269–78. Raven Press, New York.

Starr, A. and Achor, L.J. (1975). Auditory brain stem responses in neurological disease. *Arch. Neurol.*, 32, 761–8.

Stefansson, S.B., Darby, C.E., Wilkins, A.J., Binnie, C.D., Marlton, A.P., Smith, A.T. and Stockley, A.V. (1977). Television epilepsy and pattern sensitivity. *Brit. Med. J.*, 1977, 2, 88–90.

Stigsby, B., Obrist, W.D. and Sulg, I.A. (1973). Automatic data acquisition and period amplitude analysis of the EEG. *Comput. Programs Biomed.*, 3, 93–104.

Stockard, J.J. and Rossiter, V.S. (1977). Clinical and pathological correlation of brain stem auditory response abnormalities. *Neurology (Minneap.)*, 27, 316–25.

Stockard, J.J., Stockard, J.E. and Sharbrough, F.W. (1978). Nonpathologic factors influencing brainstem auditory evoked potentials. *Am. J. EEG Technol.*, 18, 177–209.

Stones, E.A., Whitehead, M.K. and MacGillivray, B.B. (1967). The nature of the eye blink artefact. *Proc. Electro-physiol. Technol. Assoc.*, 14, 208–14.

Storm van Leeuwen, W. Arntz, A., Spoelstra, P. and Wieneke, G.H. (1976). The use of computer analysis for diagnosis in routine EEG. *Rev. Electroencephalogr. Neurophysiol. Clin.*, 6, 318–27.

Strong, P. (1973). *Biophysical Measurements*. Tektronix Inc., Beaverton, Oregon.

Sugioka, K. and Davis, D.A. (1960). Hyperventilation with oxygen, a possible cause of cerebral hypoxia. *Anaesthesiology*, 21, 135–43.

Taylor, F.M. and Abraham, P. (1969). A search for a safe bentonite paste. *Proc. Electro-physiol. Technol. Assoc.*, 16, 80–3.

Townsend, H.R.A. (1968). An introducer for sphenoidal wire electrodes. *Proc. Electro-physiol. Technol. Assoc.*, 15, 67–72.

Tyner, F.S. and Knott, J.R. (1976). Amplitude asymmetries when using subdermal electrodes: is accurate head marking sufficient? *Am. J. EEG Technol.*, 15, 179–87.

Venables, P.H. and Martin, I. (Eds) (1976b). *A Manual of psychophysiological Methods*. North-Holland, Amsterdam.

Venables, P.H. and Martin, I. (1967a). Skin resistance and skin potential. In *A Manual of Psychophysiological Methods*, ed. P.H. Venables and I. Martin, pp. 53–102. North-Holland, Amsterdam.

Vera, R.S. and Blume, W.T. (1978). Technical contribution. A clinically effective spike recognition program: its use at electrocorticography. *Electroencephalogr. Clin. Neurophysiol.*, 45, 545–8.

Volavka, J., Matoušek, M., Feldstein, St., Roubiček, J., Prior, P., Scott, D.F. and Synek, V. (1973). Die Zuverlässigkeit der EEG-Beurteilung. *Z. EEG-EMG*, 4, 123–30.

Walter, D.O., Rhodes, J.M. and Adey, W.R. (1967). Discriminating among states of consciousness by EEG measurements. A study of four subjects. *Electroencephalogr. Clin. Neurophysiol.*, **22**, 22–9.

Walter, W.G. (1936). The location of cerebral tumors by electroencephalography. *Lancet*, 1936, **2**, 305.

Walter, W.G., Cooper, R., Aldridge, V.J., McCallum, W.C. and Winter, A.L. (1964). Contingent negative variation: an electric sign of sensori-motor association and expectancy in the human brain. *Nature*, **203**, 380.

Walter, W.G. and Parr, G. (1963). Recording equipment and technique. In *Electroencephalography*, ed. D. Hill and G. Parr, pp. 25–64. Macdonald, London.

Welch, L.K. and Stevens, J.B. (1971). Clinical value of the electroencephalogram following sleep deprivation. *J. Aerospace Med.*, **42**, 349–51.

Wennberg, A. and Zetterberg, L.H. (1971). Application of a computer-based model for EEG analysis. *Electroencephalogr. Clin. Neurophysiol.*, **31**, 457–68.

Wieser, H.G., Bancaud, J., Talairach, J., Bonis, A. and Szikla, G. (1979). Comparative value of spontaneous and chemically and electrically induced seizures in establishing the lateralization of temporal lobe seizures. *Epilepsia*, **59**, 20–47.

Wilkins, A.J., Darby, C.E., Binnie, C.D., Stefansson, S.B., Jeavons, P.M. and Harding, G.F.A. (1979). Television epilepsy – the role of pattern. *Electroencephalogr. Clin. Neurophysiol.*, **47**, 163–71.

Wilson, S.J. and Lloyd, D.S.L. (1973). The distribution of posterior temporal slow waves: implications of electrode placement systems. *Proc. Electro-physiol. Technol. Assoc.*, **20**, 151–8.

Zablow, L. and Goldensohn, E.S. (1969). A comparison between scalp and needle electrodes for the EEG. *Electroencephalogr. Clin. Neurophysiol.*, **26**, 530–3.

Zao, Z.Z., Gelbin, I. and Rémond, A. (1952). Le champ électrique de l'oeil. *Sem. Hop. Paris*, **36**, 1504–5.

Zivin, L. and Ajmone Marsan, C. (1968). Incidence and prognostic significant of "epileptiform" activity in the EEG of non-epileptic subjects. *Brain*, **91**, 751–778.

Zschocke, St. (1974). Technical contribution. An electronic device for continuous counting of chemically induced epileptic discharges. *Electroencephalogr. Clin. Neurophysiol.*, **37**, 191–3.

Index

Page numbers in italic refer to figures.